FRONTIERS OF INFECTIOUS DISEASES
NEW STRATEGIES IN FUNGAL DISEASE

FRONTIERS OF INFECTIOUS DISEASES

NEW STRATEGIES IN FUNGAL DISEASE

PROCEEDINGS OF AN INTERNATIONAL SYMPOSIUM
BROCKET HALL, HERTFORDSHIRE
21–24 SEPTEMBER 1991

EDITED BY

JOHN E. BENNETT

Head, Clinical Mycology Section,
Laboratory of Clinical Investigation,
National Institute of Allergy and Infectious Diseases,
Bethesda, Maryland, USA

RODERICK J. HAY

Mary Dunhill Professor of Cutaneous Medicine,
Department of Dermatology,
Guy's Hospital, London, UK

PHILLIP K. PETERSON

Professor of Medicine,
University of Minnesota Medical School;
Director, Infectious Diseases,
Hennepin County Medical Center, Minnesota, USA

ORGANIZING COMMITTEE

K.P.W.J. McADAM	H.C. NEU	S.R. NORRBY	P.K. PETERSON	J. VERHOEF
London	New York	Lund	Minneapolis	Utrecht
UK	USA	Sweden	USA	The Netherlands

The International Symposium on New Strategies in Fungal Disease was supported by
an educational grant from Glaxo Research

CHURCHILL LIVINGSTONE
EDINBURGH LONDON MADRID MELBOURNE NEW YORK AND TOKYO 1992

Distributed in the United States of America by
Churchill Livingstone Inc., 650 Avenue of the Americas, New York,
N.Y. 10011, and by associated companies, branches and
representatives throughout the world.

First Edition 1992

ISBN 0-443-04684-0

British Library Cataloguing in Publication Data
A catalogue record for this book is
available from the British Library

Library of Congress Cataloging in Publication Data
is available

Printed and bound in Great Britain by
Butler & Tanner Ltd, Frome and London

Preface

On 21 September 1991, the fourth in a series of symposia on Frontiers of Infectious Diseases convened in Hertfordshire, England. The topic of this year's meeting was mycology. Considering recent evidence that well over 1 million species of fungi inhabit the earth, the symposium was tightly focused: on the small handful of fungi that cause serious or life-threatening infections in humans. As at the previous symposia, leading basic science and clinical researchers shared their views regarding the 'state of the art' and future directions for research in the fields of pathogenesis and therapy. This book, which will be available within 5 months of the meeting, is an expression of those views and of the lively discussions which ensued. For perspective, my co-editors, Drs John Bennett and Roderick Hay, provided the keynote talks at the symposium. I highly recommend, as an editor involved mainly with organizational aspects of the project, that the reader begin with their respective contributions (Chs 1 and 12).

From the microbial side of the host–parasite interaction, *Candida albicans* and *Cryptococcus neoformans* have captured most attention in studies of pathogenesis. The priority given these two species is in no small way a reflection of their dominant role as opportunists in HIV-infected patients (*Pneumocystis carinii* was not covered at the symposium because of continued controversy as to its classification). Several *Candida* virulence factors are dealt with in this book: proteinase (Ch. 2), man-noprotein adhesins (Ch. 3), complement receptor-like molecules (Ch. 4), and genes or gene products involved in various aspects of cell wall formation or mor-phogenesis (Chs 7, 8 and 9). Several of these virulence factors are being considered as potential targets for new antifungal drugs, a possibility also raised for *Cocci-dioides immitis* (Ch. 5). Although not the sole virulence factor of *C. neoformans*, its polysaccharide capsule is clearly a key to its pathogenetic success (Ch. 10). Of great interest is the application of sexual and molecular genetics to understanding the virulence mechanisms of *C. neoformans* (Ch. 11).

From the host side of the host–parasite interaction, phagocytic cells and cyto-kines have received most attention from those interested in host defence. Alveolar macrophages and neutrophils play complementary roles in defence against patho-genic species of *Aspergillus* (Ch. 6), and studies in an animal model of cryptococcosis have revealed that two cytokines, granulocyte-macrophage colony stimulating factor and tumor necrosis factor, activate macrophages for increased phagocytosis of *C. neoformans* (Ch. 10). Other cytokines, e.g. interferon-γ (see discussion section, Ch. 5), are being considered for studies as adjunctive therapy of some fungal diseases.

Studies of the host response to invasive fungal infections have provided the foundation for immunodiagnosis. The antemortem diagnosis of deep-seated *Candida* and *Aspergillus* infections has been the bane of existence of physicians caring for patients at high risk of these infections. Initial studies focusing upon the search for diagnostic antibody levels were disappointing; however, newer approaches involving serologic assays for fungal antigens are more promising (Chs 13 and 14). While a commercially available diagnostic kit that has been proven to be sufficiently sensitive and specific for diagnosis of occult invasive candidiasis or aspergillosis does not yet exist, prospects appear hopeful.

The critical need to initiate antifungal therapy early in the course of deep-seated *Candida* and *Aspergillus* infections has prompted a large number of clinical trials aimed at their prevention (Ch. 15). While the results of most of these trials are equivocal, there are encouraging reports with newer azole drugs in prophylaxis in neutropenic patients. Along the same line are studies demonstrating clear-cut benefit with newer azoles in 'non-compromised' patients; amphotericin has taken a back shelf in certain of these infections, e.g. blastomycosis, paracoccidioidomycosis, and histoplasmosis (Ch. 16).

Finally, although there is a great deal of good news to be found within this book: many new insights into pathogenesis, hopeful diagnostic possibilities, the realization and promise of new therapies, there is also bad news – AIDS – which should serve as a potent stimulus to more rapid discovery. With improved means of prevention and treatment of *P. carinii* infection, fungi have become an increasingly important group of pathogens in HIV-infected patients, and, in areas of Africa where AIDS is most devastating, *C. neoformans* is a prominent cause of death (Ch. 17). The lessons of AIDS are important: none of our antifungal drugs are fungicidal in vivo and selection of strains resistant to currently available drugs is an emerging problem. To meet these challenges, we will rely on the innovative efforts of the contributors to this book. Given the recent accomplishments of these investigators, and their colleagues throughout the world, there is reason to be optimistic.

P. K. P.

1991

List of participants

ANDRIOLE, Vincent T, Department of Internal Medicine, Yale University School of Medicine, New Haven, Connecticut, USA

BANCROFT, Greg J, Department of Clinical Sciences, London School of Hygiene and Tropical Medicine, London, UK

BENNETT, John E, Clinical Mycology Section, Laboratory of Clinical Investigation, National Institute of Allergy and Infectious Diseases, National Institutes of Health, Bethesda, Maryland, USA

CALDERONE, Richard A, Department of Microbiology, Georgetown University School of Medicine, Washington, DC, USA

COLE, Garry T, Department of Botany, University of Texas, Austin, Texas, USA

de REPENTIGNY, Louis, Department of Microbiology and Immunology, University of Montreal, Montreal, Quebec, Canada

DIAMOND, Richard D, Department of Medicine, Boston University Medical Center, Boston, Massachusetts, USA

DISMUKES, William E, Division of Infectious Diseases, University of Alabama Medical Center, Birmingham, Alabama, USA

DOUGLAS, L Julia, Department of Microbiology, University of Glasgow, Glasgow, UK

DUPONT, Bertrand, Department of Infectious Diseases, Hôpital de l'Institut Pasteur, Paris, France

EDWARDS, Jr, John E, Department of Medicine, University of California, Los Angeles School of Medicine, Harbor UCLA Medical Center, Torrance, California, USA

GRAYBILL, J Richard, Division of Infectious Diseases, Department of Medicine, University of Texas Health Science Center, San Antonio, Texas, USA

HAY, Roderick J, Department of Dermatology, Guy's Hospital, London, UK

HAYES, Mike V, Department of Natural Products, Glaxo Group Research Ltd, Greenford, Middlesex, UK

HICKS, James B, Department of Yeast Genetics, ICOS Corporation, Seattle, Washington, USA

KOZEL, Tom R, Department of Microbiology, School of Medicine, University of Nevada, Reno, USA

KWON-CHUNG, K J, Clinical Mycology Section, Laboratory of Clinical Investigation, National Institute of Allergy and Infectious Diseases, National Institutes of Health, Bethesda, Maryland, USA

MAGEE, Beatrice, Department of Genetics and Cell Biology, University of Minnesota, St Paul, Minnesota, USA

MAGEE, Peter T, Department of Genetics and Cell Biology, University of Minnesota, St Paul, Minnesota, USA

McADAM, Keith P W J, Department of Clinical Sciences, London School of Hygiene and Tropical Medicine, London, UK

MACKENZIE, Don W R, Mycological Reference Laboratory, Central Public Health Laboratory, London, UK

MATTHEWS, Ruth C, Department of Medical Microbiology, University of Manchester Medical School, Manchester, UK

MEUNIER, Françoise, EORTC Central Office – Data Centre, Brussels, Belgium

NEU, Harold C, Infectious Diseases/Epidemiology Division, Columbia University, New York, NY, USA

NOMBELA, César, Departmento de Microbiologia II, Facultad de Farmacia, Universidad Complutense, Madrid, Spain

NORRBY, S Ragnar, Department of Infectious Diseases, University Hospital of Lund, Lund, Sweden

ODDS, Frank C, Department of Bacteriology and Mycology, Janssen Research Foundation, Beerse, Belgium

PETERSON, Phillip K, Department of Medicine, Hennepin County Medical Center, University of Minnesota, Medical School, Minneapolis, Minnesota, USA

RÜCHEL, Reinhard, Department of Medical Microbiology, Hygiene Institute, University of Göttingen, Göttingen, Germany

SCHAFFNER, Andreas, Department of Medicine, University Hospital of Zurich, Zurich, Switzerland

SHEPHERD, Maxwell G, Experimental Oral Biology Unit, School of Dentistry, University of Otago, Dunedin, New Zealand

SOBEL, Jack, Division of Infectious Diseases, Wayne State University, Detroit, Michigan, USA

SOLL, David R, Department of Biology, University of Iowa, Iowa City, USA

STEVENS, David A, Division of Infectious Diseases, Department of Medicine, Santa Clara Valley Medical Center and Stanford University Medical School, San Jose, California, USA

SYPHERD, Paul S, Department of Microbiology and Molecular Genetics, College of Medicine, University of California, Irvine, USA

TUITE, Mick F, Biological Laboratory, University of Kent, Canterbury, Kent, UK

VERHOEF, Jan, Egkman–Winkler Institute for Medical and Clinical Microbiology, University Hospital Utrecht, Utrecht, The Netherlands

WALSH, Thomas J, Infectious Diseases Section, Pediatric Branch, National Cancer Institute, National Institutes of Health, Bethesda, Maryland, USA

Contents

Plenary Lecture 1

Chairman: P. K. Peterson

1. Developing drugs for the deep mycoses: a short history

J. E. Bennett

> Diseases desperate grown
> By desperate appliances are relieved,
> Or not at all.
>
> William Shakespeare, *Hamlet* Act IV, scene 3.

As recently as 40 years ago, deep mycoses were regarded as rare diseases, difficult to diagnose, nearly impossible to treat and often fatal. Medical schools granted the subject little more than a passing nod. Even discovery of a previously undiagnosed case at post mortem examination could be dismissed with a shrug. Death could not have been prevented even were the diagnosis known. This situation was to change, first at a crawl and then at a gallop. Deep mycoses became increasingly common, diagnostic measures improved and effective therapy was finally discovered.

THE DEBUT OF AMPHOTERRIBLE

Selman A. Waksman's discovery that a soil organism produced the antibacterial antibiotic, streptomycin, prompted many others to search for antibacterial agents in the same way. Little effort was spent looking for antifungal agents until two workers at the New York City branch of the New York State Division of Laboratories and Research found nystatin. Rachel Brown and Elizabeth Hazen named the drug for the state that employed them, and the fungus, *Streptomyces noursei*, for Walter B. Nourse, who owned the farm in Warrenton, Virginia where Dr Hazen had picked up the soil (Baldwin 1981). The drug was first called fungicidin and then renamed nystatin in honour of New York State. E. R. Squibb and Sons, who had licensed the nystatin in 1951, set about to look for other antifungals produced by soil actinomycetes. Only two years later, scientists at Squibb discovered amphotericin B in soil taken from Tembladora, Venezuela, on the Orinoco River. Clinical trials were begun with oral amphotericin B, given as 100 mg capsules at a daily dose of 2–5 grams per day. Despite some limited success in clinical trials, blood levels were below 0.1 μg/ml and clinical responses were usually negligible. Clinical trials soon turned to intravenous administration, initially using a par-

3

ticulate suspension of insoluble amphotericin B. The drug was well tolerated but blood levels were low. Workers at Squibb hit upon the novel idea of preparing a colloidal suspension using the bile salt, deoxycholate. It was only when this preparation, Fungizone for Infusion, entered clinical trial that the toxicity of amphotericin B became fully apparent. In a 1960 report, 27 of 29 had fever, 25 had shaking chills and 16 had azotemia (Seabury & Dascomb 1960). For several years the renal damage was thought to be entirely temporary. Then, permanent changes in renal function and in renal histology were convincingly demonstrated. The litany of toxicity would eventually include anaemia, phlebitis, renal tubular acidosis, hypokalaemia, hypomagnesaemia, nausea, vomiting, weight loss and headache. The appellation, 'amphoterrible', was richly deserved. Claiming that the market potential of the intravenous drug was small, Squibb did very little to improve their formulation over the next 30 years.

Attempts to produce a less toxic formulation began at Rutgers University. The first derivative of amphotericin B was a series of N-acylation products that were reported by Schaffner & Borowski in 1961. N-acylation dramatically reduced antifungal activity and trials were not reported again for 11 years. Esterification of the carboxyl was to be a more promising approach. In 1972 Schaffner & Mechlinski from Rutgers reported preparation of a series of esters, of which the methyl ester had full activity in vitro. Nephrotoxicity in dogs was reduced 8–10-fold (Keim et al 1976, Parmegiani et al 1987). In mice infected with several different fungi, the methyl ester was generally less active than the deoxycholate colloidal dispersion. Whether the therapeutic ratio had been improved depended upon which toxicity endpoint was used (Gadebusch et al 1976). Dr Paul Hoeprich of the University of California, Davis, decided to pursue clinical trial of amphotericin B methyl ester (AME) (Hoeprich et al 1988). He obtained the drug as the free base in powdered form from Squibb, prepared solutions as the ascorbic salt and administered them intravenously. Later, Squibb provided AME as the powder of the aspartate salt. Between 1975 and 1980, 53 patients were given AME at doses up to five times that used with Fungizone. Renal toxicity was clearly less, but with time a new type of adverse reaction became apparent, neurotoxicity. The extent of neurological loss was obscured by the presence of meningitis in many of the patients, some of whom also received AME intrathecally as well as intravenously. When the study was terminated, Dr Hoeprich reported that in 30 patients in whom ototoxicity could be evaluated, symptomatic loss of hearing was noted in 43%, was present on audiogram but asymptomatic in 10% and absent in 47% (Hoeprich et al 1988). Dr Ellis, a neuropathologist at Dr Hoeprich's hospital, became interested in the observation that progressive loss of higher neurological function was also being seen in these patients, including some without meningitis. Dr Ellis found diffuse leukoencephalopathy in 3 of 11 autopsied patients. All seven who had received at least 9.8 g had neurological and neuropathological abnormalities (Ellis et al 1982). High pressure liquid chromatography of AME revealed eight or nine methylated compounds, raising the possibility that some of the contaminating byproducts were causing the toxicity, not AME (Hoeprich et al 1988). Full discussion of these observations was impaired initially by a malpractice suit involving the use of AME.

In 1972, Mechlinski & Schaffner (1972) from Rutgers University reported that

4

the N-acyl derivatives of AME retained the activity of the parent compound. Studies on the N-ornithyl AME, prepared by Schering-Plough, were reported during 1985–1987 (Parmegiani et al 1987). The compound proved to be much less toxic but somewhat less effective than Fungizone in experimental murine mycoses. To my knowledge, this compound never came to clinical trial, nor have other esters of N-acyl derivatives.

Table 1.1 Amphotericin B formulations

	Sculier	Lopez-Berestein	ABLC	Ambisome	Fungizone	ABCD
Content	Egg PC, cholesterol, stearylamine	DMPC, DMPG	DMPC, DMPG	DSPG, soy lecithin, cholesterol	Deoxycholate	Cholesteryl sulphate
Particle	SUV	MLV	Sheets	SUV	Micelle	Micelle

ABLC, amphotericin B lipid complex; ABCD, amphotericin B colloidal dispersion; DMPC, dimyristoylphosphatidyl choline; DMPG, dimyristoylphosphatidyl glycerol; DSPG, distearoylphosphatidyl glycerol; PC, phosphatidyl choline; SUV, simple unilamellar vesicle; MLV, multilamellar vesicle.

The next approach was to formulate amphotericin B as a liposome rather than a micelle (Table 1.1). The toxicity and efficacy of a multilamellar vesicle (MLV) formulation in murine cryptococcosis and histoplasmosis was published in 1982 by Graybill et al and Taylor et al. The following year, Juliano, Lopez-Berestein and collaborators reported preparation and mouse testing with another MLV preparation of amphotericin B (Juliano et al 1983). Description of their clinical trials was to follow in 1985. The first descriptions of a simple unilamellar vesicle (SUV) formulation of amphotericin B were by Szoka and coworkers in 1984 (Tremblay et al 1984, Panosian et al 1984). This SUV formulation contained egg phosphatidylcholine, cholesterol and tocopherol. In the years that followed, liposomal preparations of various formulations and sizes have been tried in animals. Only two institutions have prepared and administered liposomal formulations to patients with mycoses. Dr Lopez-Berestein continued his clinical trials of a MLV formulation at M.D. Anderson Hospital in Houston. In Brussels, Sculier, Meunier and Klastersky prepared and used a SUV formulation. Both groups reported a striking absence of nephrotoxicity and only occasional problems with fever or hypokalaemia (Lopez-Berestein et al 1985, Sculier et al 1988). Although no data concerning blood levels were reported with the M.D. Anderson preparation, the Jules Bordet preparation gave levels that were as high or higher than that obtained with Fungizone. The only note of warning sounded from this anecdotal use of the drug was a report of transient cardiopulmonary toxicity in a patient receiving 5 mg/kg of the M.D. Anderson preparation (Levine et al 1991).

Industry interest in liposomal formulations first appeared in the 1980s, when Lyphomed, who had been marketing generic intravenous amphotericin B, formed a development agreement with a small liposome company, Vestar, in San Demas, California. A SUV formulation was prepared with distearoyl phosphatidyl glycerol, cholesterol and egg lecithin. Later, soy lecithin was substituted for egg lecithin. This preparation had a therapeutic effect in mice with either candidiasis (Gondal et al 1989) or cryptococcosis (McManus et al 1988). Although the cooperative development with Lyphomed was later terminated, Vestar continued their efforts to market their liposomal product. Two patients at Georgetown University Hospital in Washington, D.C. were given the drug by compassionate clearance (Katz et al 1990). Blood levels in one of these were similar to those reported in the SUV formulation of Sculier. Vestar chose not to pursue clinical trials in the USA but launched compassionate clinical trials in Europe, naming the formulation Ambisome. Although organ dysfunction from underlying disease has caused some difficulties in interpretation, only 9 of 80 patients receiving Ambisome were reported to have at least a 20% increase in serum creatinine with a mean daily dose of 2.15 mg/kg (Meunier et al 1990). In another abstract concerning the European studies, 4 of 29 patients were said to have increased serum creatinine (Lazar et al 1990). Based upon these early descriptions, Ambisome appears to be less toxic than equal doses of Fungizone.

The next commercial liposomal preparation to come to clinical trial was that of Squibb, who altered the formulation used by Lopez-Berestein and colleagues by increasing the amphotericin B content from about 5–10 mol% to approximately 33 mol%. Higher amphotericin B concentrations were found to distribute the drug more evenly among the phospholipid particles and to decrease acute lethality in mice (Janoff et al 1988). Although the particle diameter remained several micrometers, the increased amphotericin B content changed the particle from a sphere to sheets and leaves. Appropriately, the preparation is called amphotericin B lipid complex (ABLC). The first clinical trials were conducted in normal volunteers, using doses up to 0.5 mg/kg. The drug was well tolerated but the area under the blood level curve was only a fifth that of Fungizone (Kan & Bennett 1991). Clinical trials are now being pursued by the manufacturer, Bristol-Myers Squibb, using doses up to 5 mg/kg daily. Elevation of aminotransferases, seen in 2 of the original 8 volunteers, has been subsequently infrequent.

The latest entry into the field of amphotericin B formulations has been a colloidal dispersion similar to Fungizone but using cholesteryl sulphate instead of deoxycholate. Liposome Technology, Inc. had named the preparation ABCD (amphotericin B colloidal dispersion). In immunosuppressed rabbits with aspergillosis, ABCD was less effective than equal doses of Fungizone but because acute lethality of intravenous ABCD was four-fold less, a superior therapeutic effect could be achieved (Patterson et al 1989). Clinical studies have just begun as of this writing.

A pervasive problem in the field of formulating amphotericin B is that we do not know what pharmacological properties favour nephrotoxicity. Nor do we know what properties favour therapeutic effect. So far, neither blood levels nor tissue levels in target organs have correlated conclusively with either nephrotoxicity or therapeutic effect in experimental murine infections (Collette et al 1991). However, promising work in this field is continuing.

THE VERSATILE DIAMIDINES

Use of diamidines for protozoal infections is well established, including the use of pentamidine for African trypanosomiasis. Physicians are also generally familiar with the use of pentamidine for *Pneumocystis carinii* pneumonia. Perhaps less well known is the antifungal activity of this class of drug. As early as 1945, aromatic diamidines, such as propamidine, were shown to be active against *Blastomyces dermatitidis*. By 1952, stilbamidine had been shown to be effective therapy in mice and in four patients with blastomycosis (Shoenbach 1952). The following year, Snapper and associates demonstrated clinical activity in blastomycosis with hydroxystilbamidine, a less toxic compound. This drug remained in use for blasto-mycosis for a decade. Use declined after a collaborative clinical trial by the Veteran's Administration found that hydroxystilbamidine was less effective than amphotericin B for the more severe forms of blastomycosis (Busey 1972). Now, hydroxystilbamidine is of historical interest only.

THE RISE AND FALL OF SARAMYCETIN

Grunberg and associates reported in 1961 that compound X5079C had activity in experimental murine mycoses. This activity had been picked up in a screening process that used animals and had not been detected in in vitro screening. X5079C, later called saramycetin, was a polypeptide antibiotic from *Streptomyces asceticus*. A small clinical trial showed activity in blastomycosis and histoplasmosis but the majority of patients relapsed (Witorsch et al 1966). Problems with purific-ation, weak therapeutic activity, the necessity for parenteral administration, allergic reactions and liver function abnormalities all combined to stop drug development.

FLUCYTOSINE: UNPLANNED PARENTHOOD

In 1962, Malbica and colleagues from Roche reported on the biological properties of 5-fluorocytosine (flucytosine). The drug was prepared following a lead by Heidelberger and colleagues that fluorinated pyrimidines might have antitumour activity (Malbica et al 1962). Although flucytosine never showed promise as a pyrimidine antagonist, Grunberg, Titsworth and Bennett from Roche discovered that the drug had activity in experimental murine candidiasis (Grunberg et al 1963). This discovery was surprising in view of the fact that no antifungal effect had been found with in vitro screening. Later, inhibitors in the culture medium were found to explain this discrepancy. Initial clinical trials were fraught with problems of weak therapeutic activity when flucytosine was used alone. A collaborative clinical trial, sponsored by the National Institute of Allergy and Infectious Disease, com-pared amphotericin B used with and without flucytosine in the treatment of cryptococcal meningitis. The combination was at least as effective as amphotericin B alone but substantial bone marrow toxicity or other toxicity ascribed to flucy-tosine occurred in a third of the patients (Bennett et al 1979). Bone marrow toxicity was clearly linked to flucytosine blood levels in excess of $100\,\mu g/ml$. Although flucytosine continues to be used as a companion drug with amphotericin B, lack of a parenteral formulation in the USA, failure of most hospital laboratories to measure blood levels and rise of alternative drugs seems likely to relegate flucytosine to obscurity. The collaborative group formed to conduct this study has persisted under NIAID sponsorship and the leadership of Dr William Dismukes, becoming a major source of collaborative research on deep mycoses.

LIPOPEPTIDE ANTIFUNGALS: DEAD OR ONLY SLEEPING?

Scientists at Lilly Research Laboratories undertook synthesis of derivatives of echinocandin B, an antifungal antibiotic from *Aspergillus* species. The search was directed towards a compound with less toxicity and retained antifungal activity. Some information on structure–function relationships already existed from work with other antifungal lipopeptides, such as echinocandins C and D, aculeacin A, mulundocandin and sporiofungin. Altering one of the acyl side chains of echinocandin B led to Ly 121019, later called cilofungin (Debono et al 1988). Although studies with cilofungin were first reported in 1984 (Gordee et al 1984), drug development was postponed because of the limited antifungal spectrum, insolubility in water, necessity for intravenous administration and very short half life. Based upon in vitro testing, susceptibility looked promising only for *Candida albicans*, *Candida tropicalis* and some isolates of other *Candida* species (Hanson & Stevens 1989). Experimental infections with *Candida albicans* gave mixed results. Results of phase 2 clinical trials, as presented in 1990, described unimpressive clinical activity and, more importantly, some cases of acidosis ascribed to the polyethylene glycol vehicle (Copley-Merriman 1990a, b). Currently, clinical trials with cilofungin have ceased. Despite the recent discovery of activity against *Pneumocystis carinii* by this class of antibiotic (Schmatz et al 1990, Current & Boylan 1990), it seems unlikely that these lipopeptides will resume clinical trial.

DAWN OF THE AZOLE ERA

In 1969 Manfred Plempel and coworkers from Bayer in Wuppertal, Germany used in vitro screening of substituted imidazoles to discover the compound called Bay 5097 (Plempel et al 1969). This drug, later named clotrimazole, was active orally in experimental murine mycoses and showed a broad spectrum of antifungal activity in vitro. In clinical trials, this compound was successful in topical therapy of mucosal candidiasis and in dermatophyte infections. Clinical trials in deep mycoses were conducted wth 100 mg/kg per day, in three or four divided doses. Despite some encouraging early reports in the treatment of aspergillosis and candidiasis, efficacy in deep mycoses was largely minimal. Blood levels were consistently below $0.5 \mu g/mi$ and often unmeasurable. Clotrimazole is now a major drug in the treatment of oral and vaginal candidiasis but is not used in deep mycoses.

In 1969–1970, reports began appearing from Janssen Pharmaceuticals about a new imidazole, miconazole. Undaunted by the drug's poor oral absorption and insolubility in water, the manufacturer prepared and marketed an intravenous formulation in polyethoxylated castor oil. This vehicle seems to be responsible for at least some adverse effects, such as phlebitis and hyponatraemia. Efficacy of intravenous miconazole was never striking and the preparation has all but disappeared from use. Along with clotrimazole, miconazole has remained a major topical drug for superficial mycoses.

The breakthrough in treatment of deep mycoses came with the discovery of ketoconazole in 1978. Good oral absorption, low toxicity and broad spectrum of activity made ketoconazole the standard against which subsequent azoles would be measured. The NIAID Mycoses Study Group's report firmly established keto-conazole as the drug of choice for most patients with blastomycosis and histo-plasmosis (National Institutes of Health Mycoses Study Group 1985). Efficacy was also established in coccidioidomycosis, paracoccidioidomycosis, chronic muco-cutaneous candidiasis, pityriasis versicolor, ringworm and vulvovaginal candi-diasis. Further development of azole antifungals centred around the search for compounds that would be more stable to metabolism and less suppressive of testosterone and cortisol synthesis, as well as the need for alternatives to ampho-tericin B in the treatment of cryptococcal meningitis, deep candidiasis and asper-gillosis. Insertion of another nitrogen into the azole ring did accomplish some of these goals by decreasing metabolism and hormonal suppression. Of the three triazoles reaching clinical trial thus far, itraconazole (Sporanox, Janssen), fluc-onazole (Diflucan, Pfizer) and SCH 39304 (Schering), all have been promising. Fluconazole has the distinction of administration by either the oral or intravenous route and of having proven activity in cryptococcal meningitis. Although itra-conazole and fluconazole are now commercially available in many countries, SCH 39304 was found to be a racemic mixture, containing equal amounts of both enantiomers, only one of which (SCH 42427) was active. This and other issues have contributed to a pause in development of SCH 42427. Current development of newer triazoles is being targeted to broaden the spectrum, particularly against *Aspergillus*.

CONCLUDING THOUGHTS: WHAT WE'VE LEARNED

1. Screening for antifungal drugs only by in vitro testing failed to discern the value of saramycetin, flucytosine and fluconazole, to name just a few. Conversely, drugs such as terbinafine have looked promising in vitro but notably inert in experimental animal testing. Despite the protestation of animal rights enthusiasts, evaluation of antifungals in experimentally infected animals remains necessary for drug develop-ment.
2. Closer scrutiny of blood levels early in drug development would have been helpful in detecting many problems, including dose-related flucytosine toxicity, the poor absorption of ketoconazole in patients taking H-receptor antagonists, the ability of rifampin to decrease blood levels of ketoconazole and itraconazole, and the accumulation of itraconazole metabolites.
3. Expanded use of multicentred trials has largely surmounted the problem of studying diseases of low prevalence. Not only have such groups been organized by pharmaceutical companies, but also groups such as the Veteran's Administration, NIAID Mycoses Study Group, AIDS Clinical Trials Group and the California Collaborative Study Group have all undertaken therapeutic trials of drugs for deep mycoses.

4. Development of drugs for deep mycoses remains a very expensive enterprise, often out of reach of smaller companies. Trials in which each centre can only contribute a few cases are particularly expensive. Similarly costly are prophylaxis trials in which many patients must be treated and followed in detail but only a few are proven to be infected.

5. Lack of experience in developing drugs for deep mycoses is a problem within many of the drug houses and often within the Food and Drug Administration, causing expensive errors in protocol design. Lack of good guidelines and inconsistent regulatory decisions have slowed and increased the cost of drug development. This situation appears to be gradually improving.

6. There are still mycoses for which no satisfactory chemotherapy trials can be devised. In these mycoses, the natural history of the infection is unpredictable and assessment of disease activity is imprecise. Deep candidiasis is the example par excellence but empiric therapy of the neutropenic patient and treatment of invasive aspergillosis are also very difficult to study.

7. The concept that deep mycoses are rare and untreatable has been so thoroughly rebuffed that the idea has become ludicrous. Both the need and the financial incentive exist for drug development.

REFERENCES

Baldwin R S 1981 The fungus fighters. Cornell University Press, Ithaca
Bennett J E, Dismukes W E, Duma R J, et al 1979 A comparison of amphotericin B alone and combined with flucytosine in the treatment of cryptococcal meningitis. New England Journal of Medicine 301: 126–131
Busey J F 1972 Blastomycosis III. A comparative study of 2-hydroxystilbamidine and amphotericin B therapy. American Review of Respiratory Disease 105: 812–818
Collette N, van der Auwera P, Meunier F, Lambert C, Sculier J P, Coune A 1991 Tissue distribution and bioactivity of amphotericin B administered in liposomes to cancer patients. Journal of Antimicrobial Chemotherapy 27: 535–548
Copley-Merriman C R, Gallis H, Graybill J R, Doebbeling B N, Hyslop D L 1990 Cilofungin treatment of disseminated candidiasis: preliminary phase II results. Abstract 582 Program and Abstracts of the Thirtieth Interscience Conference on Antimicrobial Agents and Chemotherapy
Copley-Merriman C R, Ransburg N J, Crane L R, Kerkering T M, Pappas P G, Pottage J C, Hyslop D L 1990 Cilofungin treatment of candida esophagitis: preliminary phase II results. Abstract 581 Program and Abstracts of the Thirtieth Interscience Conference on Antimicrobial Agents and Chemotherapy
Current W L, Boylan C J 1990 Anti-*Pneumocystis* activity of antifungal compounds cilofungin and echinocandin B. Abstract 558 Program and Abstracts of the Thirtieth Interscience Conference on Antimicrobial Agents and Chemotherapy
Debono M, Abbott B J, Turner J R, Howard L C, Gordee R S, Hunt A S, Barnhart M, Molloy R M, Willard K E, Fukuda D, Butler T F, Zeckner D J 1988 Synthesis and evaluation of LY121019, a member of a series of semisynthetic analogues of the antifungal lipopeptide echinocandin B. Annals of the New York Academy of Sciences 544: 152–167
Ellis W G, Sobel R A, Nielsen S L 1982 Leukoencephalopathy in patients treated with amphotericin B methyl ester. Journal of Infectious Diseases 146: 125–137
Gadebusch H H, Pansy F, Klepner C, Schwind R 1976 Amphotericin B and amphotericin B methyl ester ascorbate. I. Chemotherapeutic activity against *Candida albicans, Cryptococcus neoformans,* and *Blastomyces dermatitidis* in mice. Journal of Infectious Diseases 134: 423–427
Gondal J A, Swartz R P, Rahman A 1989 Therapeutic evaluation of free and liposome-encapsulated amphotericin B in the treatment of systemic candidiasis in mice. Antimicrobial Agents and Chemotherapy 33: 1544–1548
Gordee R S, Zeckner D J, Ellis L F, Thakkar A L, Howard L C 1984 In vitro and in vivo anti-*Candida* activity and toxicology of LY 121019. Journal of Antibiotics 37: 1054–1065

Graybill J R, Craven P C, Taylor R L, Williams D M, Magee W E 1982 Treatment of murine cryptococcosis with liposome-associated amphotericin B. Journal of Infectious Diseases 145:748–752

Grunberg E, Titsworth E, Bennett M 1963 Chemotherapeutic activity of 5-fluorocytosine. Antimicrobial Agents and Chemotherapy 3: 566–568

Grunberg E J, Berger J, Titsworth E 1961 Chemotherapeutic studies on a new anti-fungal agent, X-5079C, effective against systemic mycoses. American Review of Respiratory Diseases 84:504

Hanson L H, Stevens D A 1989 Evaluation of cilofungin, a lipopeptide antifungal agent, in vitro against fungi isolated from clinical specimens. Antimicrobial Agents and Chemotherapy 33: 1391–1392

Hoeprich P D, Flynn N M, Kawachi M M, Lee K K, Lawrence R M, Heath L K, Schaffner C P 1988 Treatment of fungal infections with semisynthetic derivatives of amphotericin B. Annals of the New York Academy of Sciences 544: 517–546

Janoff A S, Boni L T, Popescu M C et al 1988 Unusual lipid structures selectively reduce the toxicity of amphotericin B. Proceedings of the National Academy of Sciences, USA 85: 6122–6126

Juliano R, Lopez-Berestein G, Mehta R, Hopfer R, Mehta K, Lasi L 1983 Pharmacokinetic and therapeutic consequences of liposomal drug delivery: fluorodeoxyuridine and amphotericin B as examples. Biologie Cellulaire 47: 39–46

Kan V L, Bennett J E, Amantea M A et al 1991 Comparative safety, tolerance and pharmacokinetics of amphotericin B lipid complex and amphotericin B desoxycholate in healthy male volunteers. Journal of Infectious Diseases 164: 418–421

Katz N M, Pierce P F, Anzeck R A et al 1990 Liposomal amphotericin B for treatment of pulmonary aspergillosis in a heart transplant patient. Journal of Heart Transplantation 9: 14–17

Keim G R Jr, Sibley P L, Yoon Y H, Kuleska J S, Zaidi I H, Miller M M, Poutsiaka J W 1976 Comparative toxicological studies of amphotericin B methyl ester and amphotericin B in mice, rats, and dogs. Antimicrobial Agents and Chemotherapy 10: 687–690

Lazar J T, Ksionski G E, Preiss S J 1990 Efficacy of Ambisome (liposomal amphotericin B) in opportunistic pulmonary mycoses. Abstract 569 Program and Abstracts of the Thirtieth Interscience Conference on Antimicrobial Agents and Chemotherapy

Levine S J, Walsh T J, Martinez A, Eichacker P Q, Lopez-Berestein G, Nathanson C 1991 Cardiopulmonary toxicity after liposomal amphotericin B infusion. Annals of Internal Medicine 114: 664–666

Lopez-Berestein G, Fainstein V, Hopfer R et al 1985 Liposomal amphotericin B for the treatment of systemic fungal infections in patients with cancer: a preliminary study. Journal of Infectious Diseases 151: 704–710

Malbica J, Sello L, Tabenkin B et al 1962 Some biological properties of 5-fluorocytosine and its derivatives. Federation Proceedings 21: 384

McManus E J, Rahman A, Gondal J, Bennett J E 1988 Liposomal amphotericin B in murine cryptococcosis. Abstract 318 Program and Abstracts of the Twenty-Eighth Interscience Conference on Antimicrobial Agents and Chemotherapy

Mechlinski W, Schaffner C P 1972 Polyene macrolide derivatives I. N-Acylation and esterification reactions with amphotericin B. Journal of Antibiotics xxv: 256–258

Meunier F, Gorin N, Kuse E R, Prentice H G, Ringden O, Tura S, Viviani M 1990 Safety of Ambisome (liposomal amphotericin B, Vestar, USA): results from a multicenter study. Abstract 260 Program and Abstracts of the Thirtieth Interscience Conference on Antimicrobial Agents and Chemotherapy

National Institute of Allergy and Infectious Diseases Mycoses Study Group, Birmingham, Alabama and Bethesda, Maryland 1985 Treatment of blastomycosis and histoplasmosis with ketoconazole. Annals of Internal Medicine 103: 861–872

Panosian C B, Barza M, Szoka F, Wyler D J 1984 Treatment of experimental cutaneous leishmaniasis with liposome-intercalated amphotericin B. Antimicrobial Agents and Chemotherapy 25: 655–656

Parmegiani R M, Loebenberg D, Antonacci B et al 1987 Comparative in vitro and in vivo evaluation of N-D-ornithyl amphotericin B methyl ester, amphotericin B methyl ester, and amphotericin B. Antimicrobial Agents and Chemotherapy 31: 1756–1760

Patterson T F, Miniter P, Dijkstra J, Szoka F C Jr, Ryan J L, Andriole V T 1989 Treatment of experimental invasive aspergillosis with novel amphotericin B/cholesterol-sulfate complexes. Journal of Infectious Diseases 159: 717–724

Plempel M, Bartmann K, Buchel K H, Regel E 1969 Experimentelle Befunde über ein neues oral wirksames Antimykotikum mit breiten Wirkungsspecktrum. Deutsche Medizinische Wochenschrift 94: 1356–1364

Schaffner C P, Borowski E 1961 Biologically active N-acyl derivatives of polyene macrolide antifungal antibiotics. Antibiotics & Chemotherapy 11: 724–732

11

Schaffner C P, Mechlinski W 1972 Polyene macrolide derivatives II. Physical-chemical properties of polyene macrolide esters and their water soluble salts. Journal of Antibiotics 25: 259–260

Schmatz D M, Romancheck M A, Pittarelli L A et al 1990 Treatment of *Pneumocystis carinii* pneumonia with 1,3-β-glucan synthesis inhibitors. Proceedings of the National Academy of Sciences, USA 87: 5950–5954

Schoenbach E B 1952 The use of aromatic diamidines for the treatment of systemic fungal disease. Transactions of the New York Academy of Sciences 14: 272

Sculier J P, Coune A, Meunier F et al 1988 Pilot study of amphotericin B entrapped in sonicated liposomes in cancer patients with fungal infections. European Journal of Cancer and Clinical Oncology 24: 527–538

Seabury J H, Dascomb H E 1960 Experience with amphotericin B. Annals of the New York Academy of Sciences 89: 202–220

Taylor R L, Williams D M, Craven P C, Graybill J R, Drutz D J, Magee W E 1982 Amphotericin B in liposomes: a novel therapy for histoplasmosis. American Review of Respiratory Diseases 125: 610–611

Tremblay C, Barza M, Fiore C, Szoka F 1984 Efficacy of liposome-intercalated amphotericin B in the treatment of systemic candidiasis in mice. Antimicrobial Agents and Chemotherapy 26: 170–173

Witorsch P, Andriole V T, Emmons C W, Utz J P 1966 The polypeptide antifungal angent (X-5079C): further studies in 39 patients. American Review of Respiratory Diseases 93: 876–888

Discussion of paper presented by J. E. Bennett

Reported by J. E. Bennett

In the discussion following Dr Bennett's paper, Dr Soll raised the question whether or not marketing drugs which could not be patented was economically feasible. The answer received from several sources was that clinical trials of antifungal drugs were often quite expensive and were only warranted when a patent protected the product. Dr Dismukes commented that even established multicentre groups, such as the Mycoses Study Group, do not have sufficient government support to perform clinical trials free of charge to the industry.

Dr Norrby commented that flucytosine is commonly used in Sweden but that toxicity is rarely encountered. Blood levels of the drug are monitored routinely, unlike in the USA. Toxicity may be lessened not only because blood levels are kept between 25 and 100 μg/ml but also because flucytosine is often used alone.

Use of rifampin with amphotericin B was queried by Dr Schaffner who also cited data from in vitro and experimental murine infections. The response from the audience was generally negative, with little data to encourage use of this combination. Dr Peterson asked whether or not pyrogenic reactions to amphotericin B might be due to release of tumour necrosis factor, interleukin 1 and other cytokines by monocytes and macrophages. Dr Bennett replied that studies reporting this phenomenon had used generic amphotericin B contaminated with endotoxin. When the experiments were repeated with endotoxin-free amphotericin B, no such effect was found either in vitro with human monocytes or in vivo with serum from patients receiving amphotericin B.

A discussion of liposomal amphotericin B followed. Vestar's Ambisome preparation was said to cost hundreds of dollars per dose and therefore was of limited use. Preparations of large particle size, such as Bristol-Meyers Squibb's amphotericin B lipid complex, are probably taken up by fixed macrophages. However, it remains unclear whether macrophage uptake confers a therapeutic advantage or simply decreases blood levels of the drug. Optimal pharmacokinetic properties of liposomal amphotericin B remain unknown.

Session I:
Virulence factors in candidiasis
Chairman: K. P. W. J. McAdam

2. Proteinase

R. Rüchel

INTRODUCTION

In a review of the metabolic properties of *Candida albicans,* Taschdjian & Kozinn (1961) concluded that the opportunistic yeast does not break down serum proteins, and that it may subsist in the host on free amino acids as a nitrogen source. However, in 1965, Staib published his first observations on the extracellular proteolytic effect of *C. albicans* during growth in media with serum albumin as the single nitrogen source.

The proteolytic effect was subsequently related to an acid proteinase (candida proteinase, CP) by Remold et al (1968), and the enzyme was classified by specific inhibition as an aspartic proteinase (E.C.3.4.23.6) (Macdonald & Odds 1980, Rüchel 1981, Ray & Payne 1982).

CPs were found in the culture media of most isolates of the clinically relevant *Candida* species, *C. albicans, C tropicalis,* and *C. parapsilosis* (Rüchel et al 1983, Macdonald 1984). More recently, various other proteolytic enzymes of *C. albicans* were described, which are located intracellularly, such as the vacuolar proteinase B, carboxypeptidase, and high molecular weight proteinases (Rüchel et al 1985, Farley et al 1986, Portillo & Gancedo 1986, Logan 1988). An alkaline 'valyl-proteinase' was detected in culture supernatant of *C. tropicalis* (Abbasi et al 1986). Since there is still no evidence of a contribution of these enzymes to the virulence of the yeasts, interest has focused on the extracellular CPs.

During the last decade, publications on CPs appeared with an increasing frequency, adding to the general (though not undisputed) notion that CPs were important factors of virulence. This research has recently culminated in successful attempts to clone and sequence the gene of CP (Hube et al 1991, Sullivan, University of Otago, New Zealand, personal communication).

In 1985, Odds provided the first brief review on CPs. In the following, I will discuss recent findings on CPs and the present evidence for a role of CPs in different stages of mycosis. Likewise, I will point out questions concerning CPs which should be clarified in future.

EVIDENCE FOR GENERATION OF CP DURING HUMAN CANDIDIASIS

The demonstration of a microbial substance in the patient is crucial in its evaluation as a factor of virulence. Therefore, particular efforts have been made to demonstrate CP in human sera and in mycotic human tissue:

In 1980, Macdonald & Odds first demonstrated specific antibodies. Their results suggested the presence of particularly high antibody titres in sera of patients suffering from deep-seated candidiasis. We have essentially confirmed these findings (Rüchel et al 1988). However, a fifth of the patients with other signs of deep-seated infection did not respond with indicative titres, probably reflecting the inability of many high-risk patients to mount a regular immune response.

In a few cases of candidaemia due to *C. parapsilosis*, we did not find an immune response to homologous CP-antigen. However, low titres of such antibodies were detected in murine sera after experimental infection with vaginal isolates of *C. parapsilosis* (De Bernardis et al 1990b). Evidence for CP-antigen circulation in the blood stream was found in 21 out of 50 patients with signs of deep-seated candidosis. Four patients with proteinase antigen showed signs of invasive cutaneous or mucocutaneous candidiasis (Rüchel et al 1988).

The presence of CP-antigen and specific antibodies in serum without concomitant signs of truly deep-seated candidiasis was explained by monitoring CP-antigen in mycotic human tissue (Rüchel et al 1991b). This investigation includes at present 36 postmortems. Using indirect immunofluorescence, CP-antigen was consistently

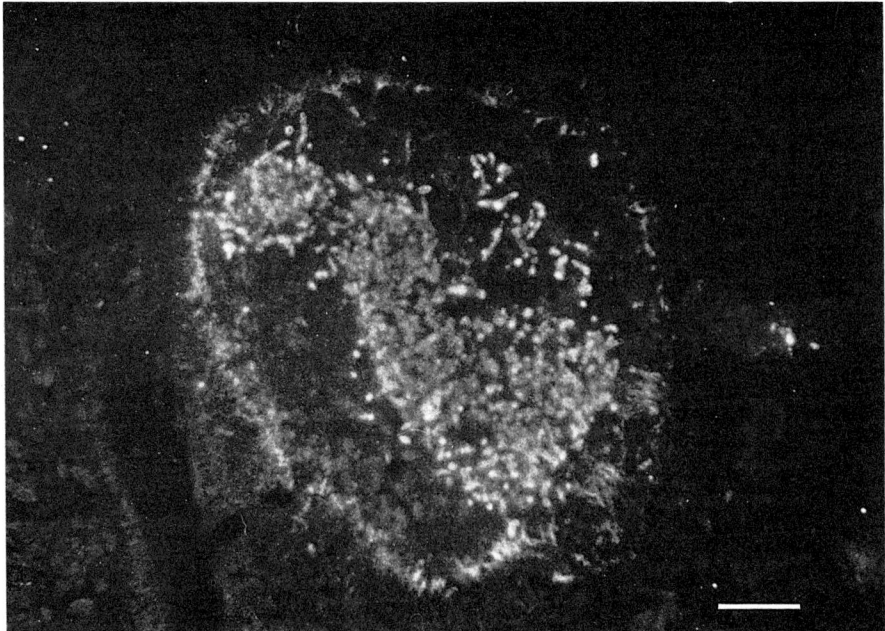

Fig. 2.1 *Candica albicans* colony in the kidney of a patient who died of disseminated mycosis. *Candida* proteinase antigen is made visible by indirect immunofluorescence using a fluorescein label. The ring of amorphous antigenic material may represent the boundary of the acid micromilieu around the colony (compare Fig. 2.3). The bar equals 20 μm. (From Rüchel 1991b, with permission of the publisher).

found in mycotic tissue from all organs investigated (including brain, lung, heart, liver, spleen, pancreas, kidney and gut). The most intriguing result, however, was the repeated demonstration of a ring of amorphous antigenic material surrounding *Candida* colonies in the kidney (Fig. 2.1). The ring of precipitated antigen is likely to represent denatured CP, and the pattern of its deposition may delineate a pH gradient which is generated by acid metabolites of the fungal cells.

However, we also found CP-antigen on fungal elements in mucosal candidiasis. This agrees with the detection of CP-antigen in vaginal fluid of patients colonized by *C. albicans* (De Bernardis et al 1990a).

So far, we have only seen tissue from two cases of candidiasis which lacked the proteinase antigen. Only yeast cells were seen in a case of nephritis, which was possibly caused by *Candida* (*Torulopsis*) *glabrata*, a non-filamentous yeast, which is considered to be non-proteolytic (Rüchel et al 1983, Macdonald 1984). In the other case, *C. albicans* was isolated postmortem from various organs of a neutropenic patient who died of disseminated candidiasis after 3 days on intravenous fluconazole. In vitro, this isolate turned proteolytic only after exposure to room temperature (Rüchel, unpublished observation).

MONITORING OF CANDIDA PROTEINASE DURING INFECTIONS IN VITRO

In 1986, Ghannoum & Abu Elteen observed a particular ability of strongly proteolytic *C. albicans* strains to adhere to human buccal epithelial cells in vitro. Subsequently, we investigated the expression of CP during experimental infection

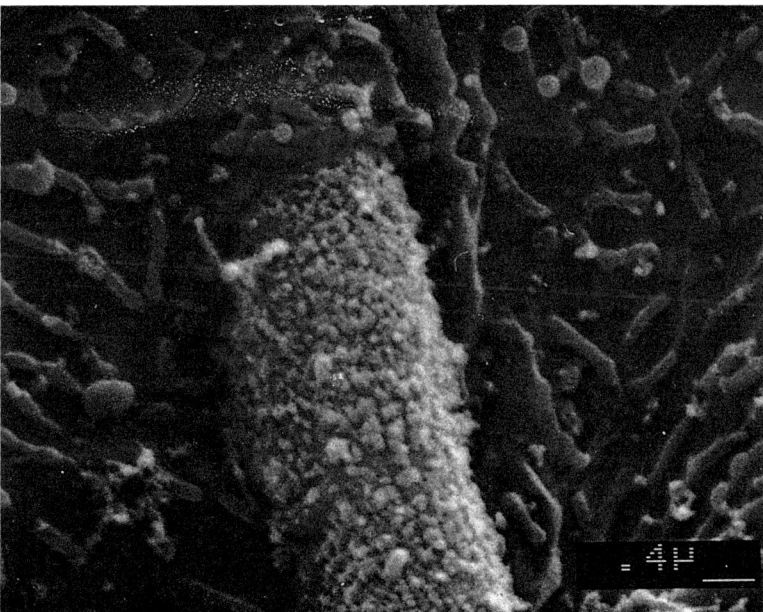

Fig. 2.2 Scanning electron micrograph of a germ tube of *C. albicans* serotype A at the point of invasion of human oral mucosa after immunoperoxidase reaction. The grainy colloids of diaminobenzidine covering the fungal surface indicate the presence of CP-antigen (from Borg & Rüchel 1988, with permission of the publisher).

of human oral mucosa (Borg & Rüchel 1988). Biopsies, after brief adaptation to tissue culture medium with 5% fetal calf serum, were infected with *C. albicans* blastoconidia. The yeasts were in the exponential growth phase but were not proteolytic at the time of infection. After 2 h in tissue culture, typical germ tubes were seen which invaded epithelial cells without causing evident damage at the site of invasion. Using immuno-scanning electron microscopy, we were able to demonstrate the CP-antigen on invading fungal elements (Fig. 2.2).

During these experiments, we detected rising concentrations of acid proteolytic activity in the culture medium if *C. albicans* or *C. tropicalis* were used for infection. Virtually no enzymatic activity was detected, however, when a particular strain of *C. parapsilosis* had been used for infection.

In the presence of 10^{-4} M of the aspartic proteinase inhibitor pepstatin-A, invasion of the proteolytic candida elements was largely suppressed, as was the adherence of fungal cells to the epithelium.

This finding correlated with the intial observation of Ghannoum & Abu Elteen (1986). It suggested a role of CP at a very early stage in the colonization of human mucosa by *Candida*. The mucosal target for CP during fungal adherence has still to be determined.

Independently, Ray & Payne (1988) published a communication on the invasion of *Candida* species in murine epidermis. They observed cavitation of the epidermal surface under attached blastoconidia only with *C. albicans*, its sucrose-negative variant *C. stellatoidea,* and *C. tropicalis*. The cavitation was inhibited by addition of pepstatin (2.5 μg/ml). Likewise the adherence of *Candida* to keratinocytes was partially inhibited by pepstatin (El-Maghrabi et al 1990).

Invasion of mucosa and dissemination of *Candida* in the host are controlled by different effectors of our defence system, as became evident from the containment of candidiasis in AIDS and its spread in leukaemic patients, who are prone to dissemination of mycosis due to a lack of phagocytic leukocytes (Matthews et al 1988).

Early in vitro observations revealed that most ingested yeasts are killed by phagocytes, but a minor fraction of candida blastoconidia were able to resist intracellular killing (Stanley & Hurley 1969). A relationship between such resistance and production of CP was suggested by Macdonald & Odds (1983), who recognized a relative resistance to phagocytic killing of proteolytically induced *C. albicans*.

Therefore, we studied the expression of CP by fungal cells after phagocytosis (Borg & Rüchel 1990). Thirty minutes after infection of cultured murine peritoneal macrophages, acid proteolytic activity became detectable in the medium, and virtually all blastoconidia were ingested after 2 h. Some of them survived and started to germinate 4 h after infection. Such intracellular germination caused the death of the phagocyte. However, the cytotoxic effect also occurred when blastoconidia only were present in the phagocyte.

Virtually all intracellular fungal elements carried the CP-antigen on their surface. The lysates from infected phagocytes showed decreasing total acid proteolytic activity (which is largely due to lysosomal cathepsin-D) and increasing concentrations of CP-antigen. These differential kinetics suggest a conflict between the microbial hydrolases and the hydrolases of the phagolysosome. The outcome of this conflict may be decisive for the progress of candidiasis. Our findings suggest that there cannot be tolerance between ingested *Candida* and the phagocyte, which would allow for intracellular persistence of candida elements over longer periods of time.

Surprisingly, several strains of the rare serotype-B of *C. albicans*, while being ingested, did express the CP-antigen on blastoconidia but not on filamentous cells (Borg & Rüchel 1990). It remains to be proven whether such differential expression of CP is a cause of the reduced virulence of serotype B, as suggested by Auger et al (1983).

Within the phagolysosome, CP may attack proteins involved in the generation of microbicidal oxygen radicals. In 1980, Sasada & Johnston, studying the generation of oxygen radicals by macrophages, recognized a strong 'respiratory burst' after ingestion of non-pathogenic *C. parapsilosis*, and a weak response to *C. albicans*. Likewise, Hilger & Danley (1980) reported an increase of the respiratory response of polymorphonuclear leukocytes (PMNs) after ingestion of killed *C. albicans* as compared with the response to viable yeasts. We have shown previously, that ingested blastoconidia of a particular strain of *C. parapsilosis* did not express the CP-antigen (Rüchel et al 1986), and this is certainly also true for killed *C. albicans*. If such ethanol-killed blastoconidia were supplemented during phagocytosis with homologous purified CP, a dose dependent reduction of the respiratory burst of PMNs was observed (M Borg-v. Zepelin & P Schuff-Werner 1991, personal communication). Hence, the paradoxically low respiratory response of phagocytes to viable *C. albicans* may indeed be due to activity of CP.

Further support for a role of CP during phagocytosis of *Candida* was lent by the results of Stutzer (1988), who infected phagocytic human tumour cells (U-937) in culture with *Candida* and recorded a cytotoxic effect which largely reflected the proteolytic activity of the yeast. Using the aspartic proteinase inhibitor pepstatin-A, he was able to demonstrate a dose-dependent protective effect on the phagocytes.

CANDIDA PROTEINASE IN EXPERIMENTAL CANDIDIASIS

During early investigations, Staib (1969) already provided circumstantial evidence for a CP-dependent virulence of *C. albicans* in mice. The first experimental evidence for proteolytic activity of *C. albicans* during experimental candidosis was presented by Macdonald & Odds (1980) who determined specific antibody titres in systemically infected rabbits and demonstrated CP-antigen on fungal elements in murine kidney. Degradation of immunoglobulins reflecting the proteolysis in mycotic murine kidneys was demonstrated by Rüchel (1984).

Later, we followed the course of systemic candidiasis in non-compromised mice by monitoring both CP-antigen and antibody titres in sequential sera (Haun et al 1987). The antigen in serum peaked around the third day after intravenous infection, thus the possibility of a transfer of the detected antigen with the inoculum could be discounted. The immune response was either boosted within the first days or it showed a typical immunization profile with a titre suddenly rising 9 days after infection. These results encouraged us to try diagnostic CP-antigen monitoring (Rüchel et al 1988).

The immunization of mice against purified CP caused a relative protection against subsequent lethal challenge with the homologous *C. albicans* strain. An inhibition of the catalytic activity of CP in vitro, though, has been accomplished neither with polyclonal antibodies, nor with monoclonal anti-CP immuno-globulins (Borg et al 1988). A comparable deficiency has been described for antibodies against the related proteinase cathepsin-D (Coetzer et al 1991).

In 1986, Ghannoum & Abu Elteen reported on a correlation of the proteolytic activity of 53 *C. albicans* isolates with strain-specific virulence in mice and adhesiveness to oral epithelia. A correlation of CP-production and invasion of the chorioallantoic membrane of infected fertilized eggs not leading to mortality was observed by Shimizu et al (1987). In a mouse model the same highly proteolytic *Candida* strains caused highest invasion and the highest mortality. These strains produced CP-antigen already at early stages of the infection (Kondoh et al 1987).

A direct assessment of the role of CP in the virulence of *C. albicans* using a virtually non-proteolytic *C. albicans* mutant and the proteolytic parental strain was first performed by Macdonald & Odds (1983), who found the mutant to be considerably less lethal for mice than the proteolytic parent.

These results were cofirmed by Kwon-Chung et al (1985), who added an observation on a proteolytic revertant, recovered from a mouse which had died after having been infected with the proteinase-deficient mutant. The revertant had regained half of the proteolytic activity of the parent and was almost as virulent as the proteolytic parent.

The virulence of another proteinase deficient mutant and its proteolytic parent were compared by Ross et al (1990), who observed a difference by a factor of thousand of the LD_{50} in favour of the proteolytic strain. This difference was confirmed in a rat model of candida vaginitis (De Bernardis et al 1990a).

The three independent investigations were performed with chemically induced mutants, and hence there have been objections, since the yeasts might have been afflicted by mutagenesis in various ways. Therefore, it is generally agreed that the results need to be confirmed by the comparison of virulence of strains which have been subjected to disruption of the CP-gene by means of molecular genetics.

In another attempt to assess the contribution of CP to the pathogenesis of candidiasis, we have investigated the effect of the aspartic proteinase inhibitor pepstatin-A on the course of lethal mycosis in mice (Rüchel et al 1990).

The inhibitor itself was slightly toxic, if applied intravenously as a suspension of micro-crystals. This detrimental effect may be due to inhibition of lysosomal cathepsin-D. The same suspension (0.1 ml at a concentration equivalent to 10^{-4} M) caused a relative protective effect if injected once prior and repeatedly after infection, thus again suggesting a role of CP in early stages of candidiasis.

Edison & Manning-Zweerink (1988) failed to demonstrate an effect of intravenous pepstatin on the course of systemic murine candidiasis. However, they used a true solution of pepstatin, which does not produce lasting inhibitory activity in serum (Rüchel et al 1990).

Likewise, we found that pepstatin is taken up in the liver, but we could not trace it in the kidneys, which are the prime targets of murine candidiasis. Therefore, future therapeutic trials with proteinase inhibitors require substances which do not react with proteinases of the host and which are taken up by the kidneys. Such substances are presently designed as therapeutic inhibitors of the related HIV-proteinases (Blundell et al 1990).

There appears to exist a particular problem with the assessment of CP-related virulence in *C. parapsilosis*. The pathogenic potential of this species in mice is considered to be much lower than that of *C. albicans* or *C. topicalis* (Bistoni et al 1984), and the extracellular proteolytic activity of most strains was correspondingly low (Rüchel et al 1983, Macdonald 1984). In a particular clinical isolate of *C. parapsilosis*, CP-activity was only induced at elevated concentrations of glucose in the medium. The strain showed low virulence in mice, and the intravenously infected animals did not mount an immune response to homologous CP. In vitro, cells of this strain were not found to express CP-antigen during phagocytosis (Rüchel et al 1986). However, vaginal isolates of *C. parapsilosis* were reported to be strongly proteolytic, though only those isolates which were derived from cases of acute vaginitis were virulent in mice (De Bernardis et al 1990b).

SECRETION OF PROTEINASE BY *CANDIDA IN CULTURE*

Extracellular acid proteolytic activity, as demonstrated by auxanographic methods, was detected by most isolates of *C. albicans, C. tropicalis,* and *C. parapsilosis* (Rüchel et al 1982, 1983, Macdonald 1984). It is generally agreed that this activity is due to truly secreted aspartic proteinase.

The assessment of proteolytic activity by exclusive use of solid media and subsequent staining of non-degraded proteins according to Staib (1965) may yield misleading results, since limited hydrolysis of the substrate protein will go unrecognized by this procedure, and strains will be falsely labelled as non-proteolytic.

By the use of liquid media with haemoglobin as nitrogen source, we have not found a truly non-proteolytic strain of *C. albicans* among 103 randomly selected clinical isolates. Testing 39 vaginal isolates of *C. albicans*, Cassone et al (1987) confirmed this result and likewise, all 35 *C. albicans* strains of a laboratory collection were proteinase positive (Howard 1987, personal communication). However, a particular strain of *C. albicans* was found to be heterozygous for the CP-gene, and CP-negative mutants of this strain occurred frequently (Crandall & Edwards 1987).

Upon electrophoresis of *C. albicans* culture supernatant, distinct patterns of degradation became apparent if bovine serum albumin was used as nitrogen source (Rüchel et al 1982). Such degradation patterns yielded the first hint of the existence of functionally different CPs.

Among 29 clinical isolates of *C. tropicalis,* we identified a single strain which proved to be virtually non-proteolytic. This strain is available from the Deutsche Sammlung von Mikroorganismen (Mascheroder Weg 1b, D-3300 Braunschweig, Germany) as DSM 4959.

All 11 clinical isolates of *C. parapsilosis* tested were moderately proteolytic, while various isolates of *C. glabrata, C. guilliermondii, C. kefyr (C. pseudotropicalis),* and *C. krusei* were negative on protein agar and produced little activity in haemoglobin broth (Rüchel et al 1983). These results were essentially in agreement with the data of Macdonald (1984) and Ray & Payne (1990).

With a single clinical isolate of *C. glabrata (Torulopsis glabrata)*, Reinholdt et al (1987) observed weak extracellular proteolytic activity. Whether this activity was truly secretory, or whether it represented the acid proteinase from the vacuoles of decaying blastoconidia, remains to be elucidated.

The conditions under which the secretion of CP is induced are critical. This was exemplified by a communication on the inhibition of CP-secretion by saliva (Germaine & Tellefson 1981). The authors used a medium with 0.1% (w/v) glucose, but in our hands, most proteolytic *Candida* strains required at least 0.3% glucose for the induction of CP-activity (Rüchel 1986). Samaranayake et al (1984) demonstrated the degradation by *C. albicans* of proteins in saliva, which was supplemented with 0.2 M glucose – a concentration which may be reached in niches of the oral cavity. Even under strictly anaerobic conditions, secretion of CP could be demonstrated, although the concentration of glucose required for induction was raised from 0.3% to 1% under these conditions (Rüchel 1986).

A sufficient concentration of degradable carbohydrate in the medium is a prerequisite for CP-activity, since organic acids derived from its incomplete degradation cause the acidification of the environment which precedes CP-activity (Fig. 2.3). It remains to be investigated whether this sequence of events is obligatory for the induction of CP or whether it rather reflects the pH-dependent profile of CP-activity.

The conditions of induction of CP secretion by particular *C. albicans* strains in the presence of keratin or BSA were described in detail by Tsuboi et al (1989) and Ross et al (1990). Media with haemoglobin, BSA, casein, collagen, or keratin were compared by Ray & Payne (1990), who found keratin-supplementation most suitable for CP-production. The growth of *C. albicans* on different types of collagen was demonstrated by Kaminishi et al (1988). Whole serum, at a concentration of, for example, 5% will also induce CP-secretion in the presence of 1% glucose.

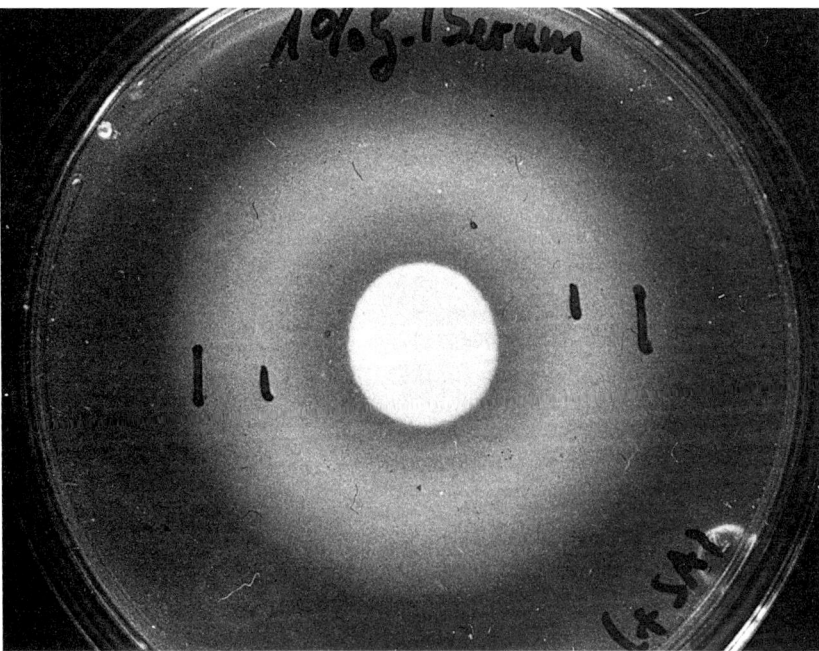

Fig. 2.3 Proteolytic candida colony on protein agar according to Staib (1965) with 5% (v/v) human serum, as the nitrogen source, and 1% glucose. Acidification causes the turbidity by precipitation of proteins. The extent of precipitation at 24 h and 48 h is shown by the marks. The resolution of turbidity directly around the colony indicates hydrolysis of the protein precipitate.

Secretion continues if carbohydrate is repeatedly supplied. With a variant of *C. albicans*, CBS-2730, we have detected up to approximately 10 mg CP per litre of medium. On depletion of glucose in the media, the pH rises due to increasing ammonia, and CP-activity disappears (Tsuboi et al 1989). Production of CP can thus be controlled. However, temperature dependence and an inoculum effect suggest a role of co-operative factors, which need to be investigated.

CHARACTERIZATION OF *CANDIDA* PROTEINASE

The first data on CP were communicated by Remold et al (1968), who purified the enzyme of *C. albicans* CBS-2730 from a BSA-broth using gel filtration and anion-exchange chromatography. They estimated the molecular weight at 40 000 and found an optimum of activity at pH 3.2. The substrate specificity was low, with an apparent preference for hydrophobic amino acid residues. None of the available inhibitors was found to act on proteinase 2730, including diazoacetylnorleucine methyl ester (DAN), which is an inhibitor of the aspartic proteinase, pepsin.

Using a different *C. albicans* strain but related techniques for purification, Macdonald & Odds (1980) showed that CP was a mannoprotein whose enzymic activity was sensitive to pepstatin-A, which is a typical inhibitor of the aspartic proteinases (E.C.3.4.23.6). This result was confirmed by Rüchel (1981), who determined the point of equivalence of the pepstatin-CP bond at 2×10^{-8} M again using CP-2730. Pepstatin proved useful as a solid phase ligand for affinity chromatography of CP. By SDS-electrophoresis, the molecular weight of the CP-2730 was estimated in the range of 45 000. An apparent molecular mass of 41 500 daltons was determined for CP of another strain by Ray & Payne (1990). CP-2730 consisted of a single polypeptide chain with an isoelectric point at pH 4.4. The enzyme was stable against freeze-thawing and non-ionic detergents. However, at room temperature above pH 8.4, the enzyme underwent rapid irreversible alkaline denaturation, which may involve dimerization as visualized during electrophoresis in a pH gradient (Rüchel & Trost 1981).

The interpretation of corresponding electropherograms was hampered by the fact that denatured CP-2730 migrated in a position of approximately 70 000 molecular weight only. This conflict may now be solved by analysis of the amino acid sequence of CP (Hube et al 1991). It contains a prepropeptide, which may still be retained in the 'monomer', which in fact could represent the proenzyme of CP. Such proenzyme (equivalent to pepsinogen) has been postulated but not yet identified. The mature monomeric enzyme may be identical with a faster migrating molecule of CP-preparations, which reacted with specific monoclonal antibodies (Borg et al 1988).

A comparison of the CP-activity of different *C. albicans* isolates suggested the existence of functionally different proteinases, with a single enzyme being secreted by any individual strain. The CP of *C. albicans* isolate 113, which hydrolysed BSA only partially, was purified and proved particularly prone to alkaline denaturation (Rüchel et al 1982). Strain 113 belongs to the rare serotype B and is available from the American Type Culture Collection as ATCC-48867. As with other strains of this serotype, expression of the CP-antigen in vitro was found only on blastoconidia (Borg & Rüchel 1990).

A functional differentiation of CPs was also detected among strains of *C. tropicalis*, when degradation of BSA and patterns of inhibition were compared (Rüchel et al 1983). Species-specific differences were suggested by reaction with rabbit antibodies, which had been elicited against purified CPs.

The patterns of BSA-degradation in vitro by clinical isolates of *C. parapsilosis* suggested a lower proteolytic activity which led to the total hydrolysis of BSA. We have purified the CP of an urinary isolate of this species; this isolate, 265, is available as DSM 4237.

CP-265 has a molecular weight in the range of 33 000 only. It is highly sensitive against alkaline pH and is not induced on blastoconidia during phagocytosis (Rüchel et al 1986).

A comparison of the reactivity with lectins of proteinase 265 and the corresponding enzymes of *C. tropicalis* 293 and *C. albicans* CBS-2730 suggested the presence of mannose residues in CP-293, but no indication of glycosylation was found with the two other CPs. This difference may again reflect the strain-specificity of CPs.

Likewise, the mature CP from *C. albicans* ATCC-10231 does not contain an obvious site for glycosylation, while CP-10261 contains two sites (Hube & Sullivan 1991, personal communications). The gene of CP-10231 was recently sequenced, and the corresponding sequence of 341 amino acids was deduced (Hube et al 1991). As a typical aspartic proteinase (Davies 1990), proteinase 10231 has two functional aspartic acid residues. Its theoretical molecular mass is 41 619 daltons. A N-terminal sequence of 50 amino acids may represent the corresponding signal peptide and a propeptide, putting the molecular mass of the mature enzyme at 36 234 daltons (Rüchel et al 1991a, in press).

At an overall homology of 72%, the sequence of CP-10231 shares many common features with the sequence of CP from *C. albicans* ATCC-10261, which has 348 amino acids (Rüchel et al 1991a, in press). The differences between the two sequences may reflect the functional differences between CPs of various strains. A high degree of genetic flexibility is also suggested by discrete differences among the N-terminal amino acid sequences of three other CPs (Odds 1991, personal communication).

Previously, a gene of an aspartic proteinase (PrA) of *C. albicans* was sequenced by Lott et al (1989). According to the EMBL-databank, the PrA gene was also derived from *C. albicans* CBS-2730. PrA was identified using the gene of the vacuolar proteinase-A of *Saccharomyces cerevisiae* as a probe. The homology of both amino acid sequences was 85%. However, it is unlikely that PrA represents the secretory proteinase of *C. albicans* CBS-2730. Certain polyclonal antibodies against purified CP of this strain did not react with *S. cerevisiae* proteinase-A, although the high homology between PrA and the enzyme from baker's yeast should have warranted such a reaction (Rüchel 1989, unpublished data). PrA may rather represent the vacuolar aspartic proteinase of *C. albicans*. There is only 25% homology between the amino acid sequences of PrA and CP-10261 (P. Sullivan, personal communication) and a 30% homology between PrA and CP-10231 (Rüchel et al 1991a, in press).

Recently, the gene of the secretory proteinase from another *C. albicans* strain was cloned. (Ganesan et al 1991) and a corresponding gene from *C. tropicalis* was sequenced (Togni et al 1991).

SUBSTRATES OF *CANDIDA* PROTEINASES

In their initial investigation, Remold et al (1968) used the insulin β-chain and serum albumin as substrates for CP of *C. albicans* CBS-2730. They observed a low specificity and a preference for peptide bonds between hydrophobic residues. Correspondingly, haemoglobin is an excellent substrate of CPs, it is not matched by any other conventional substrate. Azocoll (a red derivative of collagen) is less sensitive but particularly practical as a substrate (Rüchel 1981). Due to a lack of suitable small substrates, no reliable kinetic data on CPs are available at present.

The hydrolysis of serum albumin by most CPs is virtually total, which is surprising, since albumin is stabilized by 17 disulphides (Anderson 1979). Therefore, few proteins can be expected to resist attack by CPs. Among these are lysozyme and ferritin.

Salivary proteins such as lactoferrin, lactoperoxidase, and the protein moiety of mucin were degraded by CP (Rüchel, unpublished data). Likewise, secretory immunoglobulin-A and its constituents were degraded, including the structurally differing IgA2 (Rüchel 1986, Rüchel et al 1986), which resisted degradation by the IgA-proteinases of certain pathogenic bacteria (Kilian et al 1988). Evidence for the degradation of immunoglobulins during candidiasis was produced in mice (Rüchel 1984). It has however to be kept in mind, that such degradation can be caused in part by proteinases of the host (Neely et al 1991).

At neutral pH, no activity of CPs has been demonstrated so far. However, close to pH 6.5, limited proteolysis of a renin substrate was observed (Rüchel 1983).

At subneutral pH, CP also coverted trypsinogen to trypsin (Rüchel 1981), and a related effect was detected with the blood coagulation factor X (Rüchel 1983). The activation of factor X raises a yet unsolved question. The activated factor Xa may be atypical, since it converted whole prothrombin but did not cleave a peptide analogue at the typical activation site of prothrombin. The activation of other serine proteinases was observed by Kaminishi et al (1990), who described the activation by CP of the plasma kallikrein-kinin system.

No specific inhibitor of CP in human plasma has yet been described. Only alpha-2-macroglobulin can bind CP. However, CP may escape this trap by degradation of the inhibitor (Rüchel & Böning 1983). This mechanism was confirmed with related acid proteinases (Lah et al 1985). Antibodies inhibiting CP-activity have not yet been detected.

CONCLUSIONS

There is ample evidence for the presence of secretory acid candida proteinase (CP) in the human host during mycosis with *C. albicans* or *C. tropicalis* as causative agents. The evidence for the expression in vivo of CP by *C. parapsilosis* is still open to dispute. Likewise, the existence of CP-like activity in fresh clinical isolates of *C. glabrata* needs re-examination.

There is still no definitive answer to the question of the rank of CP as a factor of virulence. However, the available evidence suggests such a role, and confirmation may come from gene disruption experiments.

Little is known on the substrates of CP in the human host. Particularly targets of CP-activity during invasion of epithelia and in the acid milieu of the phagolysosome should be investigated. Limited proteolysis by CP at subneutral pH deserves attention, since it may alter physiological regulation.

CP is induced at an early stage of infection. The sequence of events during induction and its dependence on the secretion of protons need to be clarified. The differential expression of the CP-antigen in strains of *C. albicans* serotype B should be followed up.

The secretion of CP is a rapid process (we have, for example, not been able to trap CP in the cell wall with various specific monoclonal antibodies). Secretion and maturation of the enzyme possibly require the cleavage of a signal peptide and a propeptide. The responsible peptidases need to be identified and may yield a target for therapy like CP itself.

Therapeutic inhibitors of CP could be deduced from the compounds, which are designed for inhibition of retroviral aspartic proteinases. Such inhibitors can be based on pepstatin or could be tailored as specific substrate analogues with a modified peptide bond at the cleavage site.

Nucleotide and amino acid sequences of CPs are currently becoming available. They reveal a high degree of genetic flexibility of *Candida,* as we already suggested by functional differences among CPs. The implications of such differences (including the apparent glycosylation of some but not all CPs) for fungal virulence may open up a new field of candida research.

ACKNOWLEDGEMENT

I am indebted to my colleagues Margarete Borg-v. Zepelin and Bernard Hube for helpful discussions. Our own investigations were supported by the Deutsche Forschungsgemeinschaft.

REFERENCES

Abbasi A, Voelter W, Zaidi Z H 1986 Isolation purification and properties of a site-specific proteolytic enzyme 'valyl-proteinase' from *Candida tropicalis*. Biological Chemistry Hoppe Seyler 367: 441–445

Andersson L O 1979 Serum albumin. In: Blombäck B, Hanson L A, Winberg H (eds) Plasma proteins. John Wiley, Chichester, pp 43–54

Auger P, Dumas C, Joly J 1983 Interactions of serotypes A and B of *Candida albicans* in mice. Sabouraudia 21: 173–178

Bistoni F, Vecchiarelli A, Cenci E, Sbaraglia G, Perito S, Cassone A 1984 A comparison of experimental pathogenicity of *Candida* species in cyclophosphamide-immunodepressed mice. Sabouraudia 22: 409–418

Blundell T L, Lapatto R, Wilderspin A F et al. 1990 The 3-D structure of HIV-1 proteinase and the design of antiviral agents for the treatment of AIDS. Trends in Biochemical Sciences 15: 425–430

Borg M, Rüchel R 1988 Expression of extracellular acid proteinase by proteolytic *Candida* spp. during experimental infection of oral mucosa. Infection and Immunity 56: 626–631

Borg M, Watters D, Reich B, Rüchel R 1988 Production and characterization of monoclonal antibodies against secretory proteinase of *Candida albicans* CBS 2730. Zentralblatt für Bakteriologie und Hygiene A 268: 62–73

Borg M, Rüchel R 1990 Demonstration of fungal proteinase during phagocytosis of *Candida albicans* and *Candida tropicalis*. Journal of Medical and Veterinary Mycology 28: 3–14

Borg-v. Zepelin M, Schuff-Werner P 1991 Personal communication

Cassone A, De Bernardis F, Mondello F, Ceddia T, Agatensi L 1987 Evidence for a correlation between proteinase secretion and vulvovaginal candidosis. Journal of Infectious diseases 156: 777–783

Coetzer T H T, Elliott E, Fortgens P H, Pike R N, Dennison C 1991 Anti-peptide antibodies to cathepsins B, L and D and type IV collagenase. Journal of Immunological Methods 136: 199–210

Crandall M, Edwards J E 1987 Segregation of proteinase-negative mutants from heterozygous *Candida albicans*. Journal of General Microbiology 133: 2817–2824

Davies D R 1990 The structure and function of the aspartic proteinases. Annual Review of Biophysics and Biophysical Chemistry 19: 189–215

De Bernardis F, Agatensi L, Ross I K, et al 1990a Evidence for a role for secreted aspartate proteinase of *Candida albicans* in vulvovaginal candidiasis. Journal of Infectious Diseases 161: 1276–1283

De Bernardis F, Morelli L, Ceddia T, Lorenzini R, Cassone A 1990b Experimental pathogenicity and acid proteinase secretion of vaginal isolates of *Candida parapsilosis*. Journal of Medical and Veterinary Mycology 28: 125–137

El-Maghrabi E A, Dixon D M, Burnett J W 1990 Characterization of *Candida albicans* epidermolytic proteases and their role in yeast-cell adherence to keratinocytes. Clinical and Experimental Dermatology 15: 183–191

Edison A M, Manning-Zweerink M 1988 Comparison of the extracellular proteinase activity produced by a low-virulence mutant of *Candida albicans* and its wild-type parent. Infection and Immunity 56: 1388–1390

Farley P C, Shepherd M G, Sullivan P A 1986 The purification and properties of yeast proteinase B from *Candida albicans*. Biochemical Journal 236: 177–184

Ganesan K, Bannerjee A, Datta A 1991 Molecular cloning of the secretory acid proteinase gene from *Candida albicans* and its use as a species-specific probe. Infection and Immunity 59: 2972–2977

Germaine G R, Tellefson L M 1981 Effect of pH and saliva on protease production by *Candida albicans*. Infection and Immunity 31: 323–326

Ghannoum M, Abu Elteen K 1986 Correlative relationship between proteinase production, adherence and pathogenicity of various strains of *Candida albicans*. Journal of Medical and Veterinary Mycology 24: 407–413

Haun U, Rüchel R, Spies A 1987 A series of serological tests for the detection of antigens and specific antibodies in deep-seated candidosis: experimental aspects. Mykosen 30: 472–482

Hilger A E, Danley D L 1980 Alteration of polymorphonuclear leukocyte activity by viable *Candida albicans*. Infection and Immunity 27: 714–720

Howard D H 1987 Personal communication

Hube B, Turver C J, Odds F C et al. 1991 Sequences of the *Candida albicans* gene encoding the secretory aspartate proteinase. Journal of Medical and Veterinary Mycology 29: 129–131

Hube B, Sullivan P A 1991 Personal communication

Kaminishi H, Hagihara Y, Tanaka M, Cho T 1988 Degradation of bovine achilles tendon collagen by *Candida albicans* proteinase. Journal of Medical and Veterinary Mycology 26: 315–318

Kaminishi H, Tanaka M, Cho T, Maeda H, Hagihara Y 1990 Activation of the plasma kallikrein-kinin system by *Candida albicans* proteinase. Infection and Immunity 58: 2139–2143

Kilian M, Mestecky J, Russell M W 1988 Defense mechanisms involving Fc-dependent functions of immunoglobulin A and their subversion by bacterial immunoglobulin A proteases. Microbiological Reviews 52: 296–303

Kondoh Y, Shimizu K, Tanaka K 1987 Proteinase production and pathogenicity of *Candida albicans*. Microbiology and Immunology 31: 1061–1069

Kwon-Chung K J, Lehman D, Good C, Magee P T 1985 Genetic evidence for role of extracellular proteinase in virulence of *Candida albicans*. Infection and Immunity 49: 571–576

Lah T, Vihar M, Turk V (1985) Interaction of cathepsin D and pepsin with alpha-2-macroglobulin. In: Kostka V (ed) Aspartic proteinases and their inhibitors. Walter de Gruyter, Berlin, pp 485–490

Logan D A 1988 Regulation of intracellular carboxypeptidase activity in *Candida albicans*. Experimental Mycology 12: 386–390

Lott T J, Page L S, Boiron P, Benson J, Reiss E 1989 Nucleotide sequence of the *Candida albicans* aspartyl proteinase gene. Nucleic Acids Research 17: 1779

Macdonald F, Odds F C 1980 Inducible proteinase of *Candida albicans* in diagnostic serology and in the pathogenesis of systemic candidosis. Journal of Medical Microbiology 13: 423–435

Macdonald F, Odds F C 1983 Virulence for mice of a proteinase-secreting strain of *Candida albicans* and a proteinase-deficient mutant. Journal of General Microbiology 129: 431–438

Macdonald F 1984 Secretion of inducible proteinase by pathogenic *Candida* species. Sabouraudia 22: 79–82

Matthews R, Burnie J, Smith D et al 1988 Candida and AIDS: evidence for protective antibody. Lancet ii: 263–266

Neely A N, Childress C M, Holder I A 1991 Effect of challenge with *Candida albicans* strains with different levels of virulence on plasma proteins in burned mice. Infection and Immunity 59:1576–1578

Odds F C 1985 *Candida albicans* proteinase as a virulence factor in the pathogenesis of candida infections. Zentralblatt für Bakteriologie und Hygiene A 260:539–542

Portillo F, Gancedo C 1986 Purification and properties of three intracellular proteinases from *Candida albicans*. Biochimica et Biophysica Acta 881: 229–235

Ray T L, Payne C D 1982 Characterization of an acid protease produced by *Candida albicans* and related species. Clinical Research 30 (abstract): 801-A

Ray T L, Payne C D 1988 Scanning electron microscopy of epidermal adherence and cavitation in murine candidiasis: a role for *Candida* acid proteinase. Infection and Immunity 56: 1942–1949

Ray T L, Payne C D 1990 Comparative production and rapid purification of *Candida* acid proteinase from protein-supplemented cultures. Infection and Immunity 58: 508–514

Reinholdt J, Krogh P, Holmstrup P 1987 Degradation of IgA1, IgA2, and S-IgA by *Candida* and *Torulopsis* species. Acta Pathologica Microbiologica Immunologica Scandinavica Section C 95: 265–274

Remold H, Staib F, Fasold H 1968 Purification and characterization of a proteolytic enzyme from *Candida albicans*. Biochimica et Biophysica Acta 167: 399–406

Ross I K, De Bernardis F, Emerson G W, Cassone A, Sullivan P A 1990 The secreted aspartate proteinase of *Candida albicans*: physiology of secretion and virulence of a proteinase-deficient mutant. Journal of General Microbiology 136: 687–694

Rüchel R 1981 Properties of a purified proteinase from the yeast *Candida albicans*. Biochimica et Biophysica Acta 659: 99–113

Rüchel R, Trost M 1981 A study of the structural conversions of two carboxyl proteinases employing electrophoresis across a pH-gradient. In: All R C, Arnaud P (eds) Electrophoresis '81. Walter de Gruyter, Berlin, pp 667–676

Rüchel R, Tegeler R, Trost M 1982 A comparison of secretory proteinases from different strains of *Candida albicans*. Sabouraudia 20: 233–244

Rüchel R 1983 On the renin-like activity of candida proteinases and activation of blood coagulation in vitro. Zentralblatt für Bakteriologie und Hygiene I. Abt. Orig. A 255: 368–379

Rüchel R, Böning B 1983 Detection of *Candida* proteinase by enzyme immunoassay and interaction of the enzyme with alpha-2-macroglobulin. Journal of Immunological Methods 61: 107–116

Rüchel R, Uhlemann K, Böning B 1983 Secretion of acid proteinases by different species of the genus *Candida*. Zentralblatt für Bakteriologie und Hygiene I. Abt. Orig. A 255: 537–548

Rüchel R 1984 A variety of candida proteinases and their possible targets of proteolytic attack in the host. Zentralblatt für Bakteriologie und Hygiene A 257: 266–274

Rüchel R, Böning B, Jahn E 1985 Identification and partial characterization of two proteinases from the cell envelope of *Candida albicans* blastospores. Zentralblatt für Bakteriologie und Hygiene A 260: 523–538

Rüchel R, 1986 Cleavage of immunoglobulins by pathogenic yeasts of the genus *Candida*. Microbiological Sciences 3: 316–319

Rüchel R, Böning B, Borg M 1986 Characterization of a secretory proteinase of *Candida parapsilosis* and evidence for the absence of the enzyme during infection in vitro. Infection and Immunity 53: 411–419

Rüchel R, Böning-Stutzer B, Mari A 1988 A synoptical approach to the diagnosis of candidosis, relying on serological antigen and antibody tests, on culture, and on evaluation of clinical data. Mycoses 31: 87–106

Rüchel R, Ritter B, Schaffrinski M 1990 Modulation of experimental systemic murine candidosis by intravenous pepstatin. Zentralblatt für Bakteriologie 273: 391–403

Rüchel R, De Bernardis F, Ray T L, Sullivan P A, Cole G T 1991a. Candida acid proteinases (CAP). Journal of Medical and Veterinary Mycology, in press

Rüchel R, Zimmermann F, Böning-Stutzer B, Helmchen U 1991b Candidosis visualized by proteinase-directed immunofluorescence. Virchow's Archiv A, in press

Samaranayake K P, Hughes A, Macfarlane T W 1984 The proteolytic potential of *Candida albicans* in human saliva supplemented with glucose. Journal of Medical Microbiology 17: 13–22

Sasada M, Johnston R B Macrophage microbicidal activity. Correlation between phagocytosis-associated oxidative metabolism and the killing of *Candida* by macrophages. Journal of Experimental Medicine 152: 85–98

Shimizu K, Kondoh Y, Tanaka K 1987 Proteinase production and pathogenicity of *Candida albicans*. Microbiology and Immunology 31: 1045–1060

Staib F 1965 Serum-proteins as nitrogen source for yeastlike fungi. Sabouraudia 4: 187–193

Staib F 1969 Proteolysis and pathogenicity of *Candida albicans* strains. Mycopathologia et Mycologia Applicata 37: 345–348

Stanley V C, Hurley R 1969 The growth of *Candida* species in cultures of mouse peritoneal macrophages. Journal of Pathology 97: 357–366

Stutzer H 1988 Inhibition der Zytotoxizität von Candida-Hefen durch Antikörper und durch einen Protease-Inhibitor. MD-thesis, Faculty of Medicine, University of Göttingen, Germany

Taschdjian C L, Kozinn P J 1961 Metabolic studies of the tissue phase of *Candida albicans* induced in vitro. Sabouraudia 1: 73–82

Togni G, Sanglard D, Falchetto R, Monod M 1991 Isolation and nucleotide sequence of the extracellular acid protease gene (ACP) from the yeast *Candida tropicalis*. Federation of European Biochemical Societies Letters 286: 181–185

Tsuboi R, Matsuda K, Ko I J, Ogawa H 1989 Correlation between culture medium pH, extracellular proteinase activity, and cell growth of *Candida albicans* in insoluble stratum corneum-supplemented media. Archives of Dermatological Research 281: 342–345

Discussion of paper presented by R. Rüchel

Discussed by F. C. Odds
Reported by K. P. W. J. McAdam

In opening the discussion, Dr Odds paid tribute to Dr Rüchel's elegant experiments over the past decade all of which suggest that *Candida albicans* secreted proteinase is indeed a virulence factor of the fungus. Yet, the more that is learnt about this enzyme the more openings there are for criticism of what has been done, so that there is still not 100% proof that proteinase secretion and virulence are positively associated. For example, if it is believed that secreted proteinase of *C. albicans* is a virulence factor, then why does *Saccharomycopsis fibuligera* which also secretes a related proteinase not have similar pathological effects on patients as *C. albicans*? The answer is obviously that there is a lot more to virulence in *C. albicans* than just proteinase. Thus, this enzyme is probably just one of a panoply of virulence factors, most of which have not yet been recognized.

Dr Rüchel had mentioned some of the curious facts that seem to underpin the behaviour of *C. albicans*: for example proteinase seems to be produced only on blastospores in *C. albicans* serotype B. Dr Odds pointed out that the pseudohyphae of at least one type A strain also failed to secrete proteinase. That strain also produced much less proteinase at 37°C than at lower temperatures. This highlights the difficulty of using a single yardstick of proteolytic activity to correlate with virulence.

It was pointed out that in terms of molecular biological approaches, 1991 is the year of *Candida* proteinase since two groups, within 5 months, have published their success in cloning the *C. albicans* proteinase gene. The *C. tropicalis* secreted proteinase has also been cloned in at least two laboratories. Now that the gene is available, the obvious thing to do is to disrupt it or replace it to give a definitive mutant for virulence studies. However, mutations often involve multiple genes and, although gene deletion experiments are precise, they are technically difficult because genes must be deleted from both alleles. It would be possible to carry the gene in a less pathogenic yeast and then determine whether the virulence of that yeast has increased. There is a need to study the regulation and expression of the proteinase because *C. albicans* cells express different phenotypes, even on a cell-to-cell basis and probably within infected tissues, so there is a need to correlate the level of expression of proteinase with pathogenic situations. It would be useful to make secretion deficient mutants – mutants that synthesize the proteinase in the normal way but fail to secrete it – in order to examine how important secretion of the proteinase is, as opposed to its synthesis and appearance perhaps on the cell surface. Regulation of proteinase synthesis probably occurs at the transcriptional level but there is little hard experimental detail concerning regulation of synthesis and secretion.

It is possible to use specific monoclonal antibodies to look at cell-by-cell expression of the proteinase in vivo and in vitro, but the critical part is to do such studies in many types of *Candida* infection. Up to now the focus has been on intravenous *Candida* challenge in mice but that is rather a blunderbuss approach. There are many different forms of *Candida* infection, and since there is some evidence to suggest that the proteinase is important in initial colonization, adherence and invasion events, it is important to look at a lot more than merely lethality in a systemic infection.

One of the points raised in general discussion was that future studies need to take full account of the differences between direct proteolytic effects in pathogenesis (for example degradation of the mucin protein core and lysis of keratinaceous cells) and indirect effects (such as activation of complement and other host pro-proteins, inactivation of immunoglobulin, etc.). There is no evidence to associate the proteinase with the known tissue tropisms of *C. albicans* but future experiments could be designed to exclude such an association.

Also mentioned was that in infected tissues the proteinase may be expressed in local microniches of low pH that are created within zones of physiological pH by the acidification generated by growing *C. albicans* cells. This hypothesis may explain the apparent paradox in which an enzyme with a very low pH optimum is cited as a virulence attribute for invasion of tissues with a neutral pH.

It is possible that the secreted proteinase may be a diagnostic reagent. Dr Rüchel has shown that the antigen can be picked up in the serum of infected animals and the antibody can be detected. It seems unlikely that detection of the proteinase will act as a 'yes or no' test that would indicate if the patient has serious *C. albicans* infection, but it may be an antigen of use as a serial monitoring reagent in patients at risk. Finally, it was suggested that if the proteinase is a virulence factor, it may also be a target for drugs. This possibility is now under investigation in at least one institution. Whether inhibiting the proteinase would cure a *Candida*-infected patient remains to be seen. It seems likely that more is required than merely to block one of several virulence factors.

3. Mannoprotein adhesins of *Candida albicans*

L. J. Douglas

INTRODUCTION

The importance of adhesion as an early event in the pathogenesis of many microbial infections is now well established and adhesion mechanisms are being actively investigated at the molecular level. During the last 10 or 12 years *Candida* adhesion to a variety of surfaces has been studied in vitro. These include epithelial and endothelial cells, fibrin-platelet matrices, bacteria, neutrophils, and inert materials such as denture acrylic and Teflon (reviewed by Rotrosen et al 1986, Douglas 1987a,b). This contribution will focus primarily on the characterization of surface components involved in the interaction between *Candida albicans* and epithelial cells. The terms 'adhesin' and 'receptor' will be used to describe complementary adhesive structures on the microbial and host cell surfaces, respectively.

ADHESION AND VIRULENCE

The pathogenic *Candida* species are all opportunistic pathogens: they commonly colonize their human hosts without producing any signs of disease. Clearly, therefore, candidal adhesion is only one of a range of factors relating to pathogen or host that determine whether infection is established.

Species differences

A relationship between pathogenicity and adhesion was first demonstrated by King et al (1980) who measured *Candida* attachment to exfoliated buccal and vaginal epithelial cells. With either cell type, *C. albicans* – unquestionably the most virulent species – was also the most adherent, followed by *C. tropicalis* and *C. parapsilosis*. The less virulent species, *C. guilliermondii, C. krusei* and *C. pseudotropicalis*, showed relatively little adhesion. Similar species differences have been reported for adhesion to epidermal corneocytes (Ray et al 1984), intestinal epithelial cells (Klotz & Penn 1987), vascular endothelium (Klotz et al 1983) and fibrin-platelet matrices (Maisch & Calderone 1980) in vitro.

Strain differences

Differences in adhesion between strains of the same species are less obvious but, in the case of *C. albicans*, can often be demonstrated by growing the yeasts in medium with a high concentration of certain sugars. With some strains such conditions promote the synthesis of surface fibrils which enhance yeast adhesion (see below). Other strains do not respond in this way. In a survey of nine *C. albicans* strains (McCourtie & Douglas 1984), the adhesion and virulence of seven strains isolated from active infections were compared with those of two obtained from asymptomatic carriers. After growth in medium containing a high concentration of galactose or sucrose, all of the infective strains showed substantially enhanced adhesion and increased virulence for mice. By contrast, the carrier strains exhibited little or no increase in either property. Less pathogenic *Candida* species, as well as the non-pathogenic yeast *Saccharomyces cerevisiae*, also seem to lack the cell-surface versatility of the infective *C. albicans* strains (Critchley & Douglas 1985).

Adhesion-deficient mutants

More direct evidence for the importance of adhesion in the pathogenic process has come from studies with mutants showing a reduced ability to adhere. For example, a spontaneous cerulenin-resistant mutant of *C. albicans* adhered less readily in vitro to human vaginal epithelial cells than the parent strain, and was found to be less virulent in a mouse model of vaginal candidosis (Lehrer et al 1986). The same mutant failed to adhere to fibrin-platelet clots in vitro and was relatively avirulent in a rabbit model of endocarditis (Calderone et al 1985). Antigenic analysis revealed differences in cell-wall mannoprotein composition between mutant and wild-type strains (Calderone & Wadsworth 1988). Recently, Fukayama & Calderone (1991) have described a different type of adhesion-deficient mutant, selected on the basis of its reduced agglutination with a polyclonal anti-*Candida* antiserum, which also appears to have an altered mannoprotein composition.

THE *CANDIDA* CELL WALL

Overall composition

Since *Candida* adhesins must be located on the cell surface, their characterization requires a detailed knowledge of the fungal cell wall. The wall composition of *C. albicans* has received less attention than that of *S. cerevisiae* but it appears to be qualitatively similar, consisting mainly of mannoproteins and β-glucans. Purified walls from yeasts and germ tube-forming cells have the following composition: glucan, 48 to 60%; mannoprotein, 20 to 23%; protein, 3 to 6%; chitin, 0.6 to 2.7%; and lipid, 2% (Sullivan et al 1983). Relative amounts of alkali-soluble and insoluble glucans vary according to the growth form, and hyphae contain 3–4 times as much chitin as yeast cells. A number of germ tube-specific mannoproteins have also been identified (Sundstrom & Kenny 1985, Casanova et al 1989). Not all proteins are glycosylated, and one or more non-glycosylated proteins may be phosphorylated (Casanova & Chaffin 1991).

Wall ultrastructure

Transmission electron microscopy has shown that the wall contains five to eight distinct layers, depending on the growth conditions, growth form (yeast or hyphal) and cytochemical techniques used (Shepherd 1987). The outermost layer, which is the one most likely to be involved in adhesion, is fibrillar and sometimes discontinuous in nature (Cassone et al 1973), and there is clear evidence from both cytochemical (Tronchin et al 1981) and agglutination (Cassone et al 1978) studies with concanavalin A that it consists of mannoprotein. Its synthesis is conditioned by the composition of the growth medium (Poulain et al 1978). Growth in the presence of high concentrations of galactose or sucrose promotes its formation (McCourtie & Douglas 1981; Fig. 3.1) and simultaneously enhances yeast adhesion (Douglas et al 1981, McCourtie & Douglas 1984). Fibrils can be seen to mediate *Candida* attachment to epithelial cells in clinical samples from patients with oral candidosis (Marrie & Costerton 1981). The fibrils may represent appendages analogous to bacterial fimbriae; fimbriae have been reported in a variety of yeast species, including *C. albicans* (Gardiner et al 1982).

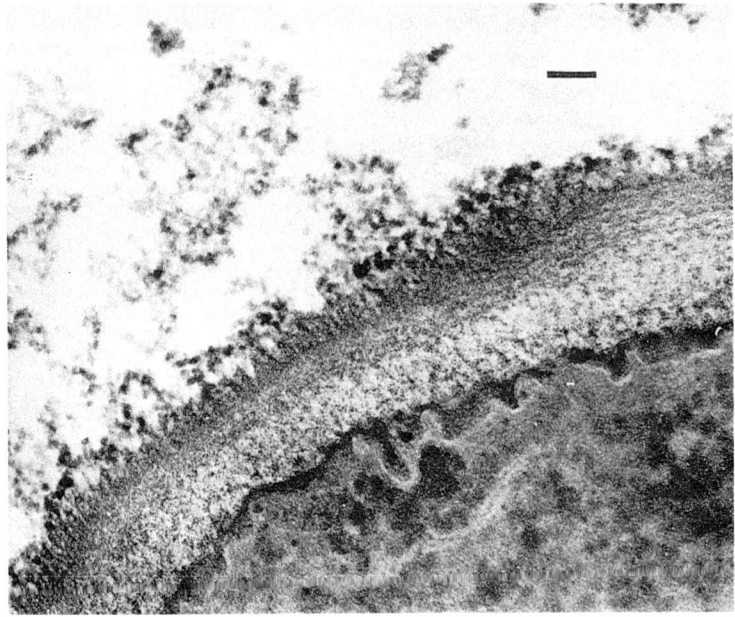

Fig. 3.1 Electron micrograph of a thin section of *C. albicans* NCPF 3153 stained with ruthenium red. Cells were harvested in the stationary growth phase from yeast nitrogen base medium containing 500 mM sucrose. Bar, 0.1 μm.

Mannoprotein structure

Yeast mannoproteins comprise a heterogeneous mixture of large molecules in which carbohydrate (mannan), accounting for as much as 95% of the overall weight, is covalently linked to protein. The basic structure of *C. albicans* mannoprotein appears to be similar to that of *S. cerevisiae* (Fig. 3.2). Carbohydrate chains are joined to protein via either O- or N-glycosidic linkages. The O-linked chains

36

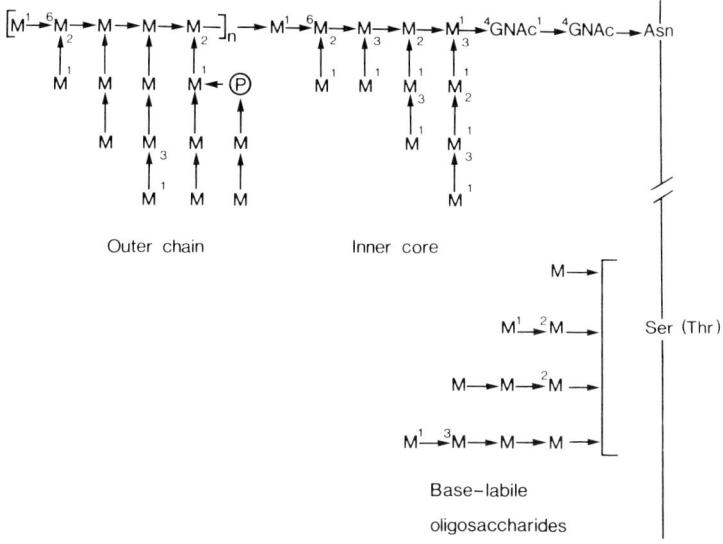

Fig. 3.2 Generalized structure for yeast mannoprotein as first proposed by Ballou (1976) for *S. cerevisiae*. M, Mannose; P, phosphate; GNAc, N-acetyl-D-glucosamine; Asn, asparagine; Ser, serine; Thr, threonine.

consist of 1 to 4 mannose residues attached to serine or threonine, from which they can be released by treatment with dilute alkali. The N-linked chains are highly branched polysaccharides joined to asparagine residues in the protein via an N-acetylglucosamine dimer bridge. They are composed of an α-1,6-linked 'backbone' with short oligomannoside side chains containing α-1,2- and α-1,3-linkages. The first segment of the polysaccharide, designated the 'inner core', can be distinguished biosynthetically from the 'outer chain' region which also contains diesterified phosphate groups (Fig. 3.2).

It appears that the mannoprotein of *C. albicans* is more highly phosphorylated than that of *S. cerevisiae*, has longer side chains, and contains some β-linked mannose residues (Nelson et al 1991). The side chains contain the epitopes that determine serospecificity (serotype A or B).

YEAST ADHESINS FOR EPITHELIAL CELLS

C. albicans adheres to different epithelial cell types in roughly comparable numbers (Botta 1981), but the adhesion mechanism may not be identical in each case. Currently, most information is available on the chemical nature of adhesins responsible for attachment to buccal and vaginal epithelial cells. Although germ-tube formation appears to promote adhesion of *C. albicans* to epithelial cells (Kimura & Pearsall 1980), the majority of investigators have used suspensions of non-germinated yeasts in adhesion assays. Possible differences in the nature or number of adhesins present in the two morphological forms have not yet been fully explored. However, it is now clear that hyphal or germ-tube-specific adhesins exist which bind to certain host proteins; these adhesins are discussed in a later section.

Evidence for mannoprotein adhesins

Although other wall components such as chitin (Segal et al 1982) and lipids (Ghannoum et al 1986) have been proposed as candidate adhesins, most experimental evidence indicates a role for mannoprotein in mediating yeast attachment to buccal and vaginal cells. Adhesion can be inhibited by pretreating the epithelial cells with a crude mannoprotein preparation obtained from culture supernatants of yeasts grown in medium containing a high concentration of galactose (McCourtie & Douglas 1985). This extracellular material is thought to originate, at least in part, from the surface fibrillar layer (Fig. 3.1) whose synthesis is promoted by growth under such conditions; its ability to inhibit adhesion indicates that it contains an adhesin capable of binding to, and thus blocking, epithelial receptors. The interaction is quite specific (McCourtie & Douglas 1985), since mannoprotein isolated from one *C. albicans* strain (GDH 2023) fails to inhibit adhesion of a second strain (GDH 2346).

Further evidence for the mannoprotein nature of the adhesin has come from experiments with tunicamycin. In yeasts, this antibiotic suppresses synthesis of mannoprotein but not that of the other major wall components, glucan and chitin (Kuo & Lampen 1974). Addition of tunicamycin to cultures of *C. albicans* in high galactose medium at the onset of stationary phase inhibited formation of the fibrillar layer, resulting in a decrease in adhesion to buccal cells of over 60% as compared with untreated yeasts (Douglas & McCourtie 1983).

Isolation and characterization of mannoprotein adhesins

Crude mannoprotein preparations obtained from culture supernatants of galacose-grown *C. albicans* contain a mixture of different components. Partial purification of adhesin has been achieved by a two-step procedure involving chromatography on concanavalin A-Sepharose and DEAE-cellulose. The purified material inhibited yeast adhesion to buccal cells 30 times more efficiently (on a weight basis) than unfractionated mannoprotein (Critchley & Douglas 1987a).

The predominant interaction between yeasts and epithelial cells seems to involve the protein portion of the mannoprotein adhesin. Pretreatment of crude adhesin with heat, dithiothreitol, or proteolytic enzymes (except papain) either partially or completely abolishes its ability to inhibit adhesion to buccal cells (Critchley & Douglas 1987a), whereas pretreatment with sodium periodate or α-mannosidase has little or no effect. Moreover, the protein-rich fraction obtained by incubating crude adhesin with endoglycosidase H inhibits adhesion to a greater extent than does the carbohydrate-rich fraction (Critchley & Douglas 1987a). These findings are consistent with earlier studies (Sobel et al 1981, Lee & King 1983) in which adhesion to vaginal cells was shown to be severely inhibited following direct treatment of yeasts with various proteolytic enzymes or reducing agents but not after treatment with glycosidases.

Recently, knowledge of receptor specificity for *C. albicans* GDH 2346 (see below) has been exploited in devising a scheme for purification of the yeast adhesin (F D Tosh & L J Douglas, unpublished results). The protocol (Fig. 3.3) involves a stepwise treatment of crude adhesin with N-glycanase, papain and dilute alkali to cleave the protein and carbohydrate portions of the mannoprotein molecule (Fig. 3.2). Fucoside-binding protein fragments are then recovered on an affinity column

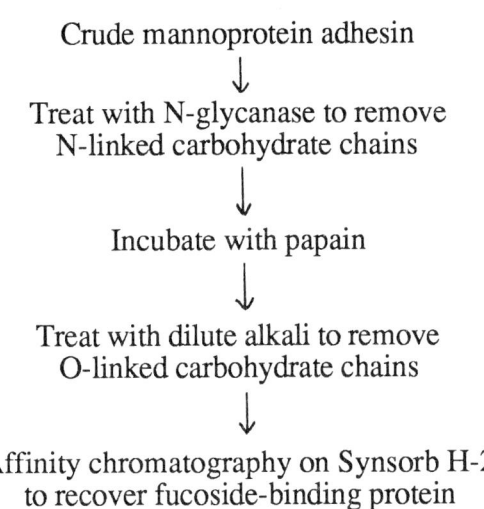

Crude mannoprotein adhesin
↓
Treat with N-glycanase to remove
N-linked carbohydrate chains
↓
Incubate with papain
↓
Treat with dilute alkali to remove
O-linked carbohydrate chains
↓
Affinity chromatography on Synsorb H-2
to recover fucoside-binding protein

Fig. 3.3 Purification of adhesin from *C. albicans* GDH 2346.

containing the trisaccharide of the H blood-group antigen which terminates in a residue of L-fucose. The purified material is devoid of carbohydrate and inhibits yeast adhesion to buccal cells 220 times more efficiently, on a protein weight basis, than crude adhesin (F D Tosh & L J Douglas, unpublished results). On an overall weight basis, inhibition is some 2000-fold greater because crude adhesin contains considerable amounts of carbohydrate. However, even this purified adhesin gives a maximum inhibition of yeast binding of only 80%, which suggests that more than one additional adhesion mechanism may operate.

Although these experiments indicate that yeasts interact with epithelial cells primarily via the protein portion of a mannoprotein adhesin, the carbohydrate chains of mannoproteins could also participate in adhesion to host surfaces. Mutants of serotype A *C. albicans* have been isolated which lack antigenic factor 6, an epitope located in the outer chain region of cell-surface mannoprotein. One such mutant adhered less readily than the parent strain to a cell line of human mouth squamous-cell carcinoma, suggesting that the factor 6 determinant may be involved in this particular interaction (Miyakawa et al 1989).

Regulation of adhesin expression

The enhanced adhesion demonstrated by many strains of *C. albicans* after growth in medium containing high concentrations of certain sugars is well documented and has been usefully exploited in studies on adhesion mechanisms (Douglas 1987a). In vivo, such sugar-mediated regulation of adhesion is probably important in the mouth, where high concentrations of sucrose and other dietary sugars are commonly found. Glucose-induced adhesion may also be significant in the pathogenesis of vaginal infections among diabetic and pregnant women whose high level of vaginal glycogen can be converted to glucose by enzymes present in the tissues or produced by the normal flora.

A recent study indicates that the availability of iron may represent an additional control mechanism in vivo (Sweet & Douglas 1991). Six strains of *C. albicans* were grown in defined medium which had been deferrated by ion-exchange chromatography and then supplemented with $FeCl_3$ to give iron concentrations ranging from $0.026\,\mu M$ (growth-limiting) to $0.8\,\mu M$ (excess). With five of the strains, adhesion to buccal epithelial cells was maximal after growth in $0.2–0.4\,\mu M$ iron, while one strain adhered best when grown in $0.026\,\mu M$ iron. There were quantitative but no qualitative differences in surface mannoprotein profiles of iron-deficient and iron-replete yeasts. Iron concentrations of $0.2–0.4\,\mu M$ are well below those found in conventional laboratory growth media and are likely to resemble those available to *C. albicans* in vivo (Sweet & Douglas, 1991).

CANDIDA SURFACE HYDROPHOBICITY

Hydrophobic interactions play a major role in microbial adhesion (Rosenberg & Kjelleberg 1986). They participate both in non-specific attachment processes and in specific adhesion between complementary adhesins and receptors. Although early studies suggested that every microbial strain possesses a fixed degree of surface hydrophobicity (van Oss 1978), more recent investigations have shown that physiological and environmental factors may modulate this property, and that components which promote (hydrophobins) or reduce (hydrophilins) hydrophobicity can co-exist on the cell surface (Rosenberg & Kjelleberg 1986). Yeast-phase cells of *C. albicans* are typically more hydrophobic when grown at room temperature (22–24°C) than are cells grown at 37°C (Hazen et al 1986). Moreover, expression of cell surface hydrophobicity by *C. albicans* is a dynamic process in which hydrophobic and hydrophilic cells can switch their status within 30 min (Hazen & Hazen 1988). Germ tubes are highly and invariably hydrophobic (Hazen & Hazen 1987).

Hydrophobicity and adhesion

Hydrophobic interactions appear to be of primary importance in the adhesion of *Candida* species to plastic surfaces in vitro (Minagi et al 1985, Klotz et al 1985, Critchley & Douglas 1985) but the extent of their involvement in epithelial cell adhesion is not entirely clear. Hazen (1989) examined expression of cell surface hydrophobicity in 19 isolates of *C. albicans* grown at 23°C and 37°C and attempted to correlate hydrophobicity with the ability of the yeasts to adhere to HeLa cells. A positive correlation was observed for cells grown at 37°C but not for cells grown at 23°C. However, there was a significantly positive correlation when results for some individual isolates were analysed. It was concluded that cell surface hydrophobicity is involved in adhesion but is not the predominant mechanism (Hazen 1989).

The importance of hydrophobic interactions is also suggested by a recent study in this laboratory that compared surface hydrophobicity of four strains of *C. albicans* after growth in medium containing either 500 mM galactose (which promotes synthesis of mannoprotein fibrils) or 50 mM glucose as the carbon source. The galactose-grown yeasts showed significantly increased hydrophobicity as well as enhanced adhesion to buccal epithelial cells (B Ener & L J Douglas, unpublished results). By contrast, Kennedy & Sandin (1988) were unable to demonstrate any correlation between cell surface hydrophobicity of *C. albicans* and adhesion to buccal cells. However, these investigators assayed hydrophobicity by the hydrocarbon adherence method of Rosenberg et al (1980); this technique is less sensitive than the polystyrene microsphere method used by Hazen (1989) and also failed to reveal differences between galactose-grown and glucose-grown yeasts in our experiments (B Ener & L J Douglas unpublished results).

Identification of hydrophobic surface components

Protein (or mannoprotein) appears to be responsible for surface hydrophobicity in *C. albicans*. When hydrophobic and hydrophilic yeast cells were exposed to various enzymes, including lipase and phospholipases, only proteases produced any change in surface hydrophobicity (Hazen et al 1990). Hydrophobic cell surfaces were sensitive to trypsin, chymotrypsin, pronase E and pepsin. Papain had no effect on hydrophobic cells but caused hydrophilic cells to appear hydrophobic. This enzyme is also the only protease whose action enhances the ability of crude mannoprotein to block yeast attachment to buccal cells (Critchley & Douglas 1987a). The proteins responsible for surface hydrophobicity could be removed by exposure to lyticase, a β-glucanase. Surface labelling of these proteins, followed by analysis by SDS-PAGE, revealed several components of low molecular mass ($< 55\,kDa$) that were associated with hydrophobic cells but were either absent or much less abundant in hydrophilic cell digests (Hazen et al 1990). When late exponential-phase hydrophilic cells were treated with tunicamycin, a high degree of surface hydrophobicity was apparent by stationary phase. Since tunicamycin is an inhibitor of protein mannosylation, this result suggests that changes in mannosylation may affect exposure of hydrophobic surface proteins (Hazen et al 1990).

EPITHELIAL CELL RECEPTORS

Elucidation of adhesion mechanisms entails not only identification of microbial adhesins but also characterization of host cell receptors. Most known receptors

Table 3.1 Proposed epithelial receptors for *Candida albicans*

Receptor	Procedures used in identification	Reference
Glycosides containing L-fucose, N-acetyl-D-glucosamine, or D-mannose	Adhesion inhibition with sugars and lectins; affinity chromatography	Critchley & Douglas 1987b
Lactosylceramide	Chromatogram overlay assay	Jimenez-Lucho et al 1990
ABO blood-group antigens	Adhesion inhibition with structurally defined oligosaccharides	Brassart et al 1991
Lewis[a] blood-group antigen	Adhesion inhibition with antiserum	May et al 1989, Tosh & Douglas 1991
Fibronectin	Direct binding of radiolabelled yeasts to fibronectin-coated surfaces	Skerl et al 1984

for micro-organisms on the surface of animal cells are carbohydrate components of membrane glycoproteins and glycolipids (Jones & Isaacson 1983). Glycosides can present a much greater range of recognition sites than can peptides. This is because the number of permutations possible with glycosidic bonding permits the formation of far more specific structures from a few monosaccharide units than can be produced from the same number of amino acids (Ofek et al 1985). Membrane glycoproteins contain the hexoses D-mannose, D-galactose, and L-fucose, together with N-acetyl-D-glucosamine, N-acetyl-D-galactosamine, and the sialic acids. D-glucose does not appear to be a constituent of glycoproteins but is present in glycolipids.

Some components of epithelial cell membranes which have been proposed as receptors for *C. albicans* are shown in Table 3.1.

Identification of glycosides as receptors

Involvement of the protein portion of a mannoprotein adhesin in the attachment process is analogous to many bacterial adhesion mechanisms in which a proteinaceous adhesin interacts in a lectin-like manner with a glycoside receptor (either glycoprotein or glycolipid) on the host cell surface. Inhibition tests with sugars and lectins have been widely used to characterize such receptors. Early tests of this type with *C. albicans* yielded apparently contradictory data (reviewed by Douglas 1987a) but more recent work indicates that there are at least two kinds of adhesion mechanism and that glycosides containing L-fucose or N-acetyl-D-glucosamine can function as epithelial cell receptors for different strains of the yeast.

The 6-deoxyhexose, L-fucose, is an important constituent monosaccharide of epithelial cell membranes, and is known to function as a receptor determinant for certain bacteria (Jones & Isaacson 1983). Addition of this sugar to in vitro adhesion assays with *C. albicans* GDH 2346 inhibited yeast attachment to buccal cells. Moreover, pretreatment of the buccal cells with lectin from *Lotus tetragonolobus* (which is specific for L-fucose), but not other lectins, also blocked adhesion (Critchley & Douglas 1987b). By contrast, adhesion of strain GDH 2023 was inhibited by N-acetyl-D-glucosamine and wheat germ agglutinin (a lectin specific for N-acetyl-D-glucosamine) but not by L-fucose or *L. tetragonolobus* lectin. Analogous results were obtained in assays with human vaginal epithelial cells (Critchley & Douglas 1987b), indicating that the mechanism of adhesion with either strain may be similar for both cell types.

Of six *C. albicans* strains tested, five appeared to bind to fucose-containing receptors (Critchley 1986). However, addition of L-fucose to assay mixtures caused only partial inhibition of adhesion with these sensitive strains, suggesting that the natural receptor is larger than an L-fucose residue or that a particular stereo-chemical configuration is necessary. It is also possible that additional adhesion mechanisms operate. Affinity chromatography has shown that crude adhesin preparations from five strains of *C. albicans* all contain lectin-like proteins (mannoproteins) capable of binding to L-fucose, D-mannose and N-acetyl-D-glucosamine although the proportion of each type varies from one strain to another (Critchley & Douglas 1987b). The relative abundance of these proteins, and more particularly their accessibility on the yeast surface, may determine the overall receptor specificity of different *C. albicans* strains.

Glycosphingolipids

Another kind of experimental approach has recently identified the glyco-sphingolipid, lactosylceramide, as a possible epithelial receptor of *C. albicans, S. cerevisiae, Cryptococcus neoformans* and other fungal species. A chromatogram overlay assay was used to measure the binding of ^{125}I-labelled organisms to individual glycosphingolipids separated on thin-layer plates (Jimenez-Lucho et al 1990). Binding required a terminal galactosyl residue since yeasts did not attach to glucosylceramide derived from lactosylceramide by treatment with β-galactosidase, nor to other neutral or acidic glycosphingolipids that contained internal lactose residues. However, the nature of the ceramide moiety also appeared to affect binding. With *C. albicans*, attachment was observed with yeasts but not hyphae. Binding was not dependent on divalent cations but seemed to require the presence of glucose (Jimenez-Lucho et al 1990). No such requirement has been demonstrated in other *Candida* adhesion systems.

Blood-group antigens

From the limited amount of information currently available, it appears that L-fucose-containing glycoside receptors may be most commonly required for *C. albicans* adhesion to epithelial cells. Among likely candidates for such receptors are the ABO and Lewis blood-group antigens, all of which possess L-fucose residues (Fig. 3.4). As described above, the adhesin from strain GDH 2346 has been purified by a protocol (Fig. 3.3) which included, as its final step, recovery of fucoside-binding protein fragments on an affinity column containing the terminal trisaccharide of the H blood-group antigen. The purified adhesin was able to block yeast attachment to buccal cells extremely effectively, suggesting that this trisaccharide closely resembles the natural receptor. Support for this notion has been provided recently by Brassart et al (1991) who investigated the ability of various glycopeptides and structurally defined oligosaccharides to inhibit *Candida* adhesion. Mixtures of glycopeptides blocked attachment by up to 55% but inhibition was completely abolished if fucose residues were removed from the compounds by mild acid hydrolysis. When oligosaccharides were used as inhibitors, the minimal structural requirement for activity was the Fuc $\alpha1 \rightarrow 2$Galβ determinant of the H-antigen which is found on all the blood-group substances of the ABO system (Fig. 3.4). However, the Lewis blood-group antigens, which are also fucosylated, were totally inactive (Brassart et al 1991).

It is well known that *C. albicans* adheres more readily to exfoliated buccal or vaginal epithelial cells from some donors than from others (King et al 1980, Sobel et al 1981), suggesting that some individuals may be more susceptible to colonization by the yeast. Burford-Mason et al (1988) reported that oral carriage of *C. albicans* in healthy subjects could be correlated with two host factors, namely blood group O and non-secretion of blood-group antigens, with the trend towards carriage being greatest in group O non-secretors. A subsequent survey revealed a significantly higher number of non-secretors among patients with oral or vaginal *Candida* infections compared with the proportion of non-secretors in the local population (Thom et al 1989). Secretors and non-secretors differ in their expression of the Lewis antigen which exists in two forms. Lewis[b] is found in the body fluids of most secretors, whereas in non-secretors it is the Lewis[a] form which

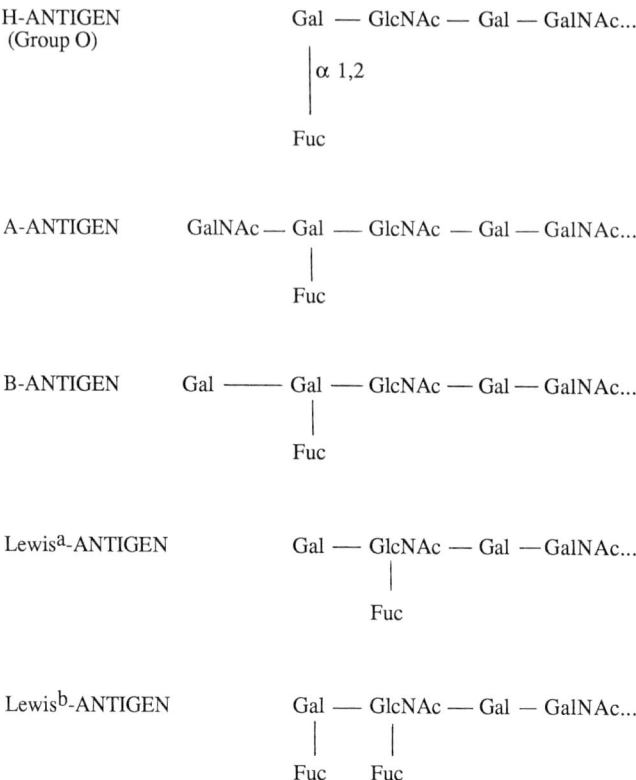

Fig. 3.4 Structure of ABO and Lewis blood-group antigens. Gal, D-galactose; Fuc, L-fucose; GlcNAc, N-acetyl-D-glucosamine; GalNAc, N-acetyl-D-galactosamine.

predominates. Recent evidence suggest that the Lewis[a] antigen, adsorbed to epithelial cell surfaces, might function as a receptor for *C. albicans*. In two separate studies, buccal cells from a secretor and a non-secretor were pretreated with anti-Lewis[a] and anti-Lewis[b] antiserum before being used in adhesion assays. In both cases, pretreatment of non-secretor buccal cells with anti-Lewis[a] antiserum had a significant inhibitory effect on yeast adhesion, while none of the other pretreatments produced statistically significant differences (May et al 1989, Tosh & Douglas 1991). These results are not consistent with those of Brassart et al (1991) who failed to observe adhesion inhibition with Lewis antigens. However, there is some evidence that the ability of *C. albicans* to bind to the Lewis[a] antigen is strain-dependent (May et al 1989).

Fibronectin

Fibronectin is a large, multifunctional glycoprotein which is found in a soluble form in blood and other body fluids, and in an insoluble form on cell surfaces and in the extracellular matrix (Proctor 1987). It is an important modulator of microbial adhesion at mucosal surfaces by acting as a receptor for some species and a blocking agent for others (Simpson et al 1982). Early studies on fibronectin binding by *Candida* produced contradictory results. In a survey of the ability of 35 microbial species to bind ^{125}I-labelled fibronectin, Myhre & Kuusela (1983) found that

C. albicans showed little or no affinity for the glycoprotein. On the other hand, Skerl et al (1984) reported significant adhesion of *C. albicans* and *C. tropicalis* to wells of tissue culture plates that had been coated (at pH 11) with fibronectin, suggesting that the glycoprotein could act as a receptor for these yeasts. Work in this laboratory has failed to demonstrate fibronectin binding by any *Candida* species at neutral pH values (Lancaster & Douglas 1986) and indicates rather that the glycoprotein may inhibit attachment to epithelial cells. However, at low or high pH values fibronectin binding is substantially increased and can reach a figure of over 80% at pH 3 with some strains (A J Lancaster & L J Douglas, unpublished results). The fibronectin molecule, which is a dimer with a molecular mass of 440 kDa, has been shown to unfold at extremes of pH (Tooney et al 1983). Presumably, therefore, most of the fibronectin present on the human vaginal mucosa (which has a pH of about 4.5) is in the unfolded form and could function as a receptor for *C. albicans*.

Vaginal epithelial cells from women of child-bearing age are primarily of two types, superficial (S) and intermediate (I). The ratio between the two types reflects hormonal status; a high level of blood oestrogen is associated with an increased number of S cells whereas a high level of progesterone correlates with an increased number of I cells. Flow cytometry has been used to demonstrate that cell populations rich in I cells have more fibronectin than those rich in S cells; they also bind *C. albicans* more avidly, and binding can be inhibited by adding exogenous fibronectin (Kalo et al 1988). These results may be relevant to clinical observations which indicate that in physiological conditions involving high progesterone levels, such as pregnancy or the premenstrual period, there is a marked predisposition to vaginal candidosis.

In addition to its presence on epithelial cell surfaces, fibronectin is an important component of the extracellular matrix (ECM) where it unfolds completely and forms multimeric fibrous strands (Proctor 1987). *C. albicans* adheres in greater numbers to subendothelial ECM than to confluent endothelium in vitro, and exposed ECM may represent an attachment target for circulating yeasts in the early stages of deep-seated infections (Klotz 1987, Klotz & Maca 1988, Klotz 1990). The attachment site for *C. albicans* on fibronectin may be the cell-binding domain which contains the amino acid sequence Arg-Gly-Asp (RGD). Klotz & Smith (1991) recently reported that specific binding of ^{125}I-labelled fibronectin to yeasts could be partially inhibited by RGD and related peptides. Many mammalian cells bind to the RGD-containing domain of fibronectin via surface glycoproteins, termed integrins, which are heterodimers composed of α and β subunits. *C. albicans* apparently possesses a protein that reacts with antiserum specific for the integrin β_1 subunit (Marcantonio & Hynes 1988). This component may therefore participate in *Candida* attachment to fibronectin and to other RGD-containing proteins such as fibrinogen, fibrin and laminin.

HYPHAL ADHESINS

Certain adhesins seem to be expressed only by hyphal forms of *C. albicans*. For example, germ tubes and hyphae bind fibrinogen (Bouali et al 1987, Page & Odds

1988), laminin (Bouchara et al 1990), and the complement (C3) conversion product C3d (Calderone et al 1988) whereas yeast cells do not. Moreover, germ-tube formation promotes adhesion to epithelial cells (Kimura & Pearsall 1980) and plastic (Tronchin et al 1988), suggesting that the morphological change is accompanied by increased synthesis of adhesins. Cytochemical methods have been used to demonstrate that germ-tube formation involves a significant reorganization of surface mannoproteins (Tronchin et al 1989).

Adhesion to plastic
Tronchin et al (1988) investigated germ-tube adhesion by incubating stationary-phase yeasts, freshly suspended in a germination medium, in a polystyrene petri dish. Electron microscopy showed that attachment to the plastic surface was mediated by fibrils which remained on the dish after mechanical removal of the germ tubes. The fibrils could be detected with concanavalin A-conjugated latex particles, indicating that they contained mannoprotein. Analysis of solubilized fibrils by SDS-PAGE revealed four components of 60, 68, 200 and > 200 kDa. These mannoproteins are obviously candidate adhesins.

Laminin binding
Laminin is a major structural glycoprotein of basement membranes. It promotes the adhesion of several mammalian cell types in vitro and binds to a number of pathogenic bacteria, including *Staphylococcus aureus* and *Streptococcus pyogenes*. Results with an immunofluorescence assay indicate that *Candida* binding of soluble laminin is restricted to germ tubes and hyphae (Bouchara et al 1990), although Klotz (1990) has reported yeast adhesion to laminin-coated surfaces. Binding sites are located in the surface fibrillar layer of germ tubes (Bouchara et al 1990).

A quantitative study using ^{125}I-labelled laminin showed that binding to germ tubes was specific and saturable, with about 8000 binding sites per cell (Bouchara et al 1990). Prior heating or trypsin treatment of germ tubes abolished binding and, of a range of different proteins and carbohydrates tested in competition experiments, only fibrinogen (and unlabelled laminin) acted as an inhibitor. Extraction of cell-wall material from germ tubes with dithiothreitol and iodoacetamide, followed by SDS-PAGE and Western blot analysis, revealed two laminin-binding components of 68 and 60–62 kDa (Bouchara et al 1990).

Fibrinogen binding
Fibrinogen plays a major role in blood clot formation via its conversion to insoluble fibrin and has been shown to interact with a number of bacteria. Its binding to *C. albicans* was first demonstrated by Bouali et al (1986) using an immuno-fluorescence assay. Subsequent studies (Bouali et al 1987, Page & Odds 1988) showed that binding was specific for germ tubes and hyphae, and was associated with the surface fibrillar layer (Tronchin et al 1987). It was decreased by pretreating germ tubes with 2-mercaptoethanol, trypsin, or α-mannosidase (Bouali et al 1987). Binding of ^{125}I-labelled fibrinogen was specific, saturable and reversible, with an average of 6000 sites per germ tube (Annaix et al 1990). When cell-wall extracts were analysed by SDS-PAGE and Western blotting, a single fibrinogen-binding component of 68 kDa was detected (Annaix et al 1990). This component may be

identical to the 68 kDa laminin-binding adhesin identified by Bouchara et al (1990).

CONCLUSIONS

The ability of *C. albicans* to adhere to a variety of host surfaces is undoubtedly an important factor in the pathogenesis of candidosis. Several types of adhesin-receptor interaction appear to exist. There is clear evidence that *Candida* adhesins are mannoproteins and are associated with the surface fibrillar layer of the fungus. Yeast adhesion to epithelial cells involves lectin-like binding of the protein portion of a mannoprotein adhesin to glycoside receptors, possibly blood-group antigens or glycosphingolipids, on the host cell membrane. *Candida* surface hydrophobicity may be a significant element in this interaction. Fibronectin, on the surface of vaginal epithelial cells or in the extracellular matrix, can also act as a receptor for the yeast. Hyphal adhesins, possibly related to the integrin family of proteins, mediate binding to other RGD-containing proteins such as laminin and fibrinogen. The relationship between all of these adhesins and *Candida* complement receptors (discussed in the following chapter) remains to be clarified.

REFERENCES

Annaix V, Bouchara J-P, Tronchin G, Senet J-M, Robert R 1990 Structures involved in the binding of human fibrinogen to *Candida albicans* germ tubes. FEMS Microbiology Immunology 64: 147–154

Ballou C E 1976 Structure and biosynthesis of the mannan component of the yeast cell envelope. Advances in Microbial Physiology 14: 93–158

Botta G A 1981 Possible role of hormones in the observed changes in adhesion of several microorganisms to epithelial cells from different body sites. FEMS Microbiology Letters 11: 69–72

Bouali A, Robert R, Tronchin G, Senet J-M 1986 Binding of human fibrinogen to *Candida albicans* in vitro: a preliminary study. Journal of Medical and Veterinary Mycology 24: 345–348

Bouali A, Robert R, Tronchin G, Senet J-M 1987 Characterization of binding of human fibrinogen to the surface of germ-tubes and mycelium of *Candida albicans*. Journal of General Microbiology 133: 545–551

Bouchara J-P, Tronchin G, Annaix V, Robert R, Senet J-M 1990 Laminin receptors of *Candida albicans* germ tubes. Infection and Immunity 58: 48–54

Brassart D, Woltz A, Golliard M, Neeser J-R 1991 In vitro inhibition of adhesion of *Candida albicans* clinical isolates to human buccal epithelial cells by fuc $\alpha 1 \rightarrow 2$ gal β-bearing complex carbohydrates. Infection and Immunity 59: 1605–1613

Burford-Mason A P, Weber J C P, Willoughby J M T 1988 Oral carriage of *Candida albicans*, ABO blood group and secretor status in healthy subjects. Journal of Medical and Veterinary Mycology 26: 49–56

Calderone R A, Cihlar R L, Lee D D-S, Hoberg K, Scheld W M 1985 Yeast adhesion in the pathogenesis of endocarditis due to *Candida albicans*: studies with adherence-negative mutants. Journal of Infectious Diseases 152: 710–715

Calderone R A, Linehan L, Wadsworth E, Sandberg A L 1988 Identification of C3d receptors on *Candida albicans*. Infection and Immunity 56: 252–258

Calderone R A, Wadsworth E 1988 Characterization of mannoproteins from a virulent *Candida albicans* strain and its derived, avirulent strain. Reviews of Infectious Diseases 10: S423–S427

Casanova M, Chaffin W L 1991 Phosphate-containing proteins and glycoproteins of the cell wall of *Candida albicans*. Infection and Immunity 59: 808–813

Casanova M, Gil M L, Cardenoso L, Martinez J P, Sentandreu R 1989 Identification of wall-specific antigens synthesized during germ tube formation by *Candida albicans*. Infection and Immunity 57: 262–271

Cassone A, Simonetti N, Strippoli V 1973 Ultrastructural changes in the wall during germ-tube formation from blastospores of *Candida albicans*. Journal of General Microbiology 77: 417–426

Cassone A, Mattia E, Boldrini L 1978 Agglutination of blastospores of *Candida albicans* by concanavalin A and its relationship with the distribution of mannan polymers and the ultrastructure of the cell wall. Journal of General Microbiology 105: 263–272

Critchley I A 1986 Mechanism of adherence of *Candida albicans* to epithelial cells. PhD Thesis, University of Glasgow

Critchley I A Douglas L J 1985 Differential adhesion of pathogenic *Candida* species to epithelial and inert surfaces. FEMS Microbiology Letters 28: 199–203

Critchley I A, Douglas L J 1987a Isolation and partial characterization of an adhesin from *Candida albicans*. Journal of General Microbiology 133: 629–636

Critchley I A, Douglas L J 1987b Role of glycosides as epithelial cell receptors for *Candida albicans*. Journal of General Microbiology 133: 637–643

Douglas L J 1987a Adhesion of *Candida* species to epithelial surfaces. CRC Critical Reviews in Microbiology 15: 27–43

Douglas L J 1987b Adhesion to surfaces. In: Rose A H, Harrison J S (eds) The Yeasts, vol. 2, 2nd edn. Academic Press, London, pp. 239–280

Douglas L J, Houston J G, McCourtie J 1981 Adherence of *Candida albicans* to human buccal epithelial cells after growth on different carbon sources. FEMS Microbiology Letters 12: 241–243

Douglas L J, McCourtie J 1983 Effect of tunicamycin treatment on the adherence of *Candida albicans* to human buccal epithelial cells. FEMS Microbiology Letters 16: 199–202

Fukayama M, Calderone R A 1991 Adherence of cell surface mutants of *Candida albicans* to buccal epithelial cells and analyses of the cell surface proteins of the mutants. Infection and Immunity 59: 1341–1345

Gardiner R, Podgorski C, Day A W 1982 Serological studies on the fimbriae of yeasts and yeast-like species. Botanical Gazette 143: 534–541

Ghannoum M A, Burns G R, Abu Elteen K, Radwan S S 1986 Experimental evidence for the role of lipids in adherence of *Candida* spp. to human buccal epithelial cells. Infection and Immunity 54: 189–193

Hazen K C 1989 Participation of yeast cell surface hyprophobicity in adherence of *Candida albicans* to human epithelial cells. Infection and Immunity 57: 1894–1900

Hazen K C, Hazen B W 1987 A polystyrene microsphere assay for detecting surface hydrophobicity variations within *Candida albicans* populations. Journal of Microbiological Methods 6: 289–299

Hazen B W, Hazen K C 1988 Dynamic expression of cell surface hydrophobicity during initial yeast cell growth and before germ tube formation of *Candida albicans*. Infection and Immunity 56: 2521–2525

Hazen K C, Plotkin B J, Klimas D M 1986 Influence of growth conditions on cell surface hydrophobicity of *Candida albicans* and *Candida glabrata*. Infection and Immunity 54: 269–271

Hazen K C, Lay J-G, Hazen B W, Chiaging Fu R, Murthy S 1990 Partial biochemical characterization of cell surface hydrophobicity of *Candida albicans*. Infection and Immunity 58: 3469–3476

Jimenez-Lucho V, Ginsburg V, Krivan H C 1990 *Cryptococcus neoformans*, *Candida albicans*, and other fungi bind specifically to the glycosphingolipid lactosylceramide (gal β1–4 glc β1–1 cer), a possible adhesion receptor for yeasts. Infection and Immunity 58: 2085–2090

Jones G W, Isaacson R E 1983 Proteinaceous bacterial adhesins and their receptors. CRC Critical Reviews in Microbiology 10: 229–260

Kalo A, Segal E, Sahar E, Dayan D 1988 Interaction of *Candida albicans* with genital mucosal surfaces: involvement of fibronectin in adherence. Journal of Infectious Diseases 157: 1253–1256

Kennedy M J, Sandin R L 1988 Influence of growth conditions on *Candida albicans* adhesion, hydrophobicity and cell wall ultrastructure. Journal of Medical and Veterinary Mycology 26: 79–92

Kimura L H, Pearsall N N 1980 Relationship between germination of *Candida albicans* and increased adherence to human buccal epithelial cells. Infection and Immunity 28: 464–468

King R D, Lee J C, Morris A L 1980 Adherence of *Candida albicans* and other *Candida* species to mucosal epithelial cells. Infection and Immunity 27: 667–674

Klotz S A 1987 The adherence of *Candida* yeasts to human and bovine vascular endothelium and subendothelial extracellular matrix. FEMS Microbiology Letters 48: 201–205

Klotz S A 1990 Adherence of *Candida albicans* to components of the subendothelial extracellular matrix. FEMS Microbiology Letters 68: 249–254

Klotz S A, Drutz D J, Harrison J L, Huppert M 1983 Adherence and penetration of vascular endothelium by *Candida* yeasts. Infection and Immunity 42: 374–384

Klotz S A, Drutz D J, Zajic J E 1985 Factors governing adherence of *Candida* species to plastic surfaces. Infection and Immunity 50: 97–101

Klotz S A, Penn R L 1987 Multiple mechanisms may contribute to the adherence of *Candida* yeasts to living cells. Current Microbiology 16: 119–122

Klotz S A, Maca R D 1988 Endothelial cell contraction increases *Candida* adherence to exposed extracellular matrix. Infection and Immunity 56: 2495–2498

Klotz S A, Smith R L 1991 A fibronectin receptor on *Candida albicans* mediates adherence of the fungus to extracellular matrix. Journal of Infectious Diseases 163: 604–610

Kuo S-C, Lampen J O 1974 Tunicamycin – an inhibitor of yeast glycoprotein synthesis. Biochemical and Biophysical Research Communications 58: 287–295

Lancaster A J, Douglas L J 1986 Role of fibronectin in the adhesion of *Candida albicans* to mucosal surfaces. In: Abstracts 14th International Congress of Microbiology, p. 170. International Union of Microbiological Societies, Manchester

Lee J C, King R D 1983 Characterization of *Candida albicans* adherence to human vaginal epithelial cells in vitro. Infection and Immunity 41: 1024–1030

Lehrer N, Segal E, Cihlar R L, Calderone R A 1986 Pathogenesis of vaginal candidiasis: studies with a mutant which has a reduced ability to adhere in vitro. Journal of Medical and Veterinary Mycology 24: 127–131

McCourtie J, Douglas L J 1981 Relationship between cell surface composition of *Candida albicans* and adherence to acrylic after growth on different carbon sources. Infection and Immunity 32: 1234–1241

McCourtie J, Douglas L J 1984 Relationship between cell surface composition, adherence and virulence of *Candida albicans*. Infection and Immunity 45: 6–12

McCourtie J, Douglas L J 1985 Extracellular polymer of *Candida albicans*: isolation, analysis and role in adhesion. Journal of General Microbiology 131: 495–503

Maisch P A, Calderone R A 1980 Adherence of *Candida albicans* to a fibrin-platelet matrix formed in vitro. Infection and Immunity 27: 650–656

Marcantonio E E, Hynes R O 1988 Antibodies to the conserved cytoplasmic domain of the integrin β_1 subunit react with proteins in vertebrates, invertebrates, and fungi. Journal of Cell Biology 106: 1765–1772

Marrie T J, Costerton J W 1981 The ultrastructure of *Candida albicans* infections. Canadian Journal of Microbiology 27: 1156–1164

May S J, Blackwell C C, Weir D M 1989 Lewis[a] blood group antigen of non-secretors: a receptor for *Candida* blastospores. FEMS Microbiology Immunology 47: 407–410

Minagi S, Miyake Y, Inagaki K, Tsuru H, Suginaka H 1985 Hydrophobic interaction in *Candida albicans* and *Candida tropicalis* adherence to various denture base resin materials. Infection and Immunity 47: 11–14

Miyakawa Y, Kagaya K, Kuribayashi T, Suzuki M, Fukazawa Y 1989 Isolation and chemical and biological characterization of antigenic mutants of *Candida albicans* serotype A. Yeast 5: S225–S229

Myhre E B, Kuusela P 1983 Binding of human fibronectin to group A, C, and G streptococci. Infection and Immunity 40: 29–34

Nelson R D, Shibata N, Podzorski R P, Herron M J 1991 *Candida* mannan: chemistry, suppression of cell-mediated immunity, and possible mechanisms of action. Clinical Microbiology Reviews 4: 1–19

Ofek I, Lis H, Sharon N 1985 Animal cell surface membranes. In: Savage D C, Fletcher M (eds) Bacterial adhesion. Plenum Press, New York, pp 71–88

Page S, Odds F C 1988 Binding of plasma proteins to *Candida* species in vitro. Journal of General Microbiology 134: 2693–2702

Poulain D, Tronchin G, Dubremetz J F, Biguet J 1978 Ultrastructure of the cell wall of *Candida albicans* blastospores: study of its constitutive layers by the use of a cytochemical technique revealing polysaccharide. Annales de Microbiologie (l'Institut Pasteur) 129: 141–153

Proctor R A 1987 Fibronectin: a brief overview of its structure, function and physiology. Reviews of Infectious Diseases 9: S317–S321

Ray T L, Digre K B, Payne C D 1984 Adherence of *Candida* species to human epidermal corneocytes and buccal mucosal cells: correlation with cutaneous pathogenicity. Journal of Investigative Dermatology 83: 37–41

Rosenberg M, Gutnick D, Rosenberg E 1980 Adherence of bacteria to hydrocarbons: a simple method for measuring cell-surface hydrophobicity. FEMS Microbiology Letters 9: 29–33

Rosenberg M, Kjelleberg S 1986 Hydrophobic interactions: role in bacterial adhesion. Advances in Microbial Ecology 9: 353–393

Rotrosen D, Calderone R A, Edwards J E 1986 Adherence of *Candida* species to host tissues and plastic surfaces. Reviews of Infectious Diseases 8: 73–85

Segal E, Lehrer N, Ofek I 1982 Adherence of *Candida albicans* to human vaginal epithelial cells: inhibition by amino sugars. Experimental Cell Biology 50: 13–17

Shepherd M G 1987 Cell envelope of *Candida albicans*. CRC Critical Reviews in Microbiology 15: 7–25

Simpson W A, Courtney H, Beachey E H 1982 Fibronectin – a modulator of the oropharyngeal bacterial flora. In: Schlessinger D (ed) Microbiology – 1982. American Society for Microbiology, Washington, DC, pp 346–347

Skerl K G, Calderone R A, Segal E, Sreevalsan T, Scheld W M 1984 In vitro binding of *Candida albicans* yeast cells to human fibronectin. Canadian Journal of Microbiology 30: 221–227

Sobel J D, Myers P G, Kaye D, Levison M E 1981 Adherence of *Candida albicans* to human vaginal and buccal epithelial cells. Journal of Infectious Diseases 143: 76–82

Sullivan P A, Chiew Y Y, Molloy C, Templeton M D, Shepherd M G 1983 An analysis of the metabolism and cell wall composition of *Candida albicans* during germ-tube formation. Canadian Journal of Microbiology 29: 1514–1525

Sundstrom P M, Kenny G E 1985 Enzymatic release of germ tube-specific antigens from cell walls of *Candida albicans*. Infection and Immunity 49: 609–614

Sweet S P, Douglas L J 1991 Effect of iron deprivation on surface composition and virulence determinants of *Candida albicans*. Journal of General Microbiology 137: 859–865

Thom S M, Blackwell C C, MacCallum C J et al 1989 Non-secretion of blood group antigens and susceptibility to infection by *Candida* species. FEMS Microbiology Immunology 47: 401–406

Tooney N M, Mosesson M W, Amrani D L, Hainfeld J F, Wall J S 1983 Solution and surface effects on plasma fibronectin structure. Journal of Cell Biology 97: 1686–1692

Tosh F D, Douglas L J 1991 Effect of blood group and secretor status on the adhesion of *Candida albicans* to mucosal surfaces. In: Tumbay E, Seeliger H P R, Ang O (eds) *Candida* and candidamycosis. Plenum Press, New York, pp. 127–130

Tronchin G, Poulain D, Herbaut J, Biguet J 1981 Cytochemical and ultrastructural studies of *Candida albicans*. II. Evidence for a cell wall coat using concanavalin A. Journal of Ultrastructure Research 75: 50–59

Tronchin G, Robert R, Bouali A, Senet J-M 1987 Immunocytochemical localization of in vitro binding of human fibrinogen to *Candida albicans* germ tube and mycelium. Annales de Microbiologie (l'Institut Pasteur) 138: 177–187

Tronchin G, Bouchara J-P, Robert R, Senet J-M 1988 Adherence of *Candida albicans* germ tubes to plastic: ultrastructural and molecular studies of fibrillar adhesins. Infection and Immunity 56: 1987–1993

Tronchin G, Bouchara J-P, Robert R 1989 Dynamic changes of the cell wall surface of *Candida albicans* associated with germination and adherence. European Journal of Cell Biology 50: 285–290

van Oss C J 1978 Phagocytosis as a surface phenomenon. Annual Reviews of Microbiology 32: 19–39

Discussion of paper presented by L. J. Douglas

Discussed by J. Sobel
Reported by K. P. W. J. McAdam

Dr Sobel pointed out that early studies of *Candida* adherence focused on the mouth, but more recent studies have moved outside the oral cavity. Building on Dr Douglas' historical perspective and personal involvement in the field of *Candida* adherence, Dr Sobel compared the adherence of *Escherichia coli* and *Candida albicans* to epithelial cells (Table 1). In *E. coli,* studies of virulence have built upon a series of gene deletion or insertion studies for genes encoding fimbriae and non-fimbrial adhesins. Dr Sobel noted the importance of establishing phase variation in *E. coli* without being able to show something comparable for *C. albicans.* Virulence factors relevant at a mucosal or epithelial surface may have no consequence during tissue invasion, whether it be the retina or the kidneys; on the contrary, the persistence of such virulence factors which may be critical for colonization may in fact constitute a disadvantage at some other site. So far little has been done to establish a genetic basis for most of the virulence factors in *Candida* and future progress will require unravelling of the molecular basis of adhesin expression on both yeast cells and hyphae.

Table 1. Comparison of *Escherichia coli* and *Candida albicans* adherence to epithelial cells

	E. coli	*C. albicans*
Putative adhesin	Fimbrial	Mannoprotein
	– Type 1	Chitin (?)
	– P	Lipids (?)
	– S	
	– Type 1c	
	– G	
	– M	
	Non-fimbrial	
	– F adhesin	
	– Dr hemagglutinin	
Genetic sequence	pil, fim, pap, sfa, afa, prs	Unknown
Virulence studies	Established	Few
Hydrophobicity	Contributory	Contributory
Phasic variation	Established	Unknown (? Switch)

Dr Sobel pointed out the flaws that might arise from studying virulence factors using isolates from patients with symptomatic infection compared with those isolates from asymptomatic patients simply colonizing the local mucosal surface.

Colonizing commensals may have the full repertoire of genetic capability for expressing virulence factors which may or may not be expressed in the carrier state, either for reasons peculiar to the organism or, more often, as a result of a variety of host factors.

Dr Sobel went on to compare *E. coli* and *C. albicans* receptors on epithelial cells (Table 2). With the establishment of a potentially dominant receptor molecule on the epithelial and hence mucosal surface, it has been tempting to postulate that enhanced susceptibility to infection in certain individuals, particularly in patients with recurrent infections, is a result of increased receptor number, density or availability, hence facilitating mucosal colonization. This has been extremely difficult to prove in epidemiological prevalence studies since many host factors influence mucosal colonization in addition to adherence to epithelial cells. Nevertheless, early epidemiological studies do suggest a correlation between blood group type and secretor status in colonization rates, hence a possible correlation with infection rates. Dr Sobel went on to recall his earlier results, comparing women with intractable recurrent vulvovaginal candiasis with a control group of women who had never experienced any *Candida* infection and who were culture negative. He had been unable to show in these studies that women who had this marked susceptibility to infection had any increased avidity in terms of adherence. These results, however were different from those obtained by Esther Segal. He pointed out that virulence factors may synergize or facilitate each other, for instance proteases may facilitate adherence and establish colonization rather than facilitating invasion. He also stressed the importance of reproductive hormones on *Candida* adhesion, including adhesin production, receptor function and availability. Despite the fact that much is known about the natural and acquired anti-adherent mechanisms with *E. coli*, little is known about anti-adherence mechanisms with regard to *Candida*, in particular the role of secretory IgA and bacterial interference.

Table 2. Comparison of *E. coli* and *C. albicans* adherence: epithelial cell receptors

	E. coli	*C. albicans*
Glycosides	D-mannose Gal a 1–4 Gal Sialyl a 2–3 Gal N-acetyl-D-glucosamine	Fuc a 1→2 Gal β
Blood group antigens	Group M (glycophorin A) Dr.	ABO (H antigen)
Secretor status	Non-secretor	Non-secretor

Dr Shepherd pointed out that another area of great interest would be the host cell response to *Candida* adherence in terms of production of cytokines and other mediators. It was questioned whether the adhesin might have sequence homology with any of the integrins or lectins but evidently purified adhesin has only recently been available for sequencing. Hicks suggested that proteases made by the *Candida* might be activating the adhesion molecule on the surface of the yeast or a receptor on the host cell.

The discussion also centred around the viability of the epithelial cells used in Dr Douglas' experiments. This is clearly one of the problems which is not present with endothelial cell monolayers where viability is high. Dr Edwards pointed out that adhesion to endothelial cells led to prostaglandin production, presumably relating to the inflammatory response that ensues. Questions were raised about whether bacterial colonization of epithelial surfaces might enhance *Candida* adherence and whether adherence to epithelial cells might be through recognized receptors such as ICAM, but these experiments remain to be done. The role of IgA defense against attachment was questioned since candidiasis is not a particular problem in patients with high IgA deficiency or even hypogammaglobulinaemia. A remarkable conclusion is that little is known about the normal defence mechanisms against adherence. Patients with AIDS have demonstrated a hierarchy of immunity to *Candida* infections. People with normal CD4 counts develop vaginal candidiasis but not necessarily oral or oesophageal candidiasis. As the CD4 count drops below 500, the risk of developing oral candidiasis is much greater. Cell-mediated immunity has a particular role to play in *Candida* colonization, although its place in preventing attachment and colonization is unclear and to date the role of cytokines has not been reported.

Although current data suggest that the major adhesin is a mannoprotein l-fucose glycoside interacting with a complementary receptor, there are likely to be other adhesion mechanisms including hydrophobicity, contributing to a lesser extent.

4. Human complement receptor-like molecules on *Candida*

J. E. Edwards Jr

HISTORICAL PERSPECTIVE

Similar to many discoveries in science, the detection of molecules resembling human complement receptors on the surface of *Candida* was not derived from prediction and testing of hypotheses; it was entirely fortuitous. Heidenreich & Dierich (1985) were using sheep erythrocytes (EA) coated with human complement degradation products of C3, C3b, and C3d, to probe for human receptors on lymphoblasts in tissue culture. Interestingly, they found the erythrocyte probes, EAC3d, and EAiC3b, adhered to the hyphae of *Candida* contaminating their preparations (Fig. 4.1). They described being surprised by the finding, since they were aware of the marked difference of the cell wall of *Candida* from the lipoprotein membrane of

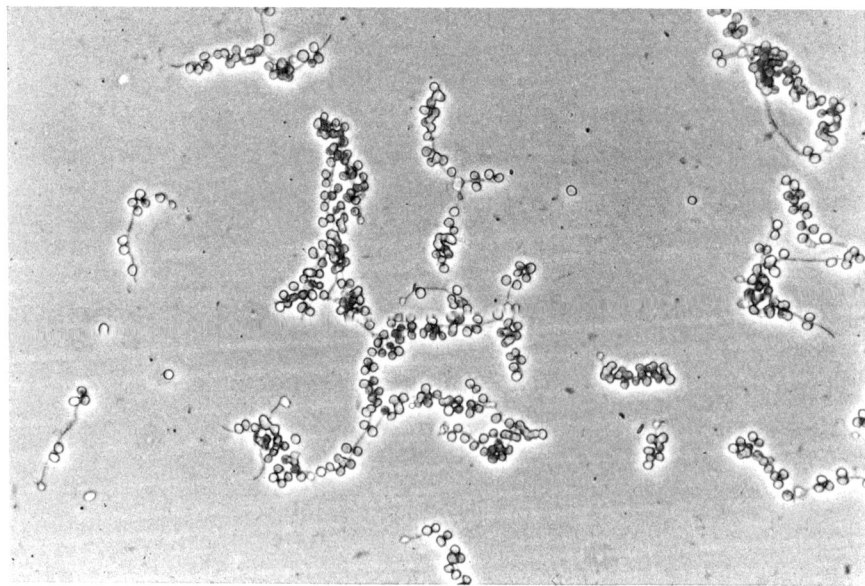

Fig. 4.1 Erythrocyes coated with human complement (EAiC3b) adhering to germinated *Candida* in vitro. Notice how the erythrocytes adhere along the length of the *Candida* hyphal structures. This preparation resembles those described by Heidenreich & Dierich (1985).

mammalian cells. Their awareness of the increasing pathogenicity of *Candida*, combined with their expertise in complement chemistry, led to pursuit of the serendipitous finding and the discovery of binding of sheep erythrocytes EAiC3b and EAC3d to the germinated portion of *C. albicans* and *C. stellatoidea*, but not to *C. tropicalis, C. parapsilosis* or *C. krusei*. Their studies of the blocking of erythrocyte adherence showed that mannan (from baker's yeast), the monosaccharides D-galactose, L-mannose, and the amino sugar N-acetylglucosamine did not block adherence, but preincubation of the erythrocytes with D-mannose and D-glucose inhibited adherence by 30%. This finding suggested a 'lectin-like' nature for the interaction of the erythrocytes and the *Candida* cell wall mannoproteins. They speculated on an anti-phagocytic potential for these molecules and a role in pathogenicity based on their restriction to pathogenic strains of *Candida*.

Almost simultaneously with the original publication of Heidenreich & Dierich, four groups independently began characterizing these human complement receptor-like molecules on *Candida*. The purpose of this discussion is to summarize and place into perspective the evolution of these studies.

INITIAL STUDIES OF THE SIMILARITY OF THE HUMAN COMPLEMENT RECEPTOR-LIKE MOLECULES ON *CANDIDA* TO HUMAN COMPLEMENT RECEPTORS

Heidenreich & Dierich (1985) showed that the sheep erythrocytes did not adhere to *Candida* until after the final stages of their preparation when human C3d and iC3b had been added, thus eliminating the possibility of the adherence being mediated non-specifically by the erythrocyte preparation process rather than the C3d and iC3b constituents themselves. Erythrocytes coated with other complement components, such as C3b, showed either very weak or no binding. Therefore, the molecules resembled most closely the human complement receptor 2 (CR2) and human CR3. The amount of adherence of EAC3d and EAiC3b was approximately equal. An additional similarity to human complement receptors has been the large number of monoclonal antibodies binding to the surface of *Candida* having specificity for human complement receptors. These antibodies have been reviewed recently (Mayer et al 1990, Calderone & Braun 1991) and are summarized in Table 4.1. Importantly, several of these monoclonals block the adherence of erythrocytes coated with iC3b and C3d.

Some controversy exists regarding whether these human iC3b-like molecules are restricted to the hyphae or are present on both yeast and hyphae. Using fluorescent-activated cell sorting, the iC3b receptors have been found on both the yeast and hyphal phases (Gilmore et al 1988). Other investigators, using immunofluorescence and light microscopy found aherence of the EAiC3b restricted to the hyphae and observed monoclonal antibodies selectively staining the hyphae. These differences may be due to sensitivity differences in the detecting systems. Frey et al (1988), using a highly sophisticated laser-activated immunofluorescence detection device, found markedly greater adherence of Mo1 monoclonal antibodies to the hyphal phase compared to the yeast phase, suggesting at least a 12-fold greater expression

Table 4.1 Selected antibodies to mammalian receptors and their reactivity with *C. albicans*

Antibody	Specificity[1]	Reactivity[2]		Blocking[3] of		Reference
		Yeast form	Hyphae	Binding	Adhesion	
OkM-1	CR3, α chain	+/−	+	+	ND	Eigentler et al 1989, Gilmore et al 1988
M522	CR3, α chain	−	+	ND	ND	Eigentler et al 1989
MO-1-94	CR3, α chain	+	+	ND	+	Gustafson et al 1991
MO-1	CR3, α chain	+/−	+	(−)	ND	Edwards et al 1986, Gilmore et al 1988
M1/70	CR3, α chain	+	+	(−)	ND	Gilmore et al 1988
BU-15	p150.95, α chain	+	+	+	ND	Hostetter et al 1989
Anti-CR2	CR2	−	−	+	ND	Edwards et al 1986
Anti-GP140	CR2	−	−	−	ND	Edwards et al 1986
Anti-CR1	CR1 (3D9)	−	−	ND	ND	Edwards et al 1986, Mayer et al 1990
60.1	CR3, α chain	−	−	ND	ND	Mayer et al 1990
Leu-15	CR3, α chain	−	−	ND	ND	Mayer et al 1990
95G8	CR3, β chain	−	−	ND	ND	Mayer et al 1990
7c3	CD15	−	+	ND	ND	Mayer et al 1990
MAB 44	CR3, α chain	+	ND	ND	+	Gustafson et al 1991
MAB 17	CR3, α chain	+	ND	ND	+	Gustafson et al 1991
MY9	CD 33	−	+	ND	ND	Mayer et al 1990
OKT4	T-cell antigen CD4	−	−	ND	ND	Mayer et al 1990
Hb55	CR2	−	−	+	ND	Edwards et al 1986

[1] Of monoclonal antibody for the mammalian receptor
[2] Determined by immunofluorescence
[3] +, Antibody blocks EAiC3b or EAC3d binding to *C. albicans* or adherence of *C. albicans* to endothelial cells; − no blocking; ND, not determined
Table adapted from Calderone & Braun (1991)

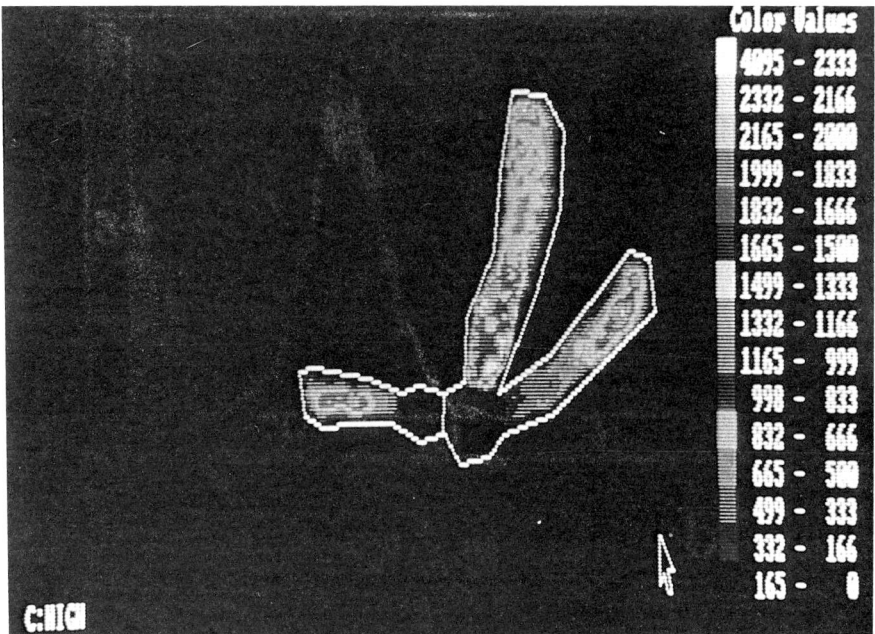

Fig. 4.2 Fluorescence emitted from the hyphae of *C. albicans* after straining with Mo1 monoclonal. Note that no signal is given from the yeast portion of the organism. The shaded areas on the hyphae represent various amounts of fluorescence detected after laser light stimulation. By courtesy of C L Frey [Frey et al (1988)].

of the receptor-like molecules on the hyphae per unit surface area (Fig. 4.2). Similar immunofluorescence studies have not been reported for the C3d-like molecules.

This binding of EAiC3b and EAC3d (prepared with human complement fragments) plus the recognition of binding sites on the organism by monoclonal antibodies specific for human complement receptors have been strongly complementary findings, establishing convincingly the presence of molecules on the surface of *Candida* closely resembling human complement receptors.

PURIFICATION AND CHARACTERIZATION OF THE HUMAN COMPLEMENT RECEPTOR-LIKE MOLECULES FOR iC3b

Efforts to purify and characterize the human CR3-like molecules are only in their early stages of evolution and the results have suggested considerable structural dissimilarity from the human CR3. Eigentler et al (1989) solubilized ^{125}I-labelled *C. albicans* and performed immunoprecipitation experiments with monoclonal antibodies OKM-1, M522, and 2G7 (an anti-CR2). Using SDS-PAGE and radioautographs of *Candida* cell surface preparations, they identified a 130kDa band specifically recognized by the OKM-1 antibody (two minor bands of 50 and 100 kDa were also found). This molecular weight differs from the dimer characterizing the human CR3 which consists of 165 and 95 kDa components. However, Hostetter et al (1989), using Western blotting, reported that Mo1 monoclonal antibody recognized a protein of 165 kDa in *Candida* cell membrane and cytosol extracts. This molecular weight is the same as the alpha chain of the CR3 (CD11b) on human neutrophils. There are no reports of protein sequencing of these immunoprecipitates to date.

Further characterization of the iC3b receptor-like site has been performed with complementary studies. IgG preparations were produced from hyperimmune serum raised in rabbits by weekly immunization with whole *Candida* cells given intravenously (Eigentler et al 1989). This specific IgG blocked adherence of EAiC3b substantially above 60 μg/ml concentrations. The blocking capacity of the IgG was restricted to the hyphal phase. Furthermore, preincubation of the IgG with germinated *Candida* caused blocking of OKM-1 recognition of the hyphal antigens. Divalent cations are not required for the binding of EAiC3b to *Candida* (equal binding in the presence or absence of 20 mmol EDTA), while they are a requirement for binding to human and mouse CR3 (Eigentler et al 1989). Gilmore et al (1988) showed that (^{3}H)iC3b, using Scatchard plot analysis, bound specifically to the yeast phase of the organisms. Expression of the molecules is temperature dependent; as the temperature in which the organisms were grown increased from 30°C to 38.5°C, the number of binding sites measured by an attachment index diminished (Eigentler et al 1989). The protein nature of the molecules has been demonstrated by the nearly 80% loss of ability to bind EAiC3b and EAC3d after treatment with trypsin (Eigentler et al 1989). Loss of binding of EAiC3b to organisms exposed to 56°C has demonstrated the heat lability of the receptor-like molecules (Eigentler et al 1989).

Expression of the molecules may also be dependent on the amount of glucose in which the organisms are grown. Hostetter et al (1989) reported a considerable increase in receptor expression (as determined by flow cytometry using Mo1 as the fluorescent marker) as organisms were grown in increasing glucose concentrations ranging from 0 to 20 mM. They described also a decrease in phagocytosis of organisms grown in 20 mM glucose compared to 20 mM glutamate. It is not clear from these studies whether change in surface area of the organisms or expression of receptors per area of surface was responsible for the flow cytometry or phagocytosis results, but apparently the organisms stayed in yeast phase during the experiments.

PURIFICATION AND CHARACTERIZATION OF THE HUMAN-LIKE COMPLEMENT RECEPTORS FOR C3d

There is considerably more structural characterization of the molecules responsible for adherence of EAC3d. Similar to the iC3b receptor-like molecules, they are sensitive to both pronase and trypsin (Saxena & Calderone 1990, Linehan et al 1988, Calderone et al 1988). Calderone et al (1988) have used complementary techniques to purify and characterize the proteins. They have passed the eluate from a DEAE-trisacryl column over a C3d-Thiol-Sepharose column and identified two proteins with silver staining after subjecting the eluate to SDS-PAGE. These proteins were 60–62 and 70 kDa in size. Their complementary method consisted of identifying a monoclonal antibody produced from spleen cells (in hybridomas) of mice immunized with *Candida* pseudohyphae cell wall preparations. The monoclonal CA-A was identified by screening antibodies produced from the mice hybridomas that blocked EAC3d adherence to *Candida*. An affinity column was made with this monoclonal antibody and a 60 kDa protein was purified from hyphal extracts passed through the column using high pressure liquid chromatography of the eluate and further purification with isoelectric focusing. However, other proteins of differing molecular weights were also isolated by this technique. They did not block adherence of EAC3d to hyphae, raising substantial questions concerning their relationship to the CR2-like molecules on the surface of the organism. Studies are underway to clarify this relationship.

A C3d-binding protein has also been isolated from cell extracts of hyphae by Calderone et al (1988). *Candida* hyphal extracts were fractionated by DEAE-trisacryl with NaCl step gradients and then isolated with a C3d-Thiol-Sepharose column. Two proteins of 60–62 kDa and 68–70 kDa were isolated with this technique.

Evidence for glycosylation of the CR2-like molecules comes from a number of experiments summarized by Calderone & Braun (1991) and includes showing that mannosylated fractions block EAC3d binding to *Candida*, that the isolated receptor-like proteins from affinity column stain with Con A on SDS-PAGE preparations, that substantive amounts of glucose and mannose have been found in HPLC analysis of purified fractions, and that glycolytic enzymes convert the purified protein to a fraction of lower molecular weight. However, the observation that hyphae saturated with Con A still bind EAC3d suggests the carbohydrate portion of the molecule may not be operative in binding EAC3d.

POSSIBLE ROLE OF THE HUMAN CR2 AND CR3-LIKE MOLECULES AS VIRULENCE FACTORS FOR *CANDIDA*

Several studies have addressed the role of the *Candida* human-like CR2 and CR3 receptors within the context of molecular mimicry and pathogenicity. However, definitive establishment of their role in pathogenicity awaits further experimentation. Gilmore et al (1988) presented indirect evidence for the iC3b receptor inhibiting phagocytosis by showing a diminished amount of phagocytosis of mycelial phase of the organism compared to yeast phase. They postulated the presence of fewer iC3b molecules on the yeast phase. Using similar reasoning, they concluded that diminished phagocytosis of organisms in media containing 50 mM glucose compared to phagocytosis in 5 mM glucose was due to increased expression of the human-like CR3 molecules by the glucose. Additionally, they blocked the human receptor-like molecules with Mo1 and found a small increase in phagocytosis. Unclear in this study is precisely what control was used for the Mo1 to determine specificity of the increase in phagocytosis.

Ollert et al (1990) examined virulence related to expression of these human-like CR2 and CR3 receptors by quantifying them on strains of *Candida* differing in pathogenicity. They found a mutant strain, m-10, with reduced capacity to adhere to fibrin platelet clots and epithelial cells and reduced capacity to cause endocarditis in a rabbit model compared to its parent strain. EAiC3b had 53% of the adherence capacity to the mutant compared to the parent strain. EAC3d adhered equally to both strains. Supporting evidence for the difference in expression of the iC3b receptor-like molecules on the two strains were bound by blocking-attachment of EAiC3b to *Candida* by cell extracts of the virulent strain and failure to block by extracts from the avirulent strain. Culture filtrates from the two strains were equal in blocking EAC3d, substantiating equal expression of the CR2 receptor-like molecules on both strains. They found also that serum from a patient with chronic mucocutaneous candidiasis recognized proteins of 68–71 kDa and 55 kDa from hyphal extracts of the virulent strain, but there was only minimal recognition of these proteins extracted from the avirulent strain. These experiments provided evidence for differing expression for the CR3 receptor molecules in the two strains differing in pathogenicity, and indirect evidence for this expression being a virulence factor.

Gustafson et al (1991) reported inhibition of the adherence of *Candida* to human vascular endothelial cells by purified iC3b and two monoclonal antibodies, mAbs 17 and 44, directed at the alpha subunit of the iC3b receptor. Frey et al (1990) reported in an abstract the blocking of adherence to endothelial cells with Mo1 antibody also.

FUTURE DIRECTIONS

Further efforts are necessary to determine precisely whether these human complement-like receptors are virulence factors. While current studies have shown a possible operative role of the CR3 in adherence to certain host cells, adherence of *Candida* has not been definitely shown to be a virulence factor. There is no definitive evidence that adherence to endothelial cells is or is not a virulence factor. While Klotz et al (1990) showed that the Arg-Gly-Asp (RGD) containing peptides block adherence to subendothelial cell matrix and that these peptides given intravenously result in less extensive infection in certain organs when intravenous challenge of *Candida* is given to experimental animals, similar studies have not been performed with endothelial cells in vitro. Intuitively, it is attractive to conclude that adherence is a virulence factor for *Candida*, but definitive proof remains to be demonstrated. The finding of a lower level of expression of these receptors on strains of *Candida* that are less virulent in vivo is supportive, but again not definitive. It is necessary to prove that these strains vary in only a single factor, the expression of the complement receptor-like molecule. The possible increased expression of these receptors in organisms grown in glucose is again indirect evidence for virulence. There is no proof that hyperglycaemia per se is associated with an increased incidence of disseminated candidiasis. While some patients on hyperalimentation may be hyperglycaemic, they may have numerous additional factors predisposing them to disseminated candidiasis which are much more important. An example would be intravenous plastic materials used to deliver the hyperalimentation fluids. Similarly, it has never been established that hyperglycaemia as an isolated factor is responsible for the increased mucocutaneous candidiasis seen in diabetic patients.

The approach most likely to relate these molecules to virulence is to sequence them and to clone their genetic programs. Then transfection vectors could be produced to be introduced into avirulent strains of *Candida*. If such studies are successful, and evidence for their virulence is established, considerable potential exists to therapeutically interact with these molecules and significantly alter the virulence they convey to the organism. Hostetter & Kendick (1989) have reported in abstract form the isolation of these immunoreactive clones in a cDNA library of *C. albicans* that have been isolated using a monoclonal antibody BU-15 that recognizes the CD11c (alpha subunit of the p150, 95) and also binds to *C. albicans*. Similar studies will accomplish the goal of defining much more accurately the role of these molecules as virulence factors.

SUMMARY

The fortuitous finding of the binding of sheep erythrocytes coated with human complement to hyphae of *Candida* has led to the discovery that the organism has molecules mimicking certain structural and functional characteristics of the CR2 and CR3 receptors of human leukocytes. Not surprisingly, there are substantial difference in these molecules from the human CR2 and CR3 in molecular weight, glycosylation, and recognition by those monoclonal antibodies that recognize human CR2 and CR3 receptors. However, substantial similarities exist in their specific binding of iC3b, recognition by monoclonal antibodies that are specific for human complement receptors and their binding of EAiC3b and EAC3d. While there is indirect evidence that they may be virulence factors, definitive evidence awaits development. Because of their potential for being operative in adherence and for being antiphagocytic, and other mechanisms for functioning as virulence factors, efforts are needed to determine their role in pathogenicity as eventual therapeutic targets.

REFERENCES

Calderone R A, Braun P C 1991 Adherence and receptor relationships of *Candida albicans*. Microbiological Reviews 55: 1–19

Calderone R A, Lineham L, Wadsworth E, Sandberg A L 1988 Identification of C3d receptors of *Candida albicans*. Infection and Immunity 56: 252–258

Edwards J E Jr, Gaither T A, O'Shea J J et al 1986 Expression of specific binding sites on *Candida* with functional and antigenic characteristics of human complement receptors. Journal of Immunology 137: 3577–3583

Eigentler A, Schulz T F, Larcher C et al 1989 C3bi-binding protein on *Candida albicans* temperature-dependent expression and relationship to human complement receptor type 3. Infection and Immunity 57: 616–622

Frey C L, Jenson B D, Drutz D J 1988 Localization and distribution of iC3b binding sites on *Candida albicans*. Abstracts of the Annual Meeting of the American Society for Microbiology 88th Annual Meeting 396

Frey C L, Barone, J M, Drutz D 1990 The role of the *Candida albicans* iC3b receptor in fungal adherence to endothelial cells. Abstracts of the Annual Meeting of the American Society for Microbiology F-101:112

Gilmore B J, Retsinas E M, Lorenz J S, Hostetter M K 1988 An iC3b receptor of *Candida albicans*: structure, function and correlates for pathogenicity. Journal of Infectious Diseases 157: 38–46

Gustafson K S, Vercellotti G M, Bendel C M, Hostetter M K 1991 Molecular mimicry in *Candida albicans*. Role of an integrin analogue in adhesion of the yeast to human endothelium. Journal of Clinical Investigation 87: 1896–1902

Heidenreich F, Dierich M P 1985 *Candida albicans* and *Candida stellatoidea* in contrast to other *Candida* species, bind iC3b and C3d but not C3b. Infection and Immunity 50: 598–600

Hostetter M K, Kendick K E 1989 Cloning and sequencing of cDNA encoding the iC3b receptor on *Candida albicans*. XIIIth International Complement Workshop 107: 348

Hostetter M K, Lorenz J S, Preus L, Kendrick K E 1989 The iC3b receptor on *Candida albicans*: subcellular localization and modulation of receptor expression by glucose. Journal of Infectious Diseases 161: 761–768

Klotz S A, Smith R L, Stewart B W 1990 RGD-containing peptide inhibits metastatic lesions arising from i.v. administration of *Candida albicans*. Program and Abstracts of the 30th Interscience Conference on Antimicrobial Agents and Chemotherapy Abstract 294, p 135

Linehan L, Wadsworth E, Calderone R A 1988 *Candida albicans* C3d receptor, isolated by using a monoclonal antibody. Infection and Immunity 56: 1981–1986

Mayer C L, Diamond R D, Edwards J E, Jr 1990 Recognition of binding sites on *Candida albicans* by monoclonal antibodies to human leukocyte antigens. Infection and Immunity 58: 3765–3769

Ollert M W, Wadsworth E, Calderone R A 1990 Reduced expression of the functionally active complement receptor for iC3b but not for C3d on an avirulent mutant of *Candida albicans*. Infection and Immunity 58: 909–913

Saxena A, Calderone R A 1990 Purification and characterization of the extracellular C3d-binding protein of *Candida albicans*. Infection and Immunity 58: 309–314

Discussion of paper presented by J. E. Edwards Jr

Discussed by R. A. Calderone
Reported by K. P. W. J. McAdam

Dr Calderone started by summarizing his own and other studies on the complement receptors of *Candida albicans*. Several different approaches have demonstrated the expression of the *Candida* CR2 in vivo. Sera from patients with different types of candidiasis, including mucocutaneous candidiasis, have reacted with purified *Candida* CR2 in Western blot assay. Lymphocytes from mice infected with *C. albicans* have proliferated in the presence of purified *Candida* CR2. Moreover, immunogold labelled rabbit monospecific antibody to purified *Candida* CR2 has stained *C. albicans* in tissue of infected mice. Dr Calderone's monoclonal antibody to *Candida* CR2 did not stain these organisms. Interestingly, the immunogold staining found the *Candida* CR2 to be localized to the cytoplasmic membrane of the fungus except for germinating organisms, where the entire cell wall was stained, including the surface.

Dr Calderone related that he had used a 1.8 kb fragment of the human B cell CR2 to screen a *C. albicans* GT11 genomic library. Southern blot had identified a 3.2 kb insert which was homologous to the human B cell DNA. This homology was localized to a 700 bp fragment obtained by digestion with Hind III. Sequencing of this fragment is underway.

Two different types of adhesion between *C. albicans* and human tissues were discussed by Drs Calderone and Edwards. One is a lectin-like interaction with the protein present on the fungus and the sugar located on the human cell. As Dr Douglas described, the fungal lectin appears to be a mannoprotein which recognizes L-fucose residues in epithelial cells. In some cases, N-acetylglucosamine residues also appear to be ligands. In another type of adhesion, *C. albicans* mannoproteins behave analogous to human CR3, binding C3bi on the surface of erythrocytes. In this protein–protein binding, amino acid sequences containing RGD (arginine-glycine-aspartic acid) are important ligands.

Dr Diamond suggested caution in the interpretation of data that have been published on *Candida* complement receptors to date. In particular, credible controls have not always been included in experiments which others have then been unable to repeat. Experiments on the upregulation of expression of surface complement receptors on blastoconidia do not always include correlative light scatter data in FACS analysis. He described expression of the *Candida* complement receptor in early germinating cells and others (Carrie Frey et al) have shown that the receptor is expressed over a specific area where the germ tube forms. Another reservation about some reported experiments has been their relevance to the in vivo situation, particularly when looking at receptor adhesion to endothelium in the presence of serum-free medium. Clearly, the luminal side of endothelium never exists in a serum-free situation and organisms appear to be coated with anti-mannan antibodies, not specifically directed against complement receptors. Dr Edwards pointed out that experiments measuring the increase in iC3b receptor expression in the presence of glucose must contain controls for the germination of the organism; it is not clear from the studies published to date that these controls have been a part of the overall design. Similarly, blocking experiments of the adherence of the organism to endothelium with iC3b need to be controlled against a molecule similar to iC3b. The notion that the *Candida* iC3b receptor may be anti-phagocytic and may be operative in adherence to endothelial cells is very intriguing and needs to be confirmed. Being able to repeat experiments in the presence of serum appears to be particularly difficult.

Dr Odds pointed out that in vivo in tissues, *C. albicans* takes on a whole variety of intermediate shapes, particularly pseudomycelial, whereas many of the experiments refer to hyphae and blastoconidia. He had noted no complement receptor expression on old parent blastoconidium as opposed to young actively growing germ tubes. Dr Edwards reported staining by monoclonal antibodies to complement receptors on the germinating form, pseudohyphae and hyphae.

In answer to a question about the identity of the recognition structures on endothelium that bind to the *Candida* CR2, Dr Edwards suggested the leucocyte-adherence molecules (LAMs) on endothelial cells. These LAMs are expressed by endothelial cells to bind neutrophils and it would be interesting to investigate whether activated endothelial cells, expressing LAMs, increase binding of *Candida*.

Dr Kozel raised the interesting possibility that the *Candida* complement receptors might have a function in regulating the complement cascade, in the same way that human CR2 contains factor H-like activity. At present, the role of the *Candida* complement receptors in pathogenesis is unknown.

Session II:
Other mycoses

Chairman: H. C. Neu

5. Targeting morphogenetic events in the parasitic cycle of *Coccidioides immitis*

G. T. Cole, D. Kruse, K. R. Seshan

INTRODUCTION

The morphogenesis of the higher fungi and to a large extent the ability of fungal pathogens to survive in the hostile environment of the host are intimately related to events of biosynthesis and modification of their cell wall components (Bartnicki-Garcia 1973, Cole & Kirkland 1991). It seems logical, therefore, that molecular targets of certain novel antifungal drugs are cell wall synthetases. Examples of such targets are β-1,3-glucan synthetase, which has been shown to be inhibited by the antifungal agent cilofungin (Taft & Selitrennikoff 1988, Drouhet et al 1990), and chitin synthetase inhibited by the nikkomycins and polyoxins (Dahn et al 1976, Hector & Pappagianis 1983, Cooper et al 1984). Since chitin is a linear β-1,4-linked polymer of N-acetylglucosamine which is not produced by mammals, compounds which inhibit its synthesis are particularly attractive for the treatment of mycoses in humans (Brillinger 1979). It should be remembered, however, that in order for these cell wall synthetase inhibitors to be effective they must penetrate the cell wall and reach the plasmalemma or cytoplasm of actively growing cells to react with their molecular targets. In certain thick-walled melanized fungi, or a pathogen like *Coccidioides immitis* which give rise to endospores (host tissue dissemination phase) within the protective envelope of the maternal cell (spherule), accessibility of the synthetase targets may be problematic. Ideally, one would like to use an antifungal agent which is readily solubilized in aqueous buffer and stable under physiological conditions, shows little or no toxicity to the host, inhibits growth of a broad diversity of pathogenic fungi, and demonstrates an adequate half-life in vivo that permits the drug to be effective at concentrations well tolerated by the patient. Evaluations of the antifungal efficacy of cilofungin in animal models and in clinical trials have revealed problems associated with its short half-life (Padula & Chambers 1989, Cole et al 1990b), limited spectrum of fungal pathogens against which the drug is directed (Hobbs et al 1988), and toxicity associated with polyethylene glycol used in its solubilization (R. S. Gordee, personal communication). Evaluation of nikkomycin Z in murine models has revealed that it is most effective against *C. immitis* and *Blastomyces dermatitidis*, less effective against yeasts with little chitin in their cell wall, and without apparent effect on *Aspergillus fumigatus* for reasons which are still unresolved (Hector et al 1990). Although results of early studies of nikkomycin hold promise, shortcomings in its application are also recognized, such as the limited spectrum of pathogenic fungi against which the drug is active and its relatively short half-life (10 to 15 min in outbred CFW mice; Hector et al 1990). In the case of experimental coccidioidomycosis, nikkomycin Z was unable totally to clear the pathogen from infected lung tissue or central nervous system (Hector et al 1990).

These relatively disappointing results from early in vivo studies of fungal wall synthetase inhibitors stimulated us to ask whether alternative cell wall-associated molecular targets exist which are also crucial for morphogenesis of the pathogen but more accessible to inhibitory compounds, To address this question, it is first necessary to return to general concepts of wall morphogenesis.

FUNGAL WALL AUTOLYSINS

It has been suggested that hyphal tip growth involves the balanced interaction of wall synthetases and wall hydrolases: together, these enzyme-driven events of wall biosynthesis and modification largely dictate the shape of the extending hyphal apex (Bartnicki-Garcia 1973). Gow (1989) has stated that 'control over the assembly of chitin and β-glucan at the tip depends not only on biosynthesis but also on controlled autolysis, with the lytic enzymes allowing the insertion of new polymers within the polysaccharide chains and maintenance of a tip of sufficient plasticity to permit turgor-driven expansion.' This same interaction between wall synthetases and hydrolases has also been suggested to influence the morphology and differentiation of fungal spores and spore-forming structures (Cole 1986). Evidence has been reported for the localization of wall autolysins in fungal hyphae, including chitinase (Gooday 1983), N-acetyl-β-D-glucosaminidase (Hoch et al 1979, Gooday 1983) and β-1,3-glucanase (Kritzman et al 1978). These first two wall autolysins are thought to perform regulatory roles in wall morphogenesis by localized breakdown of pre-existing chitin microfibrils to N,N'-diacetylchitobiose and N-acetylglucosamine, respectively. Each of these digestion products could then serve to activate chitin synthetase zymogen associated with the plasmalemma (Gooday 1983). By this mechanism, controlled intussusception of new chitin microfibrils into the expanding cell wall could take place. β-1,3-Glucanase may also participate in cell wall morphogenesis by digestion of preformed β-1,3-glucan mibrofibrils to provide for increase rate of wall growth and plasticity, by regulation of the for mation of cross-linkages between β-1,3-glucan and chitin which would otherwise increase the rigidity of the cell wall (Wessels 1986), and by other still unresolved mechanisms of localized interaction with cell wall components. Delivery of these autolysins to the hyphal wall is probably mediated by secretory vesicles derived from dictyosomal cisternae (Cole 1986, Gow 1989). Some evidence has also been presented that inhibition of the activity of such wall autolysins affects hyphal extension. For example, the presence of the β-glucanase inhibitor glucuronolactone was shown to inhibit hyphal extention and branching in *Saprolegnia monoica* and caused an atypical increase in hyphal diameter. Gow (1989) has suggested that allosamidin, shown to be a potent inhibitor of chitinase activity in *Neurospora crassa*, may be useful for examining the significance of this autolysin in morphogenesis of selected fungi.

MORPHOGENESIS OF *COCCIDIOIDES IMMITIS*

The causative agent of a respiratory disease in humans (coccidioidomycosis, San Joaquin Valley fever), *C. immitis* is the subject of the remainder of this discussion and is an appropriate model for evaluation of the roles of wall-associated autolysins in fungal morphogenesis (Cole et al 1991a,b,c, Yuan et al 1988). The parasitic cycle of *C. immitis* occurs initially in the lung by conversion of inhaled, unicellular arthroconidia (3 to 6 by 2 to 4 μm) into large multinucleate but still unicellular spherules (60 μm diameter spherules have been recorded in vivo; Cole & Sun 1985, Sun et al 1986). This morphogenetic process involves extensive synthesis and intussusception of wall microfibrils associated with relatively rapid diametric growth of the spherule envelope during the first generation of the parasitic cycle. Spherules are formed in vivo by about 48 h after intranasal inoculation of BALB/c mice with a suspension of arthroconidia (Sun et al 1986, Cole & Kirkland 1991). Transformation of arthroconidia into mature spherules typically involves an approximately 200-fold increase in total surface area of the cell (Fig. 5.1A, B). Based on concepts of hyphal growth discussed above, one would expect that wall morphogenesis in parasitic cells of *C. immitis* would necessitate a burst of wall synthetase activity as well as comparable levels of activity of wall hydrolases which modify pre-existing and nascent wall polymers and/or activate wall synthetases to accommodate the diametric expansion of the spherule. Conversion of endospores (approximately 2 μm diam; Fig. 5.1B, C) into mature spherules may involve similar

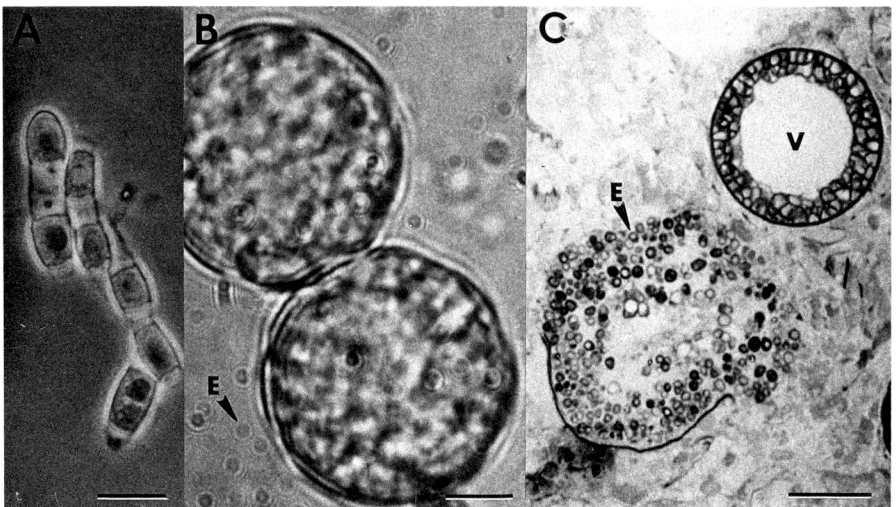

Fig. 5.1 Arthroconidia (A) and endosporulating spherules (B) of strains 634 and 735, respectively, produced in vitro. An intact, segmented spherule (strain 735) with large central vacuole (V) and ruptured spherule which has released its endospores (E) are shown in a section of infected murine lung tissue in (C). Bars represent (A) 6.0, (B) 5.0, and (C) 20.0 μm.

events of wall synthetase and hydrolase activity associated with their phase of diametric growth. Mature spherules of strains 634, 735 and Silveira grow in vitro to approximately 2/3 the diameter of spherules produced in vivo. A corresponding difference is recognized in the diameter of the central vacuole of the young spherule (c.f. Cole & Sun 1985, Fig. 5.1C). The vacuole may be important in maintenance of turgor pressure during early spherule development and, thereby, may contribute to expansion of the cell envelope.

WALL AUTOLYSINS IN C. IMMITIS

In this chapter we report the isolation and purification of a β-glucosidase from C. *immitis* and demonstrate that it is localized in cell walls of both the saprobic and parasitic phases. Preliminary evidence is presented that this enzyme may serve as a wall hydrolase and play a significant role in spherule growth. Multinucleate spherules undergo segmentation by ingrowth of septal walls. This process, like the expansion of the spherule envelope, involves extensive de novo synthesis of wall material. Segmentation first results in formation of multinucleate compartments which undergo further subdivision by branching of the endogenous septa to give rise to uninucleate compartments. The latter differentiate into endospores, each encompassed by a thin cell wall which undergoes rapid growth resulting in diametric expansion of the progeny cells even while still within the mother spherule. We present preliminary evidence in this report that a chymotrypsin-like serine proteinase may participate in wall morphogenesis associated with these phases of early endospore differentiation, diametric growth of young spherules (endospores), and differentiation of the segmentation apparatus of C. *immitis*.

A wall-associated β-glucosidase

Thin sections of young parasitic cells of C. *immitis* have revealed that the spherule envelope is composed of an outer, electron-dense (osmiophilic), hydrophobic layer which is released as membranous fragments from the cell surface both in vivo (Fig. 5.2A, B) and in vitro (Cole et al 1988a). These spherule outer wall (SOW) components were isolated from the culture supernatant and extracted with a non-ionic detergent, and the solubilized fraction was shown to react with immunoglobulin M (IgM), which has been identified as tube precipitin (TP) antibody in sera from coccidioidomycosis patients (Cole et al 1988a,b). A 120 kilodalton (kDa) glycoprotein with TP antibody reactivity (Kruse & Cole 1990) was identified in the SOW fraction and shown to be at least partly responsible for the immunoreactivity of the detergent-solubilized wall material (Cole et al 1991a). More recently, we have demonstrated that the 120 kDa glycoprotein is a β-glucosidase and produced by both the saprobic and parasitic phase (Kruse & Cole 1991). Purification of the enzyme was initially from the saprobic phase and involved isolation of a concanavalin A (Con A) bound fraction of the mycelial culture filtrate plus toluene lysate of the hyphal mat (F + L fraction; Kruse & Cole 1990). A single 120 kDa band with glucosidase activity, as detected with *p*-nitrophenol β-D-glucose substrate, was revealed in a non-reducing SDS-PAGE gel separation of the Con A fraction (Fig. 5.3A). The isoelectric point (pI) of this isolated glucosidase is

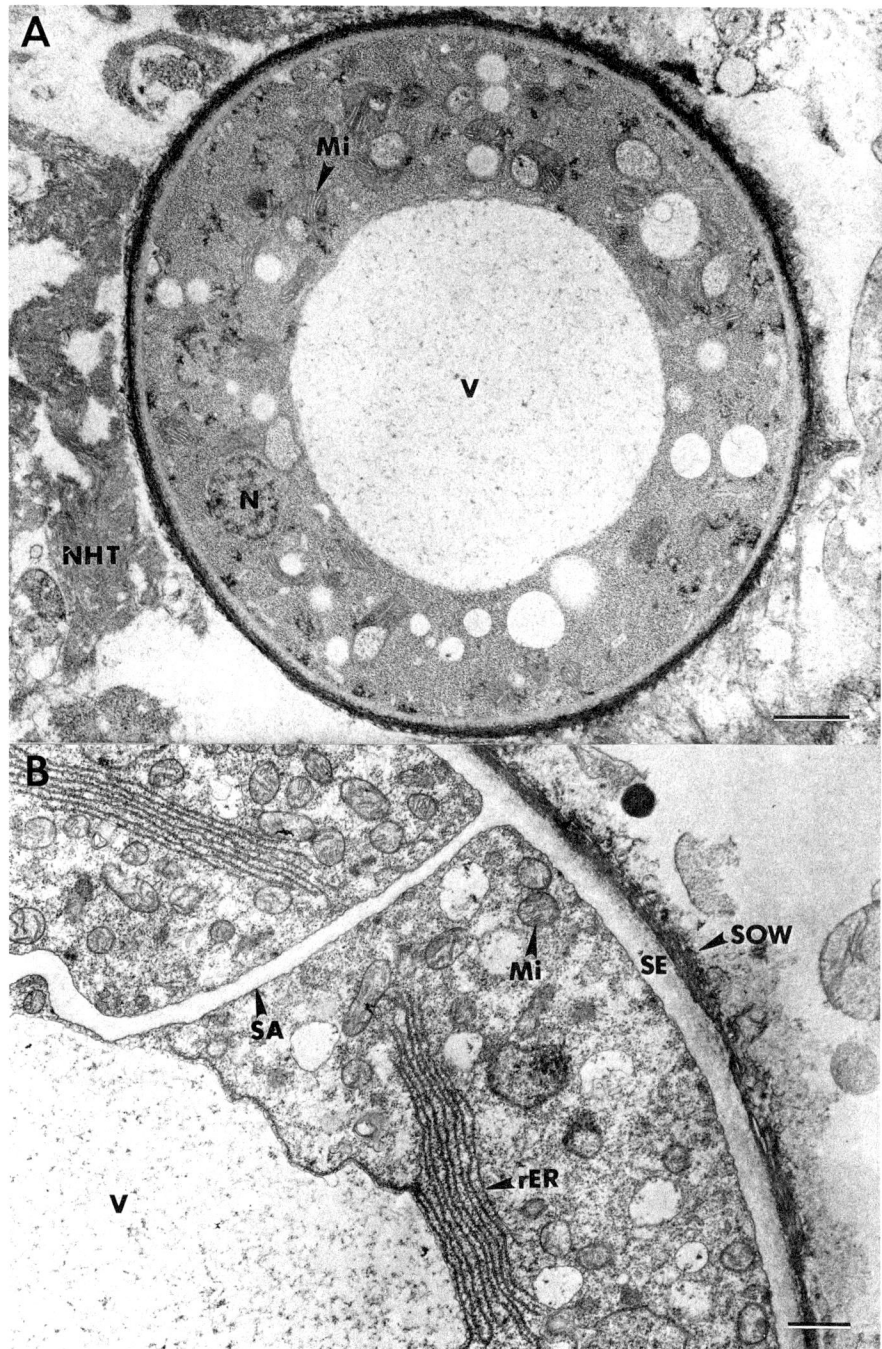

Fig. 5.2 Thin sections of young spherules in murine lung at presegmentation stage (A) and early segmentation stage (B). The latter shows invaginated wall of segmentation apparatus (SA). Mi, mitochondrion; N, nucleus; NHT, necrotic host tissue; rER, rough endoplasmic reticulum; SE, spherule envelope; SOW, spherule outer wall fragments; V, vacuole. Bars in A and B represent 1.0 μm.

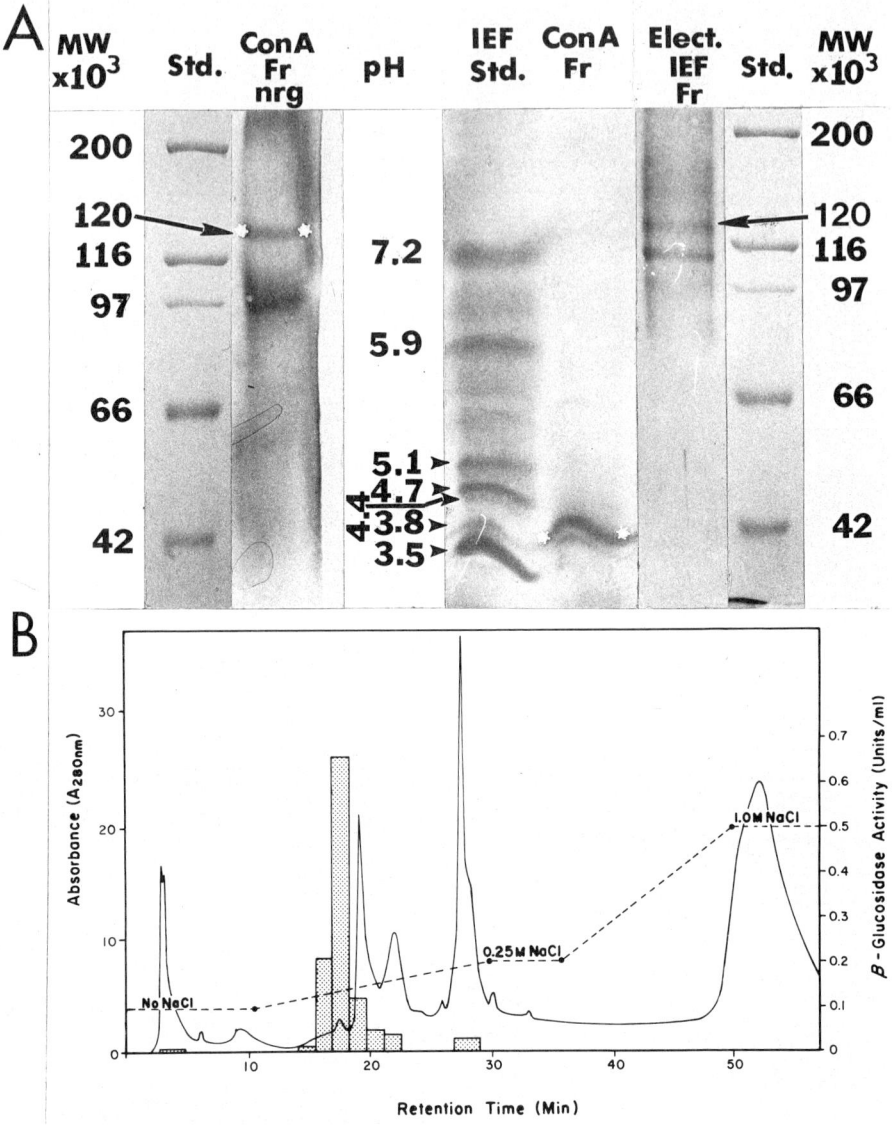

Fig. 5.3(A) Acrylamide gel electrophoresis separation of β-glucosidase. Left side: Nonreducing SDS-PAGE gel separation of ConA bound mycelial culture filtrate plus toluene lysate (F + L) which was incubated with the substrate *p*-nitrophenol(pNP)-β-D-glucopyranoside (20 min at 37°C) and the position of the band was marked. The same gel was then subjected to silver staining to visualize the bands. Right side: Isoelectric-focusing (IEF), non-denaturing gel separation of ConA bound F + L fraction (pH 3–10) followed by reaction with substrate as above. After localization of the enzyme band the gel was stained with Coomassie brilliant blue (Sigma). The band at approximately pH 3.9 of the preparative IEF gel was excised, electroeluted, and the isolated fraction was separated in a reducing SDS-PAGE gel. The bands were visualized by Coomassie stain. (B) Ion exchange (DEAE) high pressure liquid chromatographic (HPLC) separation of enzymatic band isolated from IEF gel shown in Fig. 5.3A. Fractions were eluted from the DEAE column with 10 mM phosphate buffer (pH 7.0) using indicated salt gradient. Fractions (1.0 ml) were tested for enzyme activity with 10 mM pNP-β-glucopyranoside in enzyme buffer (10 mM Tris with 0.6 mM $CaCl_2$, pH 8.0). One unit of enzyme activity equals the release of 1 μmol of pNP/min at 37°C.

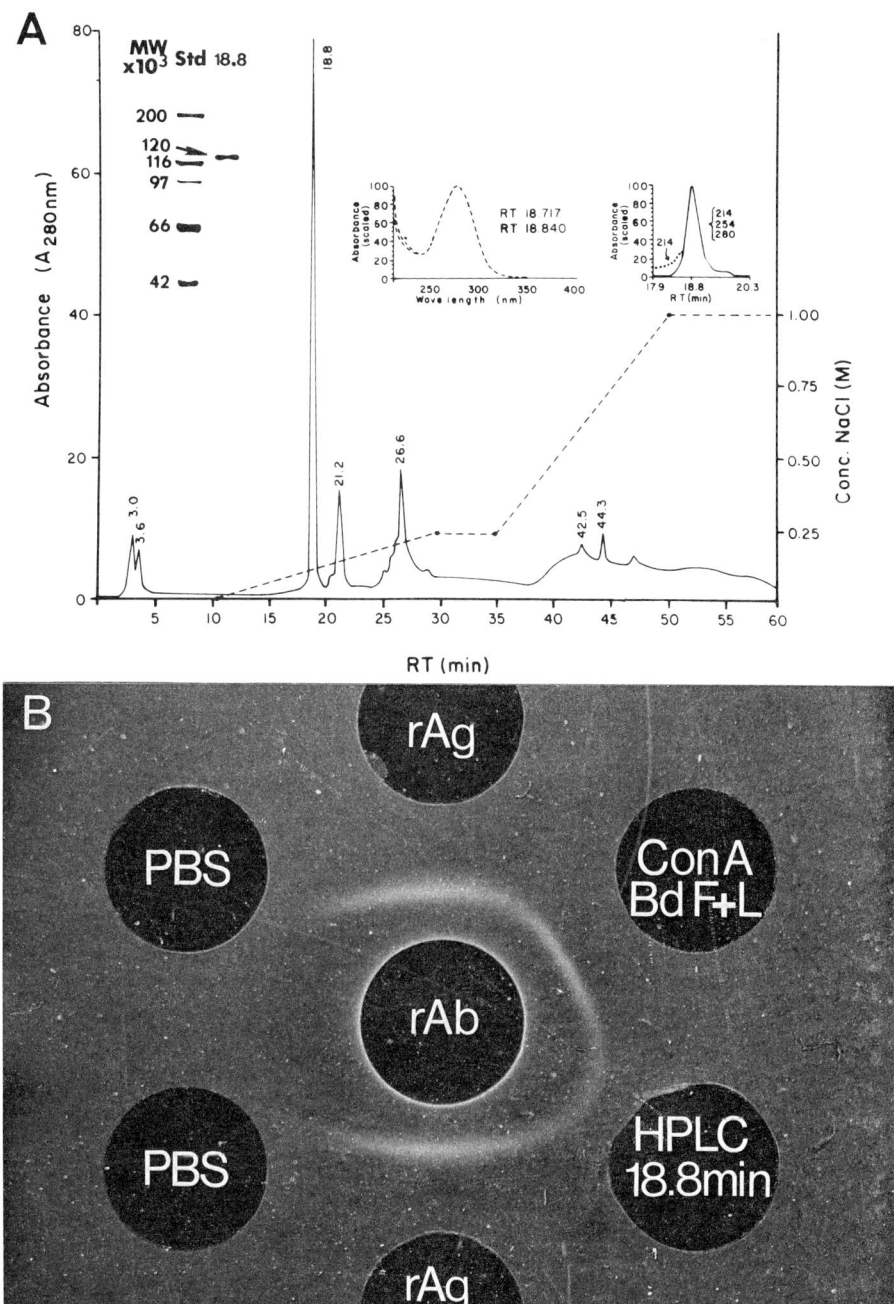

Fig. 5.4(A) DEAE-HPLC separation of the solid phase immunoadsorbed enzyme from the crude 10-day mycelial culture filtrate using guinea pig anti-120 kDa antibody. The β-glucosidase activity is at 18.8 min only. Results of analysis of absorption spectrum of 18.8 min peak (A_{210} to A_{400}) and combined elution profiles of three absorption wavelengths suggest homogeneity of fraction. Insert shows presence of single 120 kDa silver-stained band in the 18.8 min fraction (7.5% SDS-PAGE gel).
(B) Results of immunodiffusion-tube precipitin (ID-TP) assay of ConA bound F + L fraction and 18.8 min fraction shown in Fig. 5.4(A). Reference antigen (rAg) and antibody (rAb) are the same as previously described (Cole et al 1991a).

73

Table 5.1 Summary of characteristics of the β-glucosidase of *Coccidioides immitis*

pI	pH 3.8–4.0
Mol. wt. (non-red. gel)	~120 kDa
Mol. wt. (red. gel)	120 kDa
Mol. wt. (gel filt.)	120, 240, 480 kDa
pH optimum	8.0 (stability, pH 6.0 to 9.0)
Temp. optimum	37°C (stability, to 60°C for 2 h)
K_m (pNP-β-D-glucopyranoside)	0.33 mM
Carbohydrate composition 3-O-MM:Xyl:Man: Gal:Glc (monosaccharides [% ratio])	6.7 : 4.2 : 72.1 : 2.8 : 14.2

Hexosidase activity (using 10 mM p-nitrophenol substrate)[a,b]	
β-D-glucopyranoside	+ + + +
N-acetyl-β-D-galactosaminide	+ + +
N-acetyl-β-D-glucosaminide	+ +
β-D-fucopyranoside	+
N,N′-diacetyl-chitobiose[c]	+
cellobioside[c]	+
β-D-galactopyranoside	−
β-D-mannopyranoside	−
β-D-xylopyranoside	−
α-D-glucopyranoside	−
α-D-galactopyranoside	−
α-D-mannopyranoside	−
N-acetyl-α-D-glucosaminide	−
N-acetyl-α-D-galactosaminide	−
cellobiose	−

[a] Enzyme activity was detected by measure of the release of p-nitrophenol at 405 nm

[b] All substrates listed are available as p-nitrophenol conjugates from Sigma Chem. Co., St. Louis, MO.

[c] Detection of p-nitrophenol release from these substrates may not indicate hydrolysis of the disaccharides into monosaccharides.

approximately pH 3.9. The enzymatic fraction was excised from the IEF gel, electroeluted, and shown to consist of at least two components identified as 120 kDa and 110 kDa bands by SDS-PAGE (Fig. 5.3A). The 110 kDa fraction has also been shown to react with TP antibody from sera of coccidioidomycosis patients (Cole et al 1991a) but has not been shown to have any enzyme activity. Ion exchange (DEAE) chromatographic separation of the electroeluted material from the IEF gel permitted isolation of a single fraction with high glucosidase activity (Fig. 5.3B). This isolated DEAE fraction was used to raise antibody in guinea pigs for subsequent affinity purification of the enzyme from the mycelial (F + L) fraction (Fig. 5.4A). The purified enzyme was shown to elicit TP antibody response with sera from coccidioidomycosis patients (Fig. 5.4B). The enzyme has a pH optimum of 8.0 (range 6.0 to 8.5) and a temperature optimum of 35° to 40° C (stability range 25° to 60° C). The high pH optimum and broad temperature stability of the enzyme are not surprising since growth of the saprobic phase in nature occurs in hot, alkaline desert soil (Pappagianis 1988). In vitro growth of the parasitic phase has been shown to generate an alkaline environment (Cole & Sun 1985). A summary of the characteristics of the β-glucosidase is presented in Table 5.1.

In an earlier report of *C. immitis* wall composition (Cole et al 1983), we showed that the carbohydrate content of the inner conidial wall fraction was 54% by weight, approximately 22% of which was estimated to be chitin. The identity of the remaining structural carbohydrates of the conidial wall is unknown. Hector & Pappagianis (1982) proposed a model for the distribution of structural poly-saccharides in the spherule wall based on results of selected enzymatic digestion of glutaraldehyde-fixed intact cells. The authors suggested that β-glucans occur together with chitin in the inner region of the spherule envelope and segmentation apparatus, while 'interspersed throughout the wall was what appeared to be a mannan–protein complex'. Results of wheat germ agglutin (WGA) lectin and Calcofluor reactivity with prepared sections of the parasitic cells of *C. immitis* are shown in Figure 5.5. Slightly brighter fluorescence was shown in walls of spherules and endospores grown in vitro (Fig. 5.5A, B) than in fungal cells in infected lung tissue (Fig. 5.5C, D). Evidence for preferential binding of WGA lectin to polymers of GlcNAc-GlcNAc-GlcNAc is well established (Leathem & Atkins 1983). The

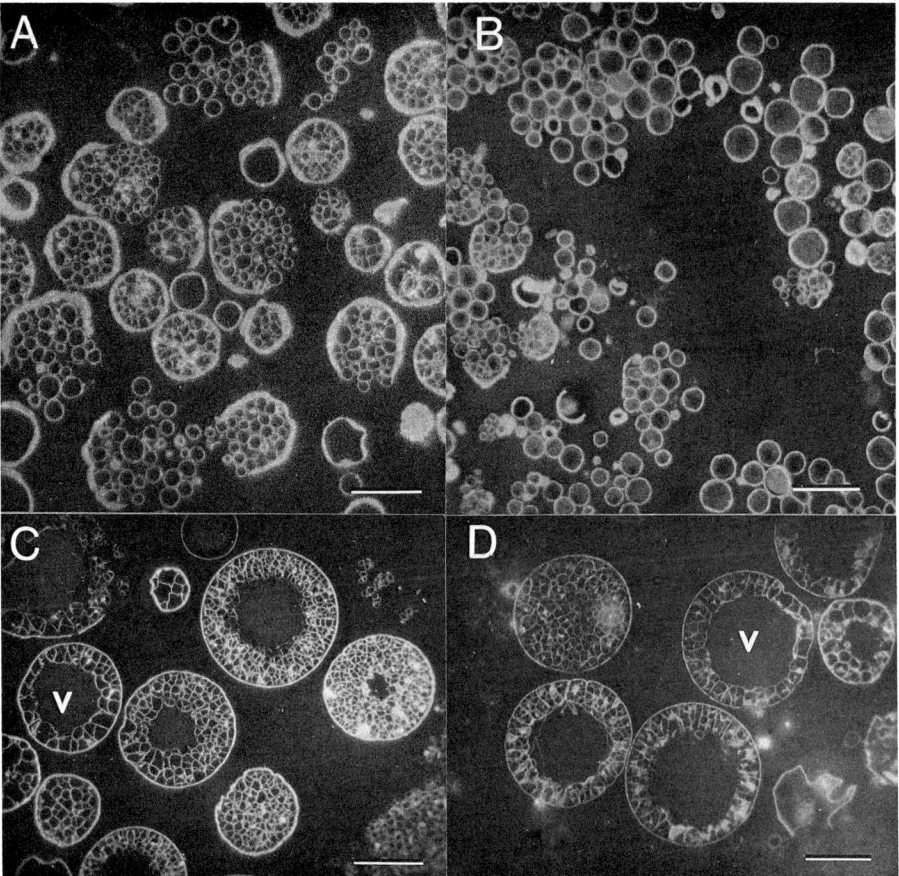

Fig. 5.5 Results of WGA-lectin binding to (A,C) and Calcofluor reactivity with (B,D) thick sections of parasitic cells of *C. immitis* grown in vitro (A,B) and in vivo (C,D). V, vacuole. Bars in A–D represent 20 μm.

specificity of Calcofluor for chitin in the fungal cell wall, on the other hand, is controversial. Pringle (1991) has concluded that 'Calcofluor is manifestly not specific for chitin in all contexts (e.g., it stains both cellulose in plant and algal cell walls and some unknown component of *Schizosaccharomyces pombe* cell walls)'. We compared reactivity of Calcofluor with commercially-available preparations of cellulose (β-1,4 linkages), pustulan (β-1,6 linkages), yeast glucan (mixed β-1,3 and β-1,6 linkages), and laminaran (primarily β-1,3 linkages). Cellulose, glucan, and laminaran showed fluorescence while pustulan showed no binding of Calcofluor. Aniline blue was shown to stain the conidial wall and the envelope of young and mature spherules. The stained walls fluoresced when examined with a FITC excitation filter. Studies of a broad range of fungi have suggested that this cyto-chemical stain is specific for β-1,3-glucan in the cell wall (Nicholas & Hunter 1991). We suggest that the results of WGA, Calcofluor, and aniline blue reactions with *C. immitis* support the earlier suggestion of the coexistence of chitin and β-1,3-glucan at least in the envelope of young and mature spherules, and in endospore walls.

Wessels (1986) has proposed that cross-linking of β-1,3-glucan and chitin by the formation of covalent bonds between chitin microfibrils and glucan can occur in fungal walls, particularly in the subapical region of hyphae. Such cross-links would contribute significantly to the rigidity of the cell wall. Chitin at the hyphal tip, on the other hand, remains loosely organized and free of cross-linkages to β-1,3-glucan, which is essential for maintenance of wall plasticity at the growing apex. Evidence has also been presented from studies of *Mucor rouxii* that nascent chitin, such as that found at hyphal tips, is much more susceptible to chitin deacetylase and chitinase activity than microfibrillar, crystalline chitin (Bartnicki-Garcia 1989). The latter consists of individual chitin chains tightly associated with one another through extensive hydrogen bonding. Crystallization of chitin, therefore, would tend to block the action of deacetylase or chitinase. With these concepts of fungal wall morphogenesis in mind, it seems unlikely that formation of glucan-chitin cross-linkages and extensive deposition of crystallized chitin would occur in the cell wall of *C. immitis* spherules during their rapid diametric growth phase. Instead, one would expect to find wall-associated hydrolases (e.g. chitinase and β-1,3-glucanase) in the envelope of spherule initials which function in concert with the corresponding synthetases to permit uninterrupted wall growth during spherule and endospore differentiation.

To test whether the 120 kDa β-glucosidase might function as a wall autolysin, we first examined its ability to digest isolated wall fractions of *C. immitis*. The wall preparations were boiled for 3 min to destroy endogenous glucosidases prior to incubation with the purified 120 kDa fraction. The results shown in Fig. 5.6A demonstrate that wall fractions from both the saprobic and parasitic phases are susceptible to digestion by the β-glucosidase, as measured by the hexokinase assay (Sigma) for glucose release (Stein 1963). We subsequently examined the ability of the *C. immitis* enzyme to digest different polysaccharide substrates of known composition to determine linkage preference of the glucosidase (Fig. 5.6B). The results suggest that the enzyme efficiently and perhaps selectively digests β-1,3-linkages and, therefore, functions as a β-1,3-glucanase.

Our next step was to determine whether the 120 kDa enzyme could be localized

76

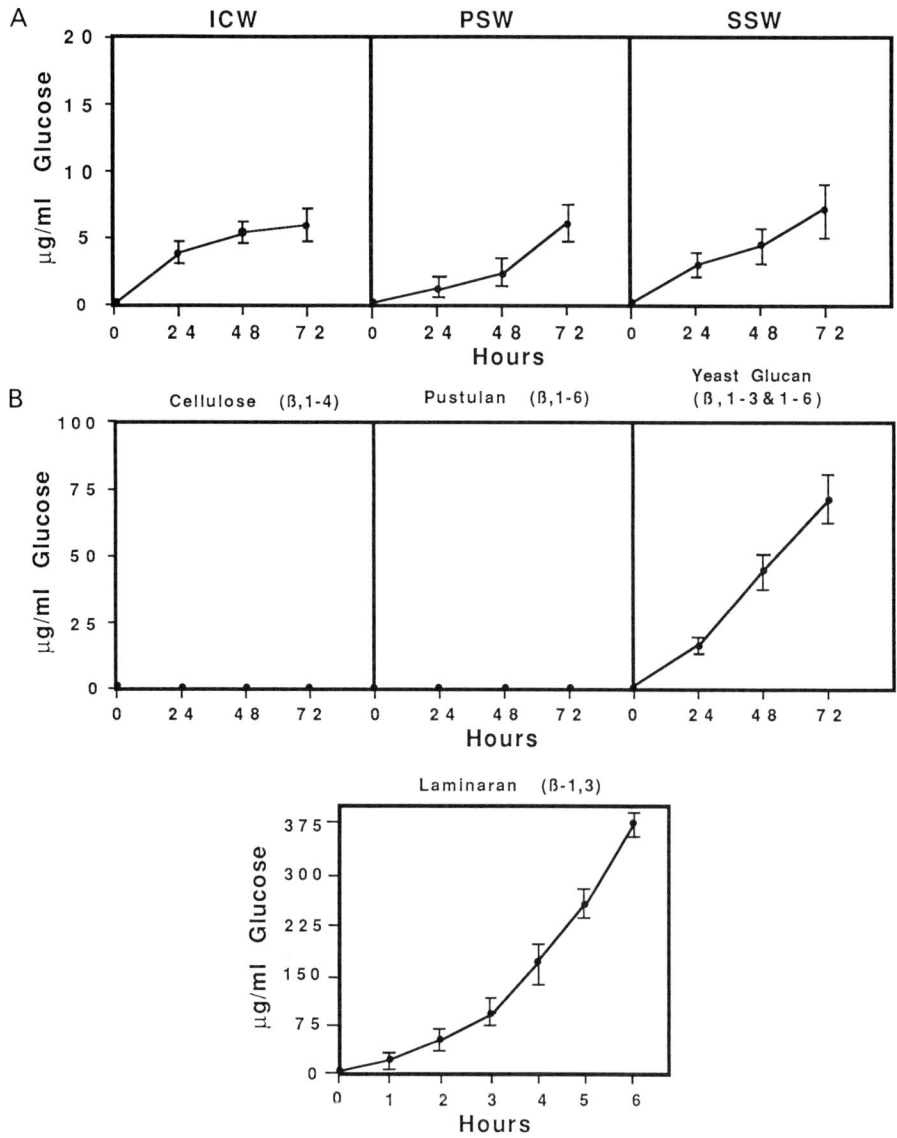

Fig. 5.6(A) Results of assays for glucose release from 1 mg samples of boiled wall substrates (ICW, inner conidial wall; PSW, presegmented spherule wall; SSW, segmented spherule wall). Purified *β*-glucosidase (0.5 units) was added to wall preparations and glucose release was monitored at 340 nm by a hexokinase/glucose-6-phosphate dehydrogenase coupled reaction (Sigma). Control without enzyme showed no glucose release. (B) Results of assays for glucose release as above from 1 mg samples of purified, natural substrates. Avicel-cellulose (EM Science), pustulan (Sigma), yeast glucan (3% *β*-1,6; Boehringer-Mannheim), and laminaran (Sigma) used to examine linkage preference in substrate digestion by *β*-glucosidase. Control without enzyme showed no glucose release.

in the cell wall at different developmental stages of *C. immitis*. We used the specific anti-120 kDa guinea pig antiserum described above as a probe for immunolabel experiments. Thin sections of conidia and spherules were reacted with the primary

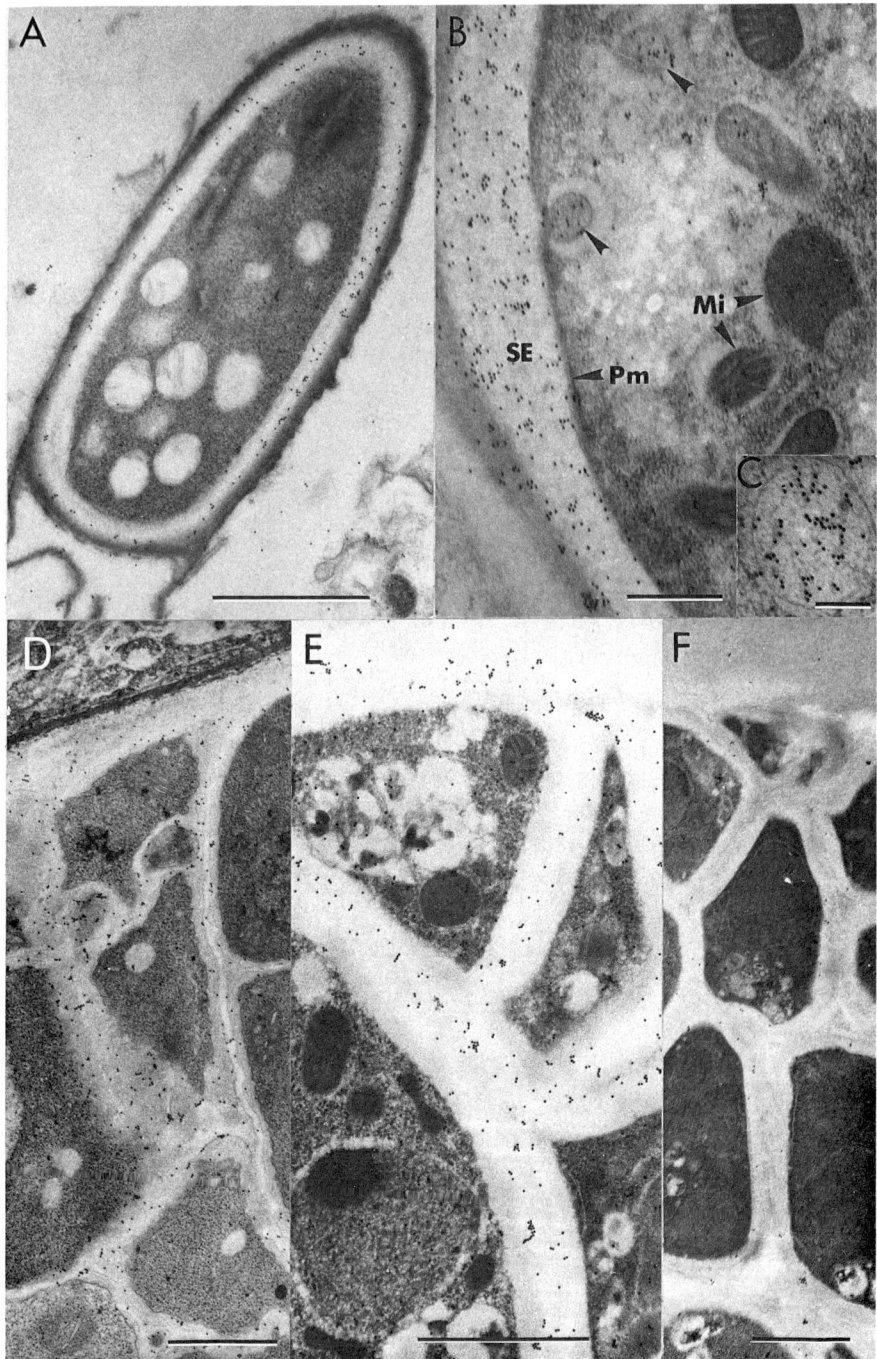

Fig. 5.7 Immunolocalization of β-glucosidase with guinea pig anti-120 kDa serum (A–D) and β-glucosidase substrate localization after incubation with enzyme-gold conjugate (E) in cell walls of *C. immitis*. Control (F) reacted with enzyme-gold conjugate which had been preincubated with 20 mM glucose. Arrowheads in (B) indicate gold-labelled vesicles, one of which is shown at higher magnification in insert (C). Mi, mitochondrion; Pm, plasmalemma; SE, spherule envelope. Bars represent (A) 1.0, (B) 0.5, (C) 0.2, (D) 1.0, (E) 1.0, and (F) 1.0 μm.

antibody followed by goat anti-guinea pig IgG/gold conjugate. In both the saprobic and parasitic cells the wall showed affinity for label (Fig. 5.7A–D) while control sections which were reacted with secondary antibody/gold conjugate alone were essentially free of label (not shown). Similar densities of immunolabel were shown on the spherule walls of *C. immitis* prepared from cultures and from infected murine lung tissue. The presegmented spherules (Fig. 5.7B) showed gold particles associated with the contents of cytoplasmic vesicles (Fig. 5.7C). We suggested in an earlier report that these organelles represent secretory vesicles which transport the 120 kDa glycoprotein from the cytoplasm to the cell wall (Cole et al 1991a). The vesicles are particularly abundant in the cytoplasm of young spherules at the developmental stage when maximum rate of diametric growth occurs. The evidence for this is derived from examination of thin sections (Cole et al 1991a) as well as immunofluorescence studies of thick sections of presegmented spherules which were reacted with the anti-120 kDa serum followed by secondary antibody/FITC conjugate (Fig. 5.8). The cells used in these investigations were grown in culture, cryofixed, subjected to freeze-substitution, and embedded in resin which was poly-merized at low temperature (Lowicryl K4M; Ted Pella Inc., Redding, CA). The secretory vesicles are most likely dictyosome-derived, although such ultrastructural relationships have not been observed in thin sections of young spherules. Upon fusion of the vesicles with the cell membrane, the products are released to the wall while the fused, vesicular membrane would contribute to expansion of the plasmalemma. We suggest that not all the product released from the vesicles remains wall-associated. In Figure 5.9 the results of indirect enzyme-linked immunosorbent assays (ELISAs) of the 120 kDa fraction in supernatants of parasitic phase cultures are shown. Each time point represents assay results of three

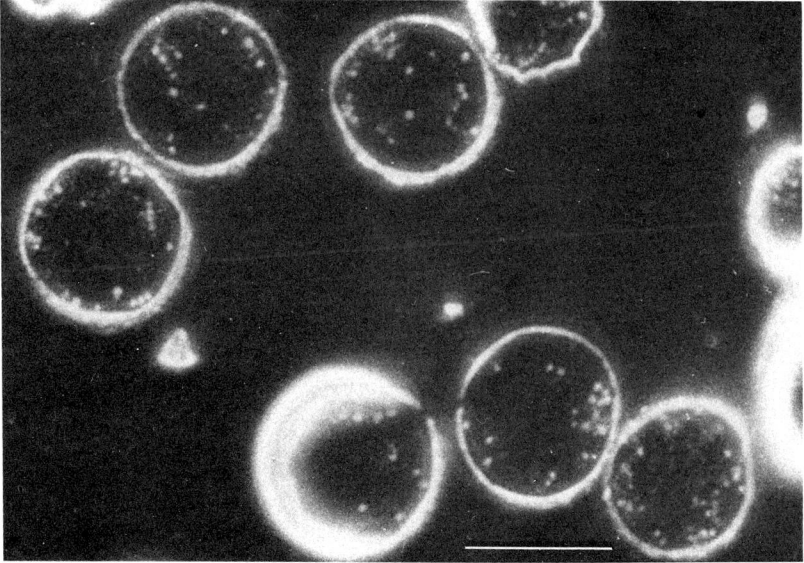

Fig. 5.8 Cryofixed and sectioned spherules (presegmentation stage) reacted with guinea pig anti-120 kDa serum followed by goat anti-guinea pig FITC conjugate. Both the spherule envelope and cytoplasmic vesicles show bright fluorescence. Bar represents 20 μm.

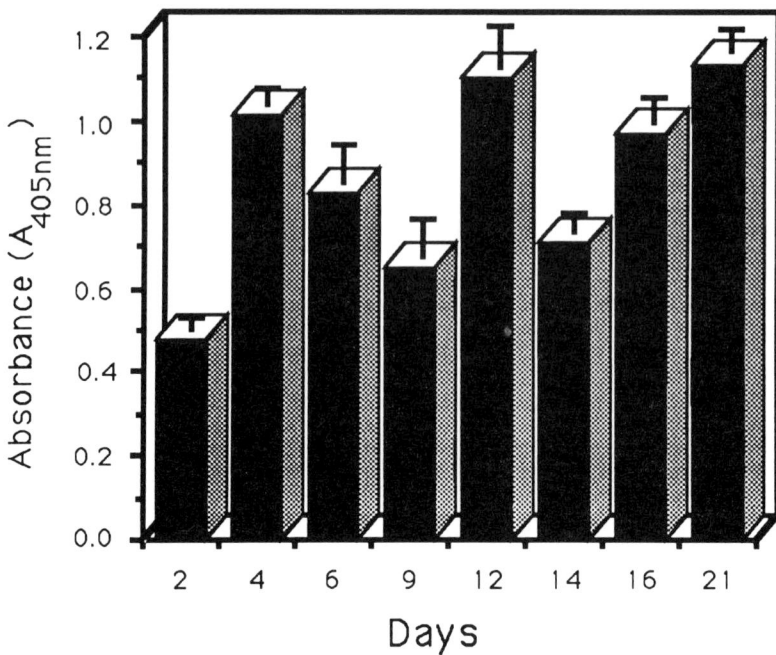

Fig. 5.9 Results of indirect ELISA of spherule culture filtrates (2–21 days) with guinea pig anti-120 kDa serum.

separate culture supernatants. Sequential rise and fall of antigen levels occurred and the absorbance maxima corresponded approximately to the time of release of endospores from the first, second, and third generations of spherules produced in vitro. The parasitic phase of strain 634 used in these studies remained fairly well synchronized in culture for the three week period of the experiments but grew rather slowly after production of the first generation of spherules. We suggest that the maxima of antigen level in Figure 5.9 actually correspond to release of the 120 kDa glycoprotein from ruptured spherules which, in turn, reflects an accumulation of active enzyme associated with the segmentation wall of maturing spherules.

To test whether this explanation of the results presented in Fig. 5.9 is plausible, we used two experimental approaches. We first determined whether the active β-glucosidase could be isolated from the wall of intact, segmented spherules by extraction with octyl-β-D-thioglucoside (OTG; Sigma) using the procedure described by Yuan et al (1988). In brief, approximately 10^0 spherules of strain 634 (72 h culture) were first washed in phosphate-buffered saline (PBS; pH 7.6), pelleted, and then resuspended in 1% OTG in PBS for 20 min at 4°C with gentle agitation. The cell suspension was centrifuged and the supernatant was dialysed against distilled water and lyophilized. The pellet was examined for cell viability and shown to be comparable to that of spherules which were suspended in PBS alone (approx. 85%). The lyophil was subjected to Con A fractionation using the same procedure described above for isolation of the β-glucosidase from the mycelial (F + L) fraction. Kinetic analysis of the Con A bound fraction was compared to that of the affinity-purified 120 kDa β-glucosidase described above. The Michaelis–Menton constants

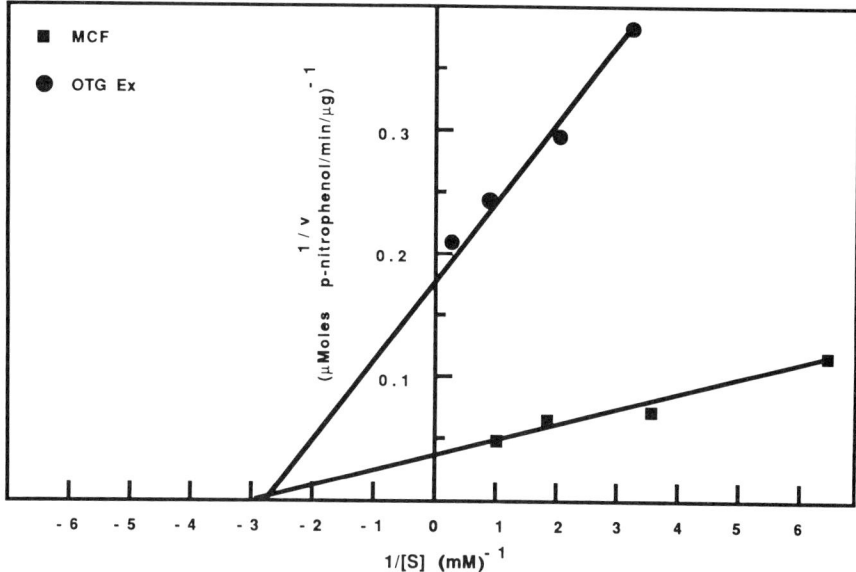

Fig. 5.10 Double-reciprocal plots of kinetic data for purified 120 kDa β-glucosidase from mycelial culture filtrate (MCF) (■) and glucosidase isolated from endosporulating spherules by octyl-β-D-thioglucopyranoside (OTG) detergent extraction and ConA affinity isolation (●). pNP-β-D-glucose was used as substrate.

(K_m) for the two preparations were determined by incubation of each fraction with the same range of concentrations of substrate ([S]), p-nitrophenol-β-D-glucose, in enzyme buffer (20mM Tris [pH 8.0] plus 0.6 mM $CaCl_2$) at 37°C. The K_m values determined from double reciprocal plots of $1/v$ against $1/[S]$ for the purified enzyme and OTG extracted fraction were 0.33 mM and 0.43 mM, respectively (Fig. 5.10). We conclude that the β-glucosidase extracted from the wall of segmented spherules with OTG is the same as the purified 120 kDa β-glucosidase. The immunolabelled 120 kDa antigen in the envelope and segmentation wall of mature spherules revealed in Fig. 5.7D at least in part represents active β-glucosidase.

A second indirect method was used to determine whether substrate for the β-glucosidase could be localized within the spherule wall. Thin sections of glutaraldehyde-fixed, low temperature resin-embedded cells were reacted with purified β-glucosidase conjugated to 15 nm gold particles according to established methods (Bendayan 1985, Bendayan & Benhamou 1987). The active enzyme–gold conjugate will bind to a specific substrate if present in the cell when the conjugate is incubated with sections of the sample at 37°C for 30 min. After reaction with the conjugate, sections were exposed to vapours of osmium tetroxide to enhance contrast and then examined by transmission electron microscopy. Label was detected in the segmentation wall and inner layer of the spherule envelope (Fig. 5.7E). Control preparations included reaction of gold particles with the enzyme followed by incubation of the conjugate with 20 mM glucose to block the reactive sites of β-glucosidase prior to its reaction with thin sections (Fig. 5.7F). Alternatively, bovine serum albumin (BSA) was adsorbed onto gold particles to test for non-specific binding of conjugate to sections. No gold label was observed after sections of mature spherules were reacted with either of these control conjugates.

Conclusions

Evidence has been presented that the TP antibody-reactive, 120 kDa glycoprotein described in earlier reports (Kruse & Cole 1990, Cole et al 1990a, 1991a) is a β-1,3-glucanase and localizes in the spherule wall. Indirect evidence that β-glucans are present in the spherule wall and probably contribute to its structural integrity have been presented here and by earlier investigators (Hector & Pappagianis 1982). Incorporation of the 120 kDa macromolecules (active enzyme?) into the wall of young spherules, presumably by fusion of secretory vesicles with the plasmalemma, appears to occur at the developmental stage when maximum plasticity would be expected to exist in the spherule envelope. The β-glucosidase, together with chitinase and other cell wall hydrolases, may be responsible for this plasticity and, thereby, play a critical role in morphogenesis of the parasitic cell types of *C. immitis*. Current research is focused on determination of the amino acid sequence of the β-glucosidase. Antibody has been raised against the deglycosylated 120 kDa fraction (Cole et al 1991a) and will be used, together with an oligonucleotide probe derived from the amino acid sequence of the enzyme, to isolate the β-glucosidase gene from a cDNA expression library of *C. immitis* constructed in lambda Zap II (Stratagene; Cole et al 1991b,c). Ultimately, we hope to use methods of recombinant DNA technology to establish the function of the enzyme in spherule morphogenesis and, thereby, critically evaluate the gene product as a potential molecular target for novel antifungal agents.

A wall-associated proteinase

We have described the isolation of a chymotrypsin-like serine proteinase from a water-soluble, conidial wall fraction (SCWF) of *C. immitis*. The enzyme was originally identified in SDS-PAGE gels as a 36 kDa polypeptide (Yuan & Cole 1987, Yuan et al 1988, Cole et al 1989, Cole & Kirkland 1991). In a recent paper we reported that the more accurate molecular size of the proteinase in SDS-PAGE reducing gels is 34 kDa (Cole et al 1991c). The molecular sizes of the active proteinase estimated by SDS-PAGE under nonreducing conditions and by gel filtration are 62 kDa and 60 kDa, respectively (Cole et al 1989). Immuno-localization of the proteinase in spherules produced in vitro (Yuan et al 1988) and in vivo (Fig. 5.11A–C) using rabbit antibody raised against the purified 34 kDa fraction (Yuan et al 1988) revealed that the antigen is concentrated in the seg-mentation wall apparatus (SA). Immunolabel is associated with the SA from its initial stage of development (Fig. 5.11C) through progressive stages of maturation of the endogenous wall complex (Fig. 5.11D, E). A consistent observation in these immunoelectron-microscopic studies was the difference in distribution of immunolabel in the young and mature segmentation wall, exemplified by Figure 5.11D and E, respectively. The gold label on the immature SA is arranged in a 'railroad track' pattern, with concentrated immunolabel adjacent to the plas-malemma which encompasses the cytoplasmic compartments. The more mature spherules (Fig. 5.11E), on the other hand, show random distribution of label on

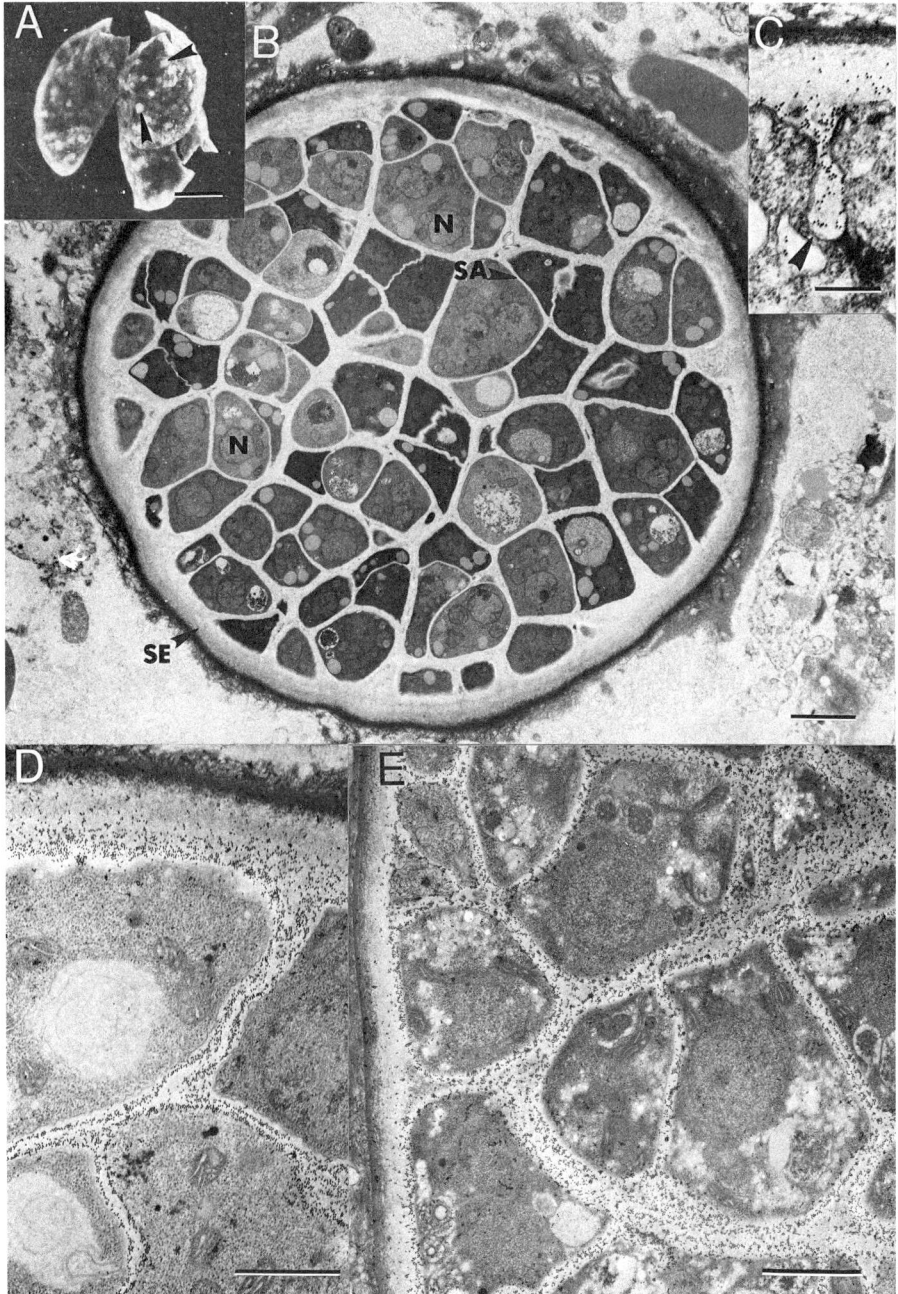

Fig. 5.11 Thin sections of segmented spherules from abscesses in infected murine lung tissue (A). Sections were reacted with rabbit anti-34 kDa antibody-gold conjugate (C–E). The control section in (B) was reacted with the secondary antibody-conjugate alone. Progressively later stages of segmentation wall development are shown in (C), (D), and (E) which reveal differences in distribution of immunolabel. Arrowheads in (A) locate abscesses. Arrowhead in (C) locates invaginated plasmalemma and segmentation wall initial. N, nucleus; SA, segmentation wall apparatus. Bars represent (A) 7.0 mm, (B) 2.0 μm, (C) 0.5 μm, (D) 1.0 μm, and (E) 1.0 μm.

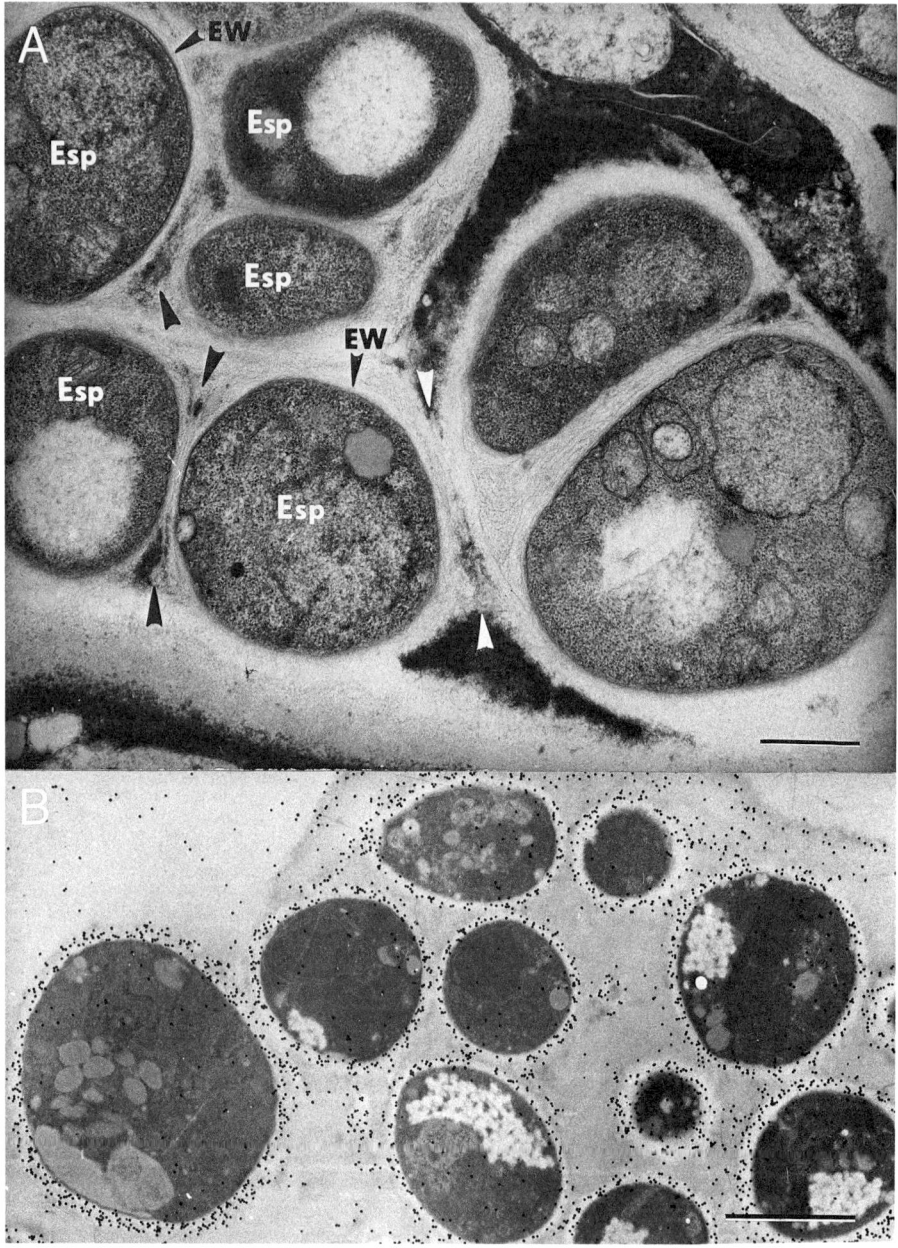

Fig. 5.12 Thin sections of mature spherules which show endospore wall differentiation (A), and presence of dense anti-34 kDa immunolabel associated with the newly-formed endospore wall (B). Remnants of the segmentation wall and spherule envelope are also immunolabelled in (B). Arrowheads in (A), region of separation between apposing endospore wall layers; Esp, endospore; EW, endospore wall. Bars in A, B represent 1.0 μm and 2.0 μm, respectively.

their segmentation wall and relatively high concentration of immunolabel on the inner layer of spherule envelope. As endospores differentiate, the segmentation wall begins to break down (autolysis?) which permits the apposing endospore walls to separate (arrowheads in Fig. 5.12A). It is tempting to speculate that the SA-associated proteinase may play a role in the autolysis of the segmentation wall and eventual release of endospores from the maternal spherule (Yuan et al 1988, Cole & Kirkland 1991). However, our current data appear to contradict this suggested role of the 34 kDa proteinase in spherule maturation.

Immunolabelled sections of endosporulating spherules indicate that the 34 kDa protein is concentrated in the young endospore wall and associated with remnants of the SA (Fig. 5.12B). When the spherule envelope finally ruptures and the contents of the maternal cell are released into the culture media, no significant increase in concentration of the 34 kDa protein was detected (Yuan et al 1988). In contrast to our report of release of the 120 kDa β-glucosidase from endosporulating spherules, results of ELISA studies of the spherule culture supernatant using monospecific anti-34kDa serum have revealed that little secretion of the protein occurred during an 18 day period of spherule growth. The antiserum may no longer recognize the antigen because it is digested by other enzymes released during the endosporulation process, and/or the protein remains bound to wall fragments. Both explanations are possible, but it is clear that the proteinase demonstrates an unusually high affinity for the wall of developing parasitic cells of *C. immitis*. We therefore set out to determine whether the active enzyme could be extracted from the walls of endosporulating spherules and if substrate for the 34 kDa proteinase was present in the isolated wall fraction of the mature cells. The active proteinase was successfully extracted by exposure of the cells to 1% OTG (Yuan et al 1988). The K_m values of the purified enzyme and endosporulating spherule wall-extracted proteinase were 0.143 mM and 0.125mM, respectively, using benzoyl tyrosine ethyl ester (BTEE) as substrate. We concluded that the purified and extracted proteinases were homologous. Different wall fractions of the parasitic and saprobic phases of *C. immitis* were tested as substrates in the presence of the purified 34 kDa protein-ase. The total wall fraction of endosporulating spherules was isolated and treated with phenylmethylsulfonyl fluoride (PMSF), an irreversible serine proteinase inhibitor used to inactivate endogenous proteinases. Preparations of mycelial and presegmented spherule walls were similarly treated and used as substrates for the purified proteinase. Only the endosporulating spherule wall was significantly digested (Yuan et al 1988).

Together, these features of the 34 kDa proteinase suggest that the enzyme participates in wall morphogenesis during the parasitic cycle of *C. immitis*, but its precise function is unknown. Results of immunolabelling experiments have indi-cated that the protein is incorporated into the spherule envelope and then the SA as invagination of the wall is initiated, which suggests that synthesis of the proteinase is maintained throughout the period of diametric growth and segmentation wall formation, respectively. The appearance of concentrated anti-34 kDa immunolabel in the newly formed endospore wall suggests a burst of synthesis of the proteinase at the endosporulation stage. To examine this relationship further, we set out to clone the 34 kDa proteinase gene and determine its temporal expression during the parasitic cell cycle. The anti 34 kDa antibody was used to isolate two cDNA

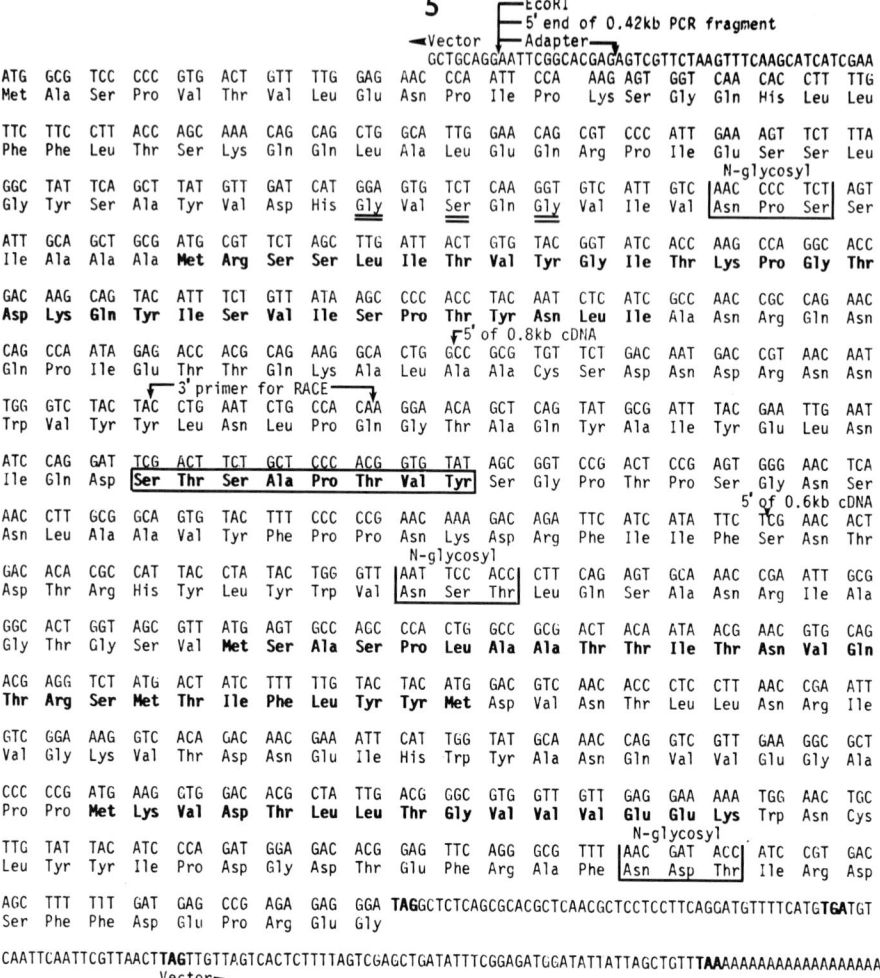

Fig. 5.13 Nucleotide and deduced amino acid sequences of 1.2 kb cDNA clone isolated from expression library by anti-34 kDa screen. Amino acid sequences containing potential sites of N-glycosyl linkages are indicated by brackets. Amino acid sequences which correspond to determined sequences of CNBr cleavage products (cf Table 5.2) are in bold type. Amino acid sequences showing partial homology with other serine hydrolases and chymotrypsin/chymotrypsinogens (cf Table 5.3) are double-underlined and indicated by bold letters with a box, respectively.

clones from the expression library of *C. immitis* (Cole et al 1991b,c). The cDNA inserts were subcloned into pBluescript SK (+/−) plasmid and shown to consist of 800 base pairs (bp) and 600 bp by agarose gel electrophoresis. The nucleotide sequences of these two subcloned cDNA fragments are shown in Fig. 5.13. The protocol of rapid amplification of cDNA ends (RACE) was employed to generate a full-length cDNA copy of the mRNA transcript of the proteinase gene (Frohman 1990). The nucleotide sequencing scheme for the cDNA clones is summarized in Fig. 5.14. The 420 bp and 800 bp fragments were ligated to each other at the

86

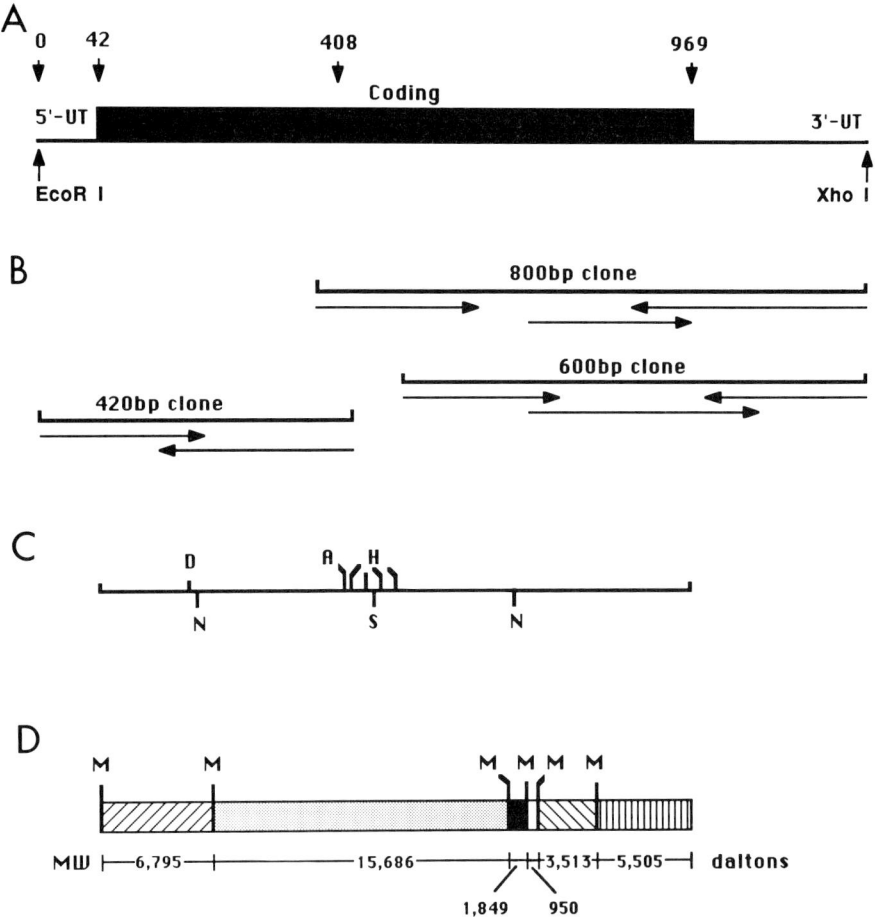

Fig. 5.14 (A) cDNA clone of 34 kDa protein showing EcoR I and Xho I restriction sites and untranslated (UT) 5' and 3' regions, respectively. (B) Sequencing strategy for cDNA clone. The arrows indicate direction and extent of sequence determination. (C) Restriction enzyme map of 1.2 kb cDNA insert (A, Acc I; D, Dpn I; H, Hinf I; N, Nla III; S, Sec I). (D) Calculated molecular weights of potential CNBr cleavage products (*Met* cleavage sites) determined from deduced amino acid sequence.

Acc I restriction site (Fig. 5.14) and subcloned into KS plasmid. The 1.2 kb cDNA clone was subsequently used as a probe in Northern hybridizations for analysis of gene expression during spherule development.

An open reading frame (ORF) of 927 nucleotide bases was obtained by sequence gel analysis of the 420 bp, 600 bp and 800 bp cDNA fragments (Fig. 5.14). The 5'-flanking region of the ORF includes a short sequence (29 nucleotides) and vector. The 3'-flanking region contains a transcription termination signal which is comparable to that reported for yeast (Yoshihisa & Anraku 1989) and identified as 5'-TAG ... TAGT ... TTT-3'. The ORF can encode a 309 amino acid polypeptide. The calculated molecular weight and isoelectric point are 34.3 and 5.1, respectively. Attempts to sequence the 34 kDa proteinase failed because of an N-terminal amino

Table 5.2 Amino acid sequences of isolated CNBr cleavage fractions of the 34 kDa proteinase

Method used for isolation of CNBr fractions	Amino acid sequence
A. Membrane immobilization and excision[a]	Met-Arg-Ser-Ser-Leu-Ile-Thr-Val-Tyr-Gly-Ile-Thr-Lys-Pro-Gly-Thr-Asp-Lys-Gln-Tyr-Ile-Ser-Val-Ile-Ser-Pro-Thr-Tyr-Asn-Leu-Ile
B. OPA-blockage[a]	Met—[**Ser-Ala-Ser**][b]-Pro-Leu-Ala-Ala-Thr-Thr-Ile-Thr-Asn-Val-Gln-Thr-Arg-Ser-Met-Thr-Ile-Phe-Leu-Tyr-Tyr-Met
C. RP-HPLC[a]	Met-Lys-**Val**-Asp-Thr-**Leu** **Leu**-Thr-Gly-**Val**-**Val**-**Val**-Glu-Glu-Lys[c]

[a] CNBr digested peptides isolated by (A) electrotransfer to Immobilon membrane (Moos et al 1988), (B) by sequence analysis in the presence of *o*-phthalaldehyde (OPA; Brauer et al 1984), and (C) by reverse phase-high pressure liquid chromatography (RP-HPLC) using a Beckman Ultrasphere-ODS C_{18} column (10 mm × 25 cm).

[b] Sequence of amino acid residues (bold type) within square brackets deduced from mixed sequence signals of unfractionated CNBr cleavage products prior to addition of OPA to reaction mixture.

[c] High percentage of hydrophobic amino acids (43%; residues indicated by bold type) contributed to affinity of CNBr fragment for C_{18} reverse phase column.

blockage. Cyanogen bromide (CNBr) cleavage of the purified 34 kDa protein yielded multiple peptide fragments (Fig. 5.15). Three fragments were isolated by different methods and subjected to sequence analysis (Table 5.2). Three regions of the deduced sequence demonstrate homology with the amino acid sequences of CNBr-generated fragments of the purified proteinase (c.f. Table 5.2 and Fig. 5.13). A correlation was demonstrated between the molecular size of the peptide fragments separated by SDS-PAGE in Fig. 5.15 and the calculated molecular size of CNBr fragments (Fig. 5.14D) based on the deduced amino acid sequence. The SDS-PAGE estimates of molecular size are slightly higher, which is probably due to glycosylation of the native proteinase. The carbohydrate content of the proteinase is estimated to be less than 10% and analysis of neutral sugar components by GC-MS revealed the presence of xylose, mannose, galactose, and glucose in a ratio of 11.6:22.1:1.4:64.9, respectively (Cole et al 1991c). Three potential N-glycosylation sites are demonstrated in the ORF (Fig. 5.13), but the occurrence of O-glycosyl linkages have not yet been ruled out. The Gly-Val-Ser-Gln-Gly sequence (residues 49–53; Fig. 5.13) shows partial homology with the conserved sequence (Gly-X-Ser-X-Gly) of all serine hydrolases (Köller 1991). Comparison between the deduced amino acid sequence of the *C. immitis* proteinase and previously recorded sequences

Table 5.3 Partial homology between deduced amino acid sequence of *C. immitis* proteinase and reported sequences of chymotrypsin and chymotrypsinogen

Enzyme	Source	Sequence		Reference
		144	151	
Chymotrypsin-like serine proteinase	*C. immitis*	**Ser-Thr-Ser**-Ala-**Pro**-Thr-**Val-Tyr**		Fig. 5.13
α-Chymotrypsin	Human	**Ser-Thr-Ser**-Thr-**Pro**-Gly-**Val-Tyr**		White et al 1978
Chymotrypsinogen 2	Dog	**Ser-Thr-Ser**-Thr-**Pro**-Gly-**Val-Tyr**		Pinsky et al 1983
Chymotrypsinogen A	Bovine	**Ser-Thr-Ser**-Thr-**Pro**-Gly-**Val**-Tyr-		Blow et al 1969
Chymotrypsinogen B	Bovine	**Ser-Thr-Ser**-Thr-**Pro**-Ala-**Val**-Tyr		Smillie et al 1968
Chymotrypsinogen B	Rat	**Ser-Thr-Ser**-Thr-**Pro**-Ala-**Val**-Tyr		Bell et al 1984

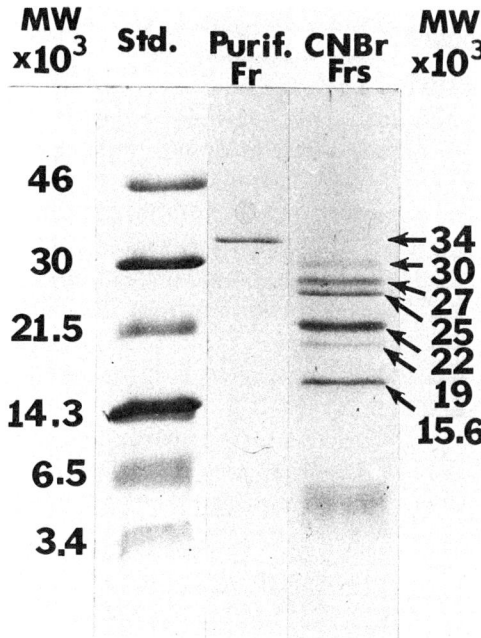

Fig. 5.15 SDS-PAGE separation of purified 34 kDa proteinase and cleavage products of cyanogen bromide (CNBr)-treated sample. Approximate molecular size of peptides are indicated.

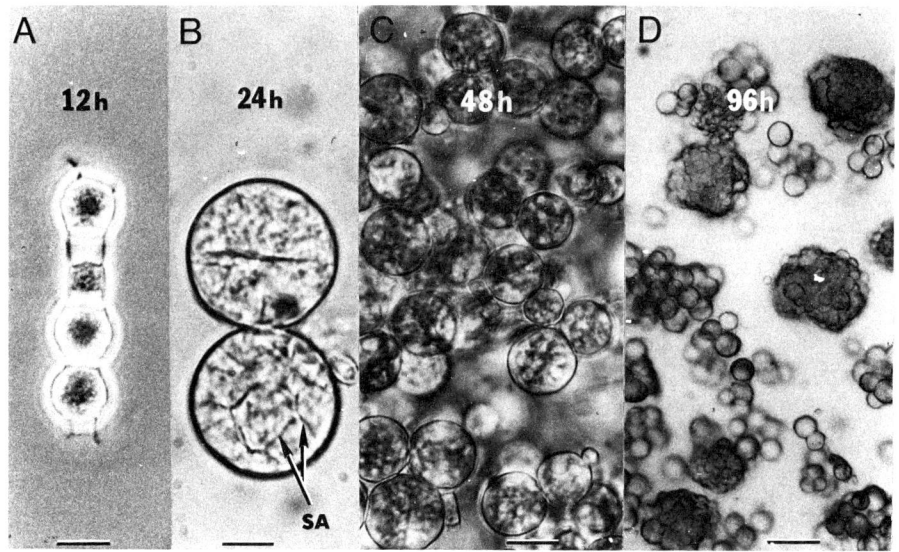

Fig. 5.16 Light micrographs of samples of cell suspensions from liquid cultures of *C. immitis* (Converse media; Cole & Sun 1985) inoculated with 30-day-old arthroconidia after 12 h(A), 24 h(B), 48 h(C), and 96 h(D) incubation. SA, wall of segmentation apparatus. Bars represent (A) 3.0 μm, (B) 10 μm, (C) 40 μm, and (D) 10 μm.

of α-chymotrypsin and chymotrypsinogens have revealed a conserved region of 75% homology (Table 5.3). It is significant that two amino acid residues in the same position in each partial sequence account for the variation observed between the *C. immitis* proteinase and reported chymotrypsins.

Converse media inoculated with arthroconidia of strain 735 produced spherule cultures which showed fairly well-synchronized development, at least through the endosporulation stage of the first generation of the parasitic cycle (Fig. 5.16). The five different time periods of spherule growth in vitro identified in Figure 5.17 represent stages of 'round cell' formation from arthroconidia and segmentation wall formation in the first generation (24 h), endospore differentiation (and endospore wall formation) in the first generation (48 h) and second generation spherules (168 h), the release of endospores from the first generation spherules (96 h) and initiation of diametric growth of second generation spherules (120 h). Cells isolated from cultures at these different time periods post-inoculation with arthroconidia were used as sources of poly (A$^+$)-containing RNA. The latter was used in Northern dot blots (White & Bancroft 1982) to estimate temporal expression of the *C. immitis* 34 kDa proteinase gene during development of the parasitic cells (Fig. 5.17). The

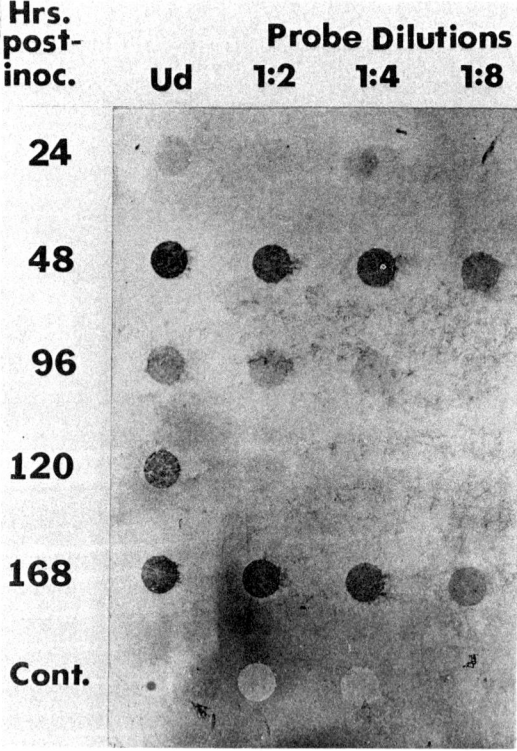

Fig. 5.17 Northern 'dot blot' hybridization of poly(A$^+$)-containing RNA isolated from spherule cultures at 24 h, 48 h, 96 h, 120 h, and 168 h (cf Fig. 5.16) with 1.2 kb cDNA probe labelled with biotin-21-dUTP by the mixed primer labelling method (Cole et al 1991c). The probe was used undiluted (Ud) or diluted 1:2 to 1:8 with reaction buffer. The negative control (cont.) was a total RNA preparation from Alaska pea (gift from S. Roux, Dept. of Botany, Univ. of Texas at Austin).

48 h spherules in Figure 5.16 showed the approximate initiation of endospore wall differentiation. This same stage was repeated in the second generation spherules at 168 h. The maximum level of hybridization between the labelled 1.2 kb gene probe and specific mRNA was detected at this early stage of endospore wall formation in both first and second generation spherules (Fig. 5.17). Lower levels of mRNA were detected at 24 h, 96 h, and 120 h. Results of hybridization of cDNA to the control RNA were negative (Fig. 5.17).

Conclusions

We have presented evidence that the 34 kDa proteinase shows affinity for the inner layer of the spherule envelope, the segmentation wall apparatus, and the endospore wall (Yuan et al 1988). High concentrations of the protein as detected by immuno-label experiments with *C. immitis* appear to correlate with stages of segmentation wall formation and endospore wall differentiation. Hector & Pappagianis (1982) have suggested that the segmentation wall contains a mannan-protein complex which is synthesized 'prior to the fracturing of the cleavage planes into endospore walls.' The protein component of this complex may represent the 34 kDa protein identified in the SA by our immunolabelling experiments. Evidence that active synthesis of the proteinase occurs at the time of incipient endospore differentiation, which correlates with its apparent accumulation in the endospore wall, is derived from recombinant DNA studies. Evidence has been presented here that we have isolated a cDNA clone from an expression library of *C. immitis* which encodes the 34 kDa proteinase. Dot blot analysis of poly(A^+)-containing RNA isolated from spherules in various stages of synchronized development in vitro has revealed that the highest detected level of specific mRNA corresponds with the initial stage of endospore wall formation. In support of this observation, the active 34 kDa proteinase was extracted from viable endosporulating spherules, the developmental stage when dense immunolabel was shown to be present in the newly-formed endospore walls (Yuan et al 1988).

Results of our studies of the 34 kDa proteinase at present suggest that the enzyme participates in wall intussusception during early stages of diametric growth of endospores and subsequent morphogenesis of the segmentation wall apparatus. A possible role of the proteinase in this process may be the activation of a wall synthetase at the surface of the plasmalemma. If one were to speculate further along this line of reasoning, the presence of an inhibitor which regulates the activity of the proteinase would be expected to exist. A peptide (approx. 5 kDa) has been isolated from the segmented spherule wall and shown to inhibit activity of the purified 34 kDa proteinase (Yuan & Cole 1989). The hydrophobic peptide is heat-stable and tolerant to a broad pH range. The inhibitor and proteinase react in a 1:1 stoichiometry and the dissociation constant (K_i) of the enzyme-inhibitor complex is 2.3×10^{-8} M. Results of kinetic studies of the proteinase-inhibitor reaction indicate that enzyme inactivation occurs by competitive inhibition. Antiserum raised in rabbits against the inhibitor was used to localize the peptide in spherules by immunoelectron microscopy. The inhibitor and proteinase were shown to be colocalized in the spherule envelope, segmentation wall apparatus, and endospore wall (Cole & Kirkland 1991). Attempts are underway to sequence and then synthesize the inhibitor peptide. If we are successful, the peptide can be tested in vitro for its ability to block activity of the proteinase during early stages of spherule growth and endosporulation.

Ultimately, we hope to develop a transformation system for *C. immitis* which, combined with construction of 34 kDa proteinase mutations by gene disruption, will allow us rigorously to assess the role of the enzyme in morphogenesis of *C. immitis*. As in the case of the β-glucosidase, results of these investigations will also permit critical evaluation of the wall-associated proteinase as a potential molecular target for novel antifungal drugs.

SUMMARY

Fungal cell wall morphogenesis is dictated largely by events of wall biosynthesis (e.g. chitin synthetase and β-1,3-glucan synthetase activities) and modification of pre-existing wall polymers by wall-associated hydrolases (e.g. chitinase and β-1,3-glucanase activities). Antifungal agents designed to target wall synthetases have been only marginally successful. One problem which may be a limiting factor in the practical use of inhibitors of wall synthetases is the difficulty of such molecules to reach their molecular targets located in the plasmalemma and cytoplasm of thick-walled fungal cells. Alternative and perhaps more accessible molecular targets proposed for still undeveloped antifungal agents are the wall-associated hydrolases, or autolysins, the function of which are also pivotal for morphogenesis of the fungal pathogen. *Coccidioides immitis* serves as a suitable model for examination of the impact of wall-associated autolysins on fungal cell development. We have focused on two wall hydrolases. The first is a glucosidase which is suggested to function as a β-1,3-glucanase in the wall of spherules during their rapid diametric growth phase and may be essential for wall plasticity. The second is a chymotrypsin-like serine proteinase which localizes in the envelope if young spherules (endo-spores) at the developmental stage when the cells undergo rapid diametric growth, in the segmentation wall from its incipient stage of morphogenesis, and is con-centrated in the wall of endospore initials contained by mature spherules. The proteinase is suggested to participate in some aspect of wall growth during early spherule development and endospore differentiation. Its precise function in the cell wall remains unknown. In both cases, inhibition of the autolysins may block morphogenesis of the parasitic cells of *C. immitis*. Evidence has been presented which supports the proposed functions of these wall-associated enzymes in spherule growth and endosporulation. The proteinase gene has been cloned which will permit future gene disruption experiments and transformation studies to assess the role of this enzyme in endospore differentiation.

Our goal in this chapter was to pursue the question of whether critical molecular functions associated with wall morphogenesis can be identified in the fungal patho-gen other than wall synthetase activities, which have been targeted with only moderate success by currently available antifungal drugs. We hope that we have at least been successful in providing the framework for discussion and exper-imentation in this quest to identify potential molecular targets for future develop-ment of novel antifungal agents.

ACKNOWLEDGEMENTS

This investigation was supported by Public Health Service grant AI19149 from the National Institute of Allergy and Infectious Diseases.

REFERENCES

Bartnicki-Garcia S 1973 Fundamental aspects of hyphal morphogenesis. In: Ashworth J M, Smith J E (eds) Microbial differentiation: Twenty-third symposium of the Society for General Microbiology. Cambridge University Press, London, pp 245–267

Bartnicki-Garcia S 1989 The biochemical cytology of chitin and chitosan synthesis in fungi. In: Skjak-Braek G, Thorleif A, Sanford P (eds) Chitin and chitosan. Sources, chemistry, biochemistry, physical properties and applications. Elsevier Publishing, New York, pp 23–35

Bell G I, Quinto C, Quiroga M, Valenzuela P, Craik C S, Rutter W J 1984 Isolation and sequence of a rat chymotrypsin B gene. Journal of Biological Chemistry 295: 14265–14270

Bendayan M 1985 The enzyme-gold technique: a new cytochemical approach for the ultrastructural localization of macromolecules. In: Bullock G R, Petrusz P (eds) Techniques in immunocytochemistry, vol 3. Academic Press, New York, pp 179–201

Bendayan M, Benhamou N 1987 Ultrastructural localization of glucoside residues on tissue sections by applying the enzyme-gold approach. Journal of Histochemistry and Cytochemistry 35: 1149–1155

Blow B M, Birktoft J J, Hartley B S 1969 Role of a buried acid group in the mechanism of action of chymotrypsin. Nature (London) 221: 337–341

Brauer A W, Oman C L, Margolies M N 1984 Use of o-phthalaldehyde to reduce background during automated Edman degradation. Analytical Biochemistry 137: 134–142

Brillinger G U 1979 Metabolic products of microorganisms. 181. Chitin synthase from fungi, a test model for substances with insecticidal properties. Archiv für Mikrobiologie 121: 71–74

Cole G T, Pope L M, Huppert M, Sun S H, Starr P 1983 Ultrastructure and composition of conidial wall fractions of Coccidioides immitis. Experimental Mycology 7: 297–318

Cole G T, Sun S H 1985 Arthroconidium-spherule-endospore transformation in Coccidioides immitis. In: Szaniszlo P J (ed) Fungal dimorphism, with emphasis on fungi pathogenic for humans. Plenum Press, New York, pp 281–333

Cole G T 1986 Models of cell differentiation in conidial fungi. Microbiological Reviews 50: 95–132

Cole G T, Kirkland T N 1991 Conidia of Coccidioides immitis: their significance in disease initiation. In: Cole G T, Hoch H C (eds) The fungal spore and disease initiation in plants and animals. Plenum Press, New York, pp 403–443

Cole G T, Seshan K R, Franco M, Bukownik E, Sun S H, Hearn V M 1988a Isolation and morphology of an immunoreactive outer wall fraction produced by spherules of Coccidioides immitis, Infection and Immunity 56:2685–2694

Cole G T, Kirkland J N, Franco M, Zhu S, Yuan L, Sun S M, Hearn V M 1988b Immunoreactivity of a surface wall fraction produced by spherules of Coccidioides immitis. Infection and immunity 56: 2695–2701

Cole G T, Zhu S, Pan S, Yuan L, Kruse D, Sun SH 1989 Isolation of antigens with proteolytic activity from Coccidioides immitis. Infection and Immunity 57: 1524–1534

Cole G T, Kruse D, Zhu S, Seshan K R, Wheat R W 1990a Composition, serologic reactivity, and immunolocalization of a 120-kilodalton tube precipitin antigen of Coccidioides immitis. Infection and Immunity 58: 179–188

Cole G T, Lynn K T, Seshan K R 1990b Evaluation of a murine model of hepatic candidiasis. Journal of Clinical Microbiology 28: 1828–1841

Cole G T, Kruse D, Seshan K R 1991a Antigen complex of Coccidioides immitis which elicits a precipitin antibody response in patients. Infection and Immunity 59: 2434–2446

Cole G T, Pan S, Zhu S, Seshan K R 1991b Cell wall-associated proteinases of Coccidioides immitis. In: Latgé J P, Boucias D G (eds) The fungal cell wall and immune response. Springer-Verlag, Heidelberg, pp 269–284

Cole G T, Zhu S, Hsu L, Kruse D, Seshan K R, Wang F 1991c Isolation and expression of a gene which encodes a wall-associated proteinase of Coccidioides immitis. Infection and Immunity 59 (in press)

Cooper C R, Harris J L, Jacobs C W, Szaniszlo P J 1984 Effects of polyoxin AL on cellular development in Wangiella dermatitidis. Experimental Mycology 8: 349–363

Dahn U, Hagenmaier H, Hohne H, Konig W A, Wolf G, Zahner H 1976 Nikkomycin, ein nuer Hemmstoff der Chitin synthese bei Pilzen. Archive für Mikrobiologie 107: 143–160

Drouhet E, Dupont B, Improvisi L, Lesourd M, Prevost M C 1990 Activity of cilofungin (LY121019), a new lipopeptide antibiotic, on the cell wall and cytoplasmic membrane of *Candida albicans*. Structural modifications in scanning and transmission electron microscopy. Journal of Medical and Veterinary Mycology 28: 425–436

Frohman M A 1990 RACE: rapid amplification of cDNA ends. In: Innis M A, Gelfand D H, Sninsky J J, White T J (eds) PCR protocols. A guide to methods and applications. Academic Press, New York, pp 28–38

Gooday G W 1983 The hyphal tip. In: Smith J E (ed) Fungal differentiation. A contemporary synthesis. Marcel Dekker, New York, pp 315–356

Gow N A R 1989 Control of extension of the hyphal apex. In: McGinnis M R, Borgers M (eds) Current topics in medical mycology, vol. 3. Springer-Verlag, New York, pp 109–152

Hector R F, Pappagianis D 1982 Enzymatic degradation of the wall of spherules of *Coccidioides immitis*. Experimental Mycology 6: 136–152

Hector R F, Pappagianis D 1983 Inhibition of chitin synthesis in the cell walls of *Coccidioides immitis* by polyoxin D. Journal of Bacteriology 154: 488–498

Hector R F, Zimmer B L, Pappagianis D 1990 Evaluation of nikkomycins X and Z in murine models of coccidioidomycosis, histoplasmosis, and blastomycosis. Antimicrobial Agents and Chemotherapy 34: 587–593

Hobbs M, Perfect J, Durack D 1988 Evaluation of in vitro antifungal activity of LY121019. European Journal of Clinical Microbiology and Infectious Diseases 7: 77–80

Hoch H C, Hanssler G, Reisener H J 1979 Cytochemical localization of N-acetyl-β-D-glucosaminidase in hyphae of *Mucor racemosus*. Experimental Mycology 3: 164–173

Köller W 1991 The plant cuticle: a barrier to be overcome by fungal plant pathogens. In: Cole G T, Hoch H C (eds) The fungal spore and disease initiation in plants and animals. Plenum Press, New York, pp 219–246

Kritzman G, Chet I, Henis Y 1978 Localization of β-(1,3)-glucanase in the mycelium of *Sclerotium rolfsii*. Journal of Bacteriology 134: 470–475

Kruse D, Cole G T 1990 Isolation of tube precipitin antibody-reactive fractions of *Coccidioides immitis*. Infection and Immunity 58: 169–178

Kruse D, Cole G T 1991 A β-glucosidase of *Coccidioides immitis* which demonstrates tube precipitin antibody reactivity. Abstract, 91st General Meeting of American Society for Microbiology, ASM Publication, Washington, D.C., F62, p 418

Leathem A J C, Atkins N J 1983 Lectin binding to paraffin sections. In: Bullock G R, Petrusz P (eds) Techniques in immunochemistry, vol 1. Academic Press, New York, pp 39–69

Moos M, Nguyen N Y, Liu T-Y 1988 Reproducible high yield sequencing of proteins electrophoretically separated and transferred to an inert support. Journal of Biological Chemistry 263: 6005–6008

Nicholas R O, Hunter P A 1991 Study of fungal cell walls using fluorochromes. Abstract, XI Congress of the International Society of Human and Animal Mycology, Montreal, Canada, psi. 28, p 69

Padula A, Chambers H F 1989 Evaluation of cilofungin (LY121019) for treatment of experimental *Candida albicans* endocarditis in rabbits. Antimicrobial Agents and Chemotherapy 33: 1822–1823

Pappagianis D 1988 Epidemiology of coccidioidomycosis. In: McGinnis M R (ed) Current topics in medical mycology, vol 2. Springer-Verlag, New York, pp 199–238

Pinsky S D, LaForge K S, Luc V, Scheele G 1983 Identification of cDNA clones encoding secretory isoenzyme forms: sequence determination of canine pancreatic prechymotrypsinogen 2 mRNA. Proceedings of the National Academy of Sciences (USA) 80: 7486–7490

Pringle J R 1991 Staining of bud scars and other cell wall chitin with calcofluor. Methods in Enzymology 194: 732–735

Smillie L B, Furka A, Nagabhushan N, Stevenson K J, Parkes C O 1968 Structure of chymotrypsinogen B compared with chymotrypsinogen A and trypsinogen. Nature (London) 218: 343–346

Stein M W 1963 D-glucose, determination with hexokinase and glucose-6-phosphate dehydrogenase. In: Bergemeyer H U (ed) Methods in enzymatic analysis. Academic Press, New York, p 117

Sun S H, Cole G T, Drutz D J, Harrison J L 1986 Electron-microscopic observations of the *Coccidioides immitis* parasitic cycle in vitro. Journal of Medical and Veterinary Mycology 24: 183–192

Taft C S, Selitrennikoff C P 1988 LY121019 inhibits *Neurospora crassa* growth and (1–3)-β-glucan synthase. Journal of Antibiotics 41: 697–701

Wessels J G H 1986 Cell wall synthesis in apical hyphal growth. International Review of Cytology 104: 37–79

White A, Handler P, Smith E L, Hill R L, Lehman I R 1978 Principles of biochemistry. McGraw-Hill, New York, p 246

White B A, Bancroft F C 1982 Cytoplasmic dot hybridization. Simple analysis of relative mRNA levels in multiple small cell or tissue samples. Journal of Biological Chemistry 257: 8569–8572

Yoshihisa Y, Anraku Y 1989 Nucleotide sequence of *AMSI*, the structure gene of vascular α-mannosidase of *Saccharomyces cerevisiae*. Biochemical and Biophysical Research Communications 163: 908–915

Yuan L, Cole G T 1987 Isolation and characterization of an extracellular proteinase of *Coccidioides immitis*. Infection and Immunity 55: 1970–1978

Yuan L, Cole G T 1989 Characterization of a proteinase inhibitor isolated from the fungal pathogen *Coccidioides immitis*. Biochemical Journal 257 729–736

Yuan L, Cole G T, Sun S H 1988 Possible role of a proteinase in endosporulation of *Coccidioides immitis*. Infection and Immunity 56: 1551–1559

Discussion of paper presented by G. T. Cole

Discussed by D. A. Stevens
Reported by H. C. Neu

Dr Stevens focused his discussion on the ability of *Coccidioides immitis* to thwart host defenses in several ways by each of its morphological forms. He reviewed some studies with J. Galgiani on the effect of cilofungin. He reported that cilofungin is a β 1,3 glucan synthetase inhibitor, which inhibited the N-acetylglycosamine uptake in vitro in *C. immitis* but had no effect on developing spherules (the parasitic form of the organism) compared with a substantial effect on arthroconidia.

Stevens reviewed interactions between *Coccidioides* and the host. Spherulin, which is a lysate of spherules, was a more potent agent to detect delayed-type hypersensitivity in epidemiological studies in endemic areas than the mycelial filtrate which had been the classic test reagent. Both spherulin and mycelial filtrate are chemotactic, although at high concentrations spherulin has an inhibitory effect on leukocytes. Both of these substances are able to activate the classical and alternate pathways of complement so it has been difficult to explain the inhibition of chemotaxis at high concentrations of spherulin.

When *C. immitis* is forced to replicate in its parasitic phase in vitro it produces antigens which are referred to as endosporulation antigens. These antigens are 500-times more potent than spherulin in stimulating blastogenesis, and when the material is heated or dialysed, its potency is further increased. Conversely, concentrated material depresses lymphocyte blastogenesis. When endosporulation antigens are produced in avirulent isolates, the antigens stimulate blastogenesis of lymphocytes, but in a concentrated form are less inhibitory. Thus, during endosporulation, antigens are produced which in vitro can be stimulating or suppressive to host–cell response.

Stevens reported that in studies of patients with disseminated and progressive *C. immitis* infection, autologous serum from some patients contained immune complexes which depressed their lymphocyte transformation to the parasitic phase *Coccidioides* antigens, and this seemed to correlate with worse disease.

Polymorphonuclear neutrophils (PNMs) attach poorly to arthroconidia and do not kill them. Macrophages do not kill arthroconidia unless immune lymphocytes are present. There is failure of macrophage phagolysosomal fusion. Cationic peptides can kill arthroconidia and PNMs can inhibit N-acetylglucosamine incorporation into arthroconidia; this inhibition can be reproduced by hydrogen peroxide suggesting this as a mechanism. If the outer wall layer of arthroconidia is stripped away, phagocytosis of conidial particles is improved, but soluble components from the inner layers suppress superoxide production by macrophages and suppress T-cell proliferation.

Spherules present another problem to phagocytosis since as they increase in size the ability of PMNs to inhibit N-acetylglucosamine incorporation and killing is decreased. However, this is not just a phenomenon of size since as the spherules increase in size the inhibition of N-acetylglucosamine by hydrogen peroxide is less. Fibrillar material on the surface of spherules inhibits contact by leukocytes.

When spherules rupture, their endospores are released in a packet of material derived from the inner spherule wall which inhibits PMN contact. PMNs kill endospores poorly, and when macrophages encounter endospores there is failure of phagolysosomal fusion.

There are defenses against the endospores. Gamma interferon can transform PMNs into effective destroyers of endospores but not of arthroconidia. This later failure is not due to a failure of an oxidative burst and indicates that some other property of arthroconidia protect them from activated PMNs.

In reviewing Dr Cole's data on the effect of the inhibition of 1,3 β glucosidase, concern was expressed by participants that the cells of *Coccidioides* would still be viable. Bacilli that lack autolysins undergo profound morphological changes, but the cells are viable and can ultimately produce disease. Thus, it might be incorrect to view the β-glucosidase as a real target. It was agreed that it will be of value to screen other fungi for the glucosidase and to pursue the role of the enzyme by cloning and antibody studies.

6. Host defence in aspergillosis

A. Schaffner

INTRODUCTION

Aspergilli have emerged as important human pathogens over the last three decades, causing a progressive number of infections or contributing otherwise to various pathological conditions after colonization of the host (Table 6.1). Because *Aspergillus* had been discovered in the 18th century (Micheli 1729), and because there is no reason to suspect that it has become more abundant, or has changed its virulence since that time, it is apparent that it must be the host defences which have been impaired more than previously and now offer the fungus the opportunity to cause infection more often. Nevertheless, before examining host defence mechanisms operative against aspergilli, it is appropriate to look first at the offensive pathogenic potential of the fungus in order to appreciate the defensive tasks of the host.

Table 6.1 Types of diseases associated with invasion by or colonization with *Aspergilli*

Colonization of bronchial tree
Fungal bronchitis
Aspergilloma in preformed cavity (lungs, paranasal sinus)
Chronic necrotizing pulmonary aspergillosis
Invasive fungal sinusitis
Invasive pulmonary aspergillosis
Disseminated aspergillosis
Primary non-respiratory invasive aspergillosis (skin, GI-tract)
Hypersensitivity syndromes:
   Allergic bronchopulmonary aspergillosis
   Extrinsic allergic alveolitis
   Eosinophilic pneumonia

THE PATHOGENIC PERSONALITY OF *ASPERGILLUS*

Aspergilli are ubiquitous saprobic fungi living on an amazing spectrum of organic subtrates and under a wide range of conditions. Aspergilli do not appear, however, to have the ability to gain an ecological advantage by causing infection. Colonization or invasion of a host must therefore rather be seen as an accident. Some mechanisms which aspergilli have evolved in the competition for new ecological niches under competitive conditions have, however, contributed to their ability to cause infection. It has even been proposed that some of the more specific pathogenic mechanisms may have evolved in response to the ecological pressure of phagocytic protozoa such as amoebae (Seaton & Robertson 1989) which feed on fungal spores in soil (Old & Darbyshire 1978).

The major role of *Aspergillus* as an opportunistic fungal pathogen appears unthinkable without the impressive propagative apparatus, which can easily release 50 000 conidia from a single sporing head into the air. This prolificity, together with the omnipresence of pathogenic *Aspergillus* spp. on decaying organic material and the optimal size of conidia for inhalation and deposition in the terminal airways, forms the basis of the pathogenic profile of species such as *A. fumigatus* (Table 6.2)

Table 6.2 The pathogenic features of *Aspergillus*

Prolific sporulation
Omnipresence
Size compatible with deposition in alveoli
Growth at 37–38°C
Spore wall
Modest nutritional requirements
Digestive enzymes: elastase, proteinases
Toxic metabolites (e.g. gliotoxin)
Complement-inhibitory phospholipids
Angiotropism

It is a prerequisite for a pathogen causing deep infections to possess enzyme systems which function at temperatures above 37°C in order to be able to colonize the airways and invade the warm-blooded host. Many aspergilli are thermophilic, and are, therefore, in contrast to numerous other moulds, able to adapt to extreme temperatures, and even grow preferentially at elevated temperatures such as those encountered in a febrile patient.

A property of *A. fumigatus* which contributes to its pathogenic potential is its ability to germinate and grow in extremely simple media. Spores swell in distilled water, and germinate and grow in phosphate-buffered dextrose in the absence of additional nutritives (Fig. 6.1). It is therefore difficult to imagine that by sequestering nutrients from the fungus, the host can build up an efficient defence system of 'nutritional immunity'.

Among their many digestive enzymes, aspergilli produce proteinases of all four classes (Cohen 1977). Furthermore *A. fumigatus* and *A. flavus* regularly exhibit elastase activity (Kothary et al 1984, Rhodes et al 1988, 1990). It has been proposed, by comparison with other pathogens, that production of general proteinases and elastases is correlated to virulence. There is evidence for both assumptions (Miyaji & Nishimura 1977, Kothary et al 1984, Zhu et al 1990) but these observations require confirmation of a causal relationship between enzyme production and pathogenicity. It seems logical that release of proteinases into their surroundings can contribute to the ability of aspergilli to invade the host and cross anatomical barriers such as vessel walls. Observations that spores from strains of *A. fumigatus* that do not produce elastase fail to germinate in the lungs of cortisone-treated mice (Kothary et al 1984) point to other pathogenic mechanisms of elastase.

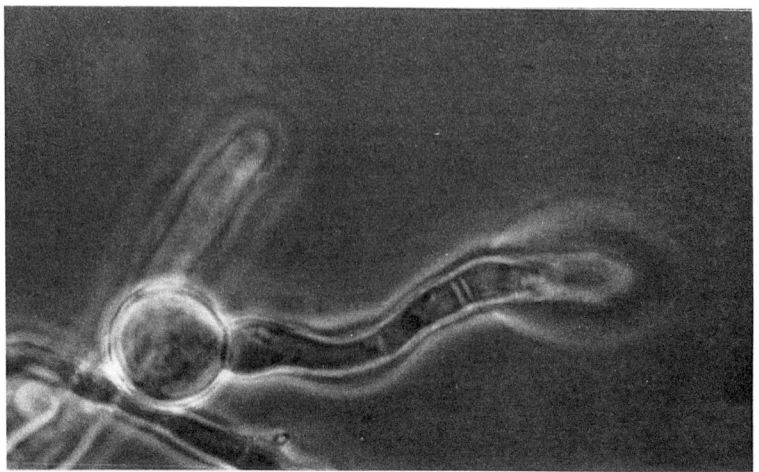

Fig. 6.1 Spore from *A. fumigatus* germinating in 1% dextrose buffered with 0.2 M Soerensens phosphate buffer pH 7.2.

Attention has been drawn to other metabolic products released by pathogenic aspergilli into their environment that might contribute to their virulence. Thus, hyphae from *A. fumigatus* produce lipophilic material, possibly phospholipids, which inhibit complement activity, particularly of the alternative pathway (Washburn et al 1986, 1990). Other metabolites and toxins, such as gliotoxin, which interfere in vitro with phagocyte function (Müllbacher et al 1985, Eichner et al 1986) may contribute to the virulence of aspergilli, but confirmation that such toxins reach effective concentrations and are active in vivo are lacking. Antiphagocytic materials are apparently also released from spores (Robertson et al 1987). Furthermore, poly- and oligosaccharides can interfere with the recognition and binding of non-opsonized fungal particles by phagocytes (Kan & Bennett 1991), pointing to the possibility that cell-wall material shed from hyphae might prevent phagocytes from attacking the fungus in tissue.

Finally, the ability of aspergilli to track and invade blood vessels should be mentioned because it determines part of the pathology of aspergillosis. Aspergilli share this talent with other moulds pathogenic to man, animals, and plants. Despite the broad importance of angiotropism, no insight into the mechanisms by which moulds are attracted to blood vessels has been gained so far. A better understanding of such mechanisms, which have devastating consequences, might provide a means of preventing complications such as the characteristic infarcts of aspergillosis or the rapid dissemination of hyphae to the brain and other organs after they have gained access to pulmonary blood vessels.

CLINICAL AND EPIDEMIOLOGICAL ASPECTS OF THE HOST

Observations on the epidemiology of aspergillosis have provided much insight into host defences against *Aspergillus* and markedly influenced experimental studies of this mycosis. The key information gained from these observations is that, despite the continuous inhalation of conidia by persons breathing non-filtered air, aspergillosis is very uncommon and mainly affects immunocompromised individuals. It is therefore evident that host defence mechanisms reliably protect normal people from aspergilli. It is noteworthy that inhalation of even large numbers of spores, such as that occurring in farmers turning or stacking mouldy hay, only very exceptionally causes invasive infection (Meeker et al 1991).

Aspergillosis has emerged as a problem only after the introduction of aggressive immunosuppressive regimens into clinical practice, and after improvements were made in the control of opportunistic bacterial infections, prolonging the life of many immunocompromised individuals. Both advances have put patients, more often and for longer periods, at risk of developing aspergillosis.

Established risk factors predisposing to invasive aspergillosis are: (1) intensive glucocorticoid therapy (Gustafson et al 1983) or endogenous hypercorticoidism (Graham & Tucker 1984); (2) severe neutropenia, particularly if lasting longer than 18 to 20 days (Gerson et al 1984); and (3) inherited phagocyte defects, in particular chronic granulomatous diseases of childhood (Cohen et al 1981), in which phagocytes fail to produce normal amounts of reactive oxygen intermediates. Thus, at the time of autopsy, aspergillosis can be found in up to 30% of patients with acute leukaemia in whom no preventative measures have been taken (Bodey & Vartiverian 1989). Up to one-third of patients with chronic granulomatous disease will develop serious, frequently lethal aspergillosis, and 2–4% of solid organ transplant recipients will acquire invasive aspergillosis, particularly in relation to immunosuppression with glucocorticoids (Gustafson et al 1983).

Other risk factors have been proposed but not documented adequately. Thus, therapy with broad spectrum antibiotics has been found to be a contributing factor and not an independent risk factor, in a careful study of invasive pulmonary aspergillosis (Gerson et al 1984), a fact which is not surprising if one considers that there is no competing bacterial flora at the point of entry for this most common form of aspergillosis. It has not been excluded, however, that antibiotics might play a role as cofactors in neutropenic cancer patients with sinusitis caused by *Aspergillus* (Viollier et al 1986). It has been proposed that graft-versus-host disease renders the host vulnerable to invasive aspergillosis but such reports have usually overlooked the fact that patients with grade III–IV GvHD receive high doses of methylprednisolone daily, explaining the increased risk for aspergillosis. Reports proposing that cytomegalovirus infection predisposes to aspergillosis have also failed so far to provide a statistically valid association between the viral and the fungal infection. Furthermore, since the two infections may coexist in transplant recipients, it is conceivable that also in this situation immunosuppressive therapy with glucocorticoids was the common denominator for the vulnerability of patients to both infections.

The number of patients with clinically manifest HIV infection is ever increasing, and now by far exceeds those with acute leukaemias, but aspergillosis appears not to be a major problem in patients with the acquired immune deficiency syndrome (Jaffe & Selik 1984). Furthermore, the established risk factors (granulocytopenia and glucocorticoids) appear to be important in this population of patients (Denning et al 1991). It is possible that pneumocystis pneumonia, particularly if associated with structural damage such as cavitation, might predispose to pulmonary aspergillosis (Denning et al 1991).

Finally, it is important to realize that in some patients no factors known to predispose to invasive aspergillosis can be identified, despite careful evaluation, and that the mycosis is encountered in common conditions such as influenza, alcoholism or cystic fibrosis (Karam & Griffin 1986), which are not commonly associated with opportunistic fungal infections and do not provide a link between fungal invasion and a particular defect in host defence systems.

EXPERIMENTAL STUDIES ON HOST DEFENCES AGAINST *ASPERGILLUS* IN ANIMAL MODELS

The early experimental studies on aspergillosis were prompted by the increasing numbers of opportunistic mycoses, including infections caused by aspergilli, reported in the late 50s and 60s (Sideransky & Friedman 1959, Sideransky & Verney 1962). In accordance with clinical observations, it became rapidly clear that normal laboratory animals were highly resistant to the inoculation of conidia by various routes. Accordingly, mice or guinea pigs challenged with high doses of aerosolized spores eliminated conidia from *A. fumigatus* or *A. flavus* within a few days. Elimination curves followed first order kinetics, an observation suggesting that acquired immunity does not explain the high degree of resistance of laboratory animals to aerogenous conidia (Sideransky & Verney 1962, Chernez-Rieux et al 1967, Schaffner et al 1982). Animal models of opportunistic mycoses were however rapidly established in the laboratory by immunosuppressive regimens held responsible for the clinically observed increase in the number of fungal infections (Syverton et al 1952, Mankowski & Littelton 1954, Roth et al 1957).

Aspergillosis was most successfully provoked in rodents with glucocorticoids (Sideransky & Friedman 1959, Turner et al 1976). In a series of important publications, Sideransky and his group documented that alveolar macrophages play an important role in resistance to aspergilli, by phagocytosing inhaled spores, and preventing their germination. Furthermore, these authors showed that in mice treated with a single dose of cortisone the ability of alveolar macrophages to inhibit germination of spores was impaired (Sideransky & Friedman 1959, Sideransky & Verney 1962, Sideransky et al 1965, Epstein et al 1967, Merkow et al 1968, 1971). However, in contradiction to these observations, which helped to explain why mice immunosuppressed with cortisone were more vulnerable to aspergilli, the same immunosuppressive regimen with a single dose of cortisone did not slow down the rapid elimination of inhaled fungi from the lung (Sideransky & Verney 1962).

Similarly, experimental neutropenia, clinically the most important risk factor for aspergillosis, had only a disappointingly small effect on natural resistance of mice to a challenge with conidia from *A. flavus* (Sideransky et al 1965) or *A. fumigatus* (Kish et al 1977), raising the question whether host defence systems of small rodents were representative of human aspergillosis.

In our own studies (Schaffner et al 1982) we confirmed that neutropenia did not significantly lower the resistance of mice to *A. fumigatus* injected i.v. or to a sizeable challenge of aerosolized conidia (Table 6.3). In contrast to neutropenia, cortisone

Table 6.3 Effect of immune defects on susceptibility of mice to 'resting' and 'activated' spores (difference between LD_{50} in normal and immunocompromised mice)

Type of host	Difference in LD_{50} ($\log_{10}$)	
	'Resting' spores	'Activated' spores
Cortisone (CA) 1×5 mg	-1.7	-1.5
Cortisone 6×2.5 mg	-3.9	-3.5
Neutropenia	-0.5^*	-1.2
Athymic	$+0.4$	-0.2^*
Athymic, 5 mg CA	-1.8	not done
'Reinfected'†	-0.2^*	not done
'Reinfected', 5 mg CA	-1.6	not done

Adapted from Schaffner et al (1982).

* Not significantly different from control mice.

† Reinfected mice were rechallenged after a strong humoral immune reaction had developed.

increased the susceptibility of mice to *A. fumigatus* in a dose-dependent manner, and resulted in lethal aspergillosis after a challenge with only few spores. Such an immunosuppressive regimen, which consisted of daily injections of cortisone acetate, in contrast to the aforementioned immunosuppression with a single dose of the glucocorticoid, also resulted in an impaired clearance of spores from the lungs (Fig. 6.2).

Taken together, these observations suggested that a single dose of cortisone given prior to challenge with conidia (Sideransky & Friedman 1959) affects the ability of macrophages to prevent germination of spores, but that continuous immuno-suppression with glucocorticoids, in addition to an effect on mononuclear cells, impairs other defence systems. Cortisone is well known for its effects on acquired T-cell-mediated immunity (Fauci et al 1976). But T-cell-mediated immunity appeared not to be the target for cortisone in lowering resistance to *Aspergillus*, because T-cell-deficient mice were not more susceptible to spores, and cortisone affected athymic mice comparable to normal mice (Fig. 6.2, Table 6.3).

The observation that spores, preincubated in broth to the point of germination, could no longer be prevented from germination by mouse peritoneal macrophages (Sideransky et al 1972) led us to reevaluate the role of cortisone, T-cell deficiency, and neutropenia in mice challenged with such 'activated' spores (Schaffner et al 1982). These experiments confirmed the assumption that host defence against *A. fumigatus* consisted of two independent defence lines. It appeared that the first line of defence, which was rendered ineffective by a single dose of cortisone, was formed by macrophages, and was directed against spores. However, after germination and transformation into hyphae, another defence system became operative against *Aspergillus*. This line was apparently formed by neutrophil granulocytes because neutropenia which failed to render mice susceptible to 'resting' spores led to lethal aspergillosis in mice challenged with 'activated' spores which could not be prevented from germination by macrophages (Table 6.3). Also other findings were in agree-ment with such an assumption. Multiple doses of cortisone, continued after a challenge with spores, in addition to impairing macrophages prevented the mobi-lization of neutrophil granulocytes around hyphae. Accordingly, multiple doses of cortisone, by breaching both defence lines, rendered mice equally susceptible to 'activated' and 'resting' spores (Table 6.3). Further support for this concept is

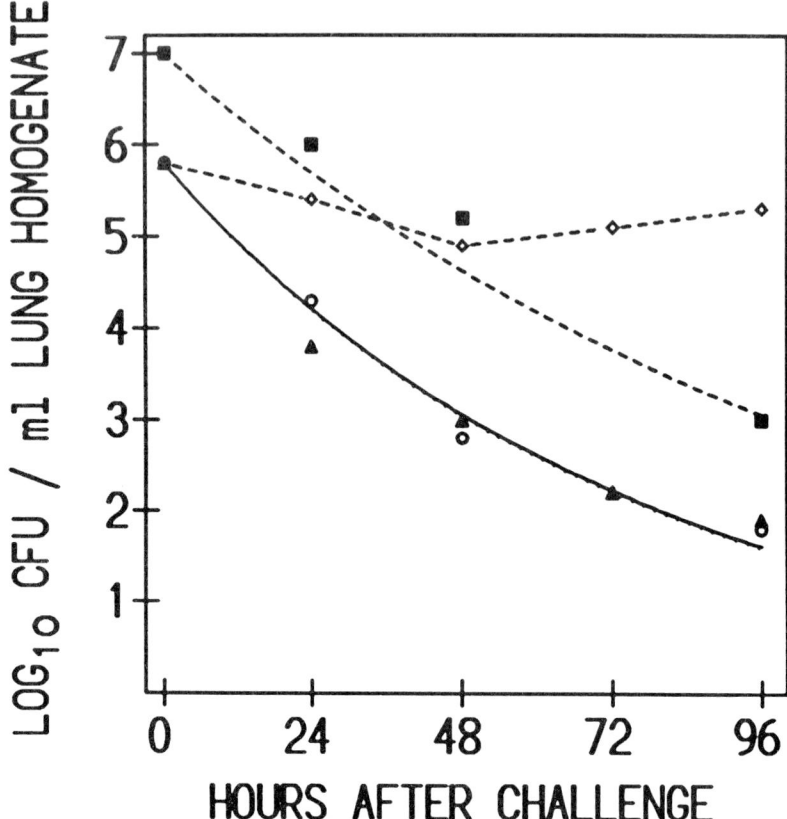

Fig. 6.2 Clearance of conidia from *A. fumigatus* from the lung of normal (○), neutropenic (▲), athymic (■), and cortisone (◇) treated (6 × 2.5 mg cortisone acetate) mice. Adapted from Schaffner et al 1982. Note that the challenge dose with aerosolized spores was 10 times higher in athymic nu/nu mice.

provided by the recent observation that to establish aspergillosis in DBA/2N mice, which lack the C5 component of the complement system, a defect resulting in impaired mobilization of neutrophils, requires, in contrast to control mice, only a single cortisone dose to succumb to lethal pulmonary aspergillosis (Hector et al 1990).

Experiments with 'resting' or 'activated' spores gave no indication that acquired immunity, which depends on antibody production, or T-cell-mediated immunity are relevant to resistance to *Aspergillus* (Table 6.3).

In conclusion, studies in animal models have established that the host can call upon two independent phagocytic cell lines, that form graded defence systems and provide independently reliable protection against aspergilli in the absence of a specific immune response, which seems superfluous to the control and elimination of these fungi.

EXPERIMENTAL STUDIES ON HOST DEFENCE AGAINST
ASPERGILLUS HYPHAE AT THE CELLULAR LEVEL

Even before animal models were developed which permitted the demonstration in vivo of the major role of neutrophil granulocytes in host defences against hyphae from *Aspergillus*, in vitro studies with human granulocytes and hyphae had established that neutrophils attack and metabolically and ultrastructurally damage, and most probably kill, hyphae from *A. fumigatus* despite its size, which precludes its ingestion (Diamond et al 1978). Meanwhile it has been confirmed that human neutrophils indeed kill hyphae from *A. fumigatus* (Schaffner et al 1982, Levitz & Diamond 1985a) and other *Aspergillus* spp. (Schaffner et al 1986).

Neutrophils attack hyphae, which are too large to be completely enclosed in a phagosome, and intimately adhere to the surface of the mycelia. This contact of neutrophils with hyphae triggers the respiratory burst, the secretion of reactive oxygen intermediates, and results in degranulation (Diamond et al 1978). Neither the complement system nor antibodies are required to bring about this interaction between granulocytes and hyphae (Diamond et al 1978, Schaffner et al 1982, 1986). It is however conceivable that opsonins improve the efficacy of neutrophils. Hyphae activate the complement cascade, and C3 is deposited on the surface of mycelia after incubation in fresh serum. The classical, as well as the alternate, pathway appears to be involved in the process (Kozel et al 1989).

Studies of the effects of inhibitors of antimicrobial oxygen metabolites on killing of hyphae, with cells from patients with defective oxidative killing systems or with cell-free killing systems, suggest that oxidative mechanisms are primarily responsible for neutrophil-mediated damage to hyphae (Diamond et al 1978, Diamond & Clark 1982, Rex et al 1990). Non-oxidative killing systems such as the defensins, natural antimicrobial peptides found in abundance in human granulocytes are also active against hyphae and germinating spores (Levitz et al 1986). In addition to granulocytes, mononuclear phagocytes are able to kill mycelia (Diamond et al 1983, Schaffner et al 1983a, 1986), a finding which is not surprising in view of the similarity between some killing systems in the two kinds of phagocytes. The efficacy of phagocytes, granulocytes as well as mononuclear phagocytes, in killing hyphae in the absence of a specific immune reaction, point out that antibodies or activation of phagocytes by lymphokines are superfluous for the elimination of hyphae.

EXPERIMENTAL STUDIES OF HOST DEFENCE AGAINST
ASPERGILLUS SPORES AT THE CELLULAR LEVEL

Aerosolized spores appear to be the infective particle of aspergilli in most instances. Their size of $2.5-4.5\,\mu m$ allows their deposition in the terminal part of the respiratory tract. Spores are, in contrast to some bacterial respiratory pathogens such as pneumococci (Coonrod & Yoneda 1983), resistant to alveolar lining material which even supports their germination (author's unpublished observation). The first effective line of defence spores therefore encounter, after they have reached the terminal portion of the respiratory tract, is formed by resident alveolar macrophages. Alveolar macrophages from rodents (Schaffner et al 1983a) and human alveolar macrophages (Schaffner 1985) readily ingest conidia even in the absence of opsonins. Lectin-like attachment sites on mononuclear phagocytes such as the mannosyl-fucosyl receptor possibly mediate attachment and phagocytosis of spores in the absence of antibody and complement (Kan & Bennett 1988, 1991), opsonins which are probably not readily available in the normal lung.

Alveolar and blood-derived macrophages, from mice, rabbits and man, but not their resident peritoneal macrophages, prevent spores from germination and kill conidia from all pathogenic aspergilli. Killing of spores is comparable under aerobic and strictly anaerobic conditions, and blood-derived macrophages from children with chronic granulomatous disease of childhood handle spores from *A. fumigatus* as well as cells from normal blood donors (Schaffner et al 1983a, Schaffner 1985), showing that killing of spores ingested in their resting state is independent of oxidative mechanisms. This is not surprising because resting spores are much more resistant to oxidants than the hyphal phase of the fungus or germinating spores (Levitz & Diamond 1985b). This observation also explains why conidia are resistant

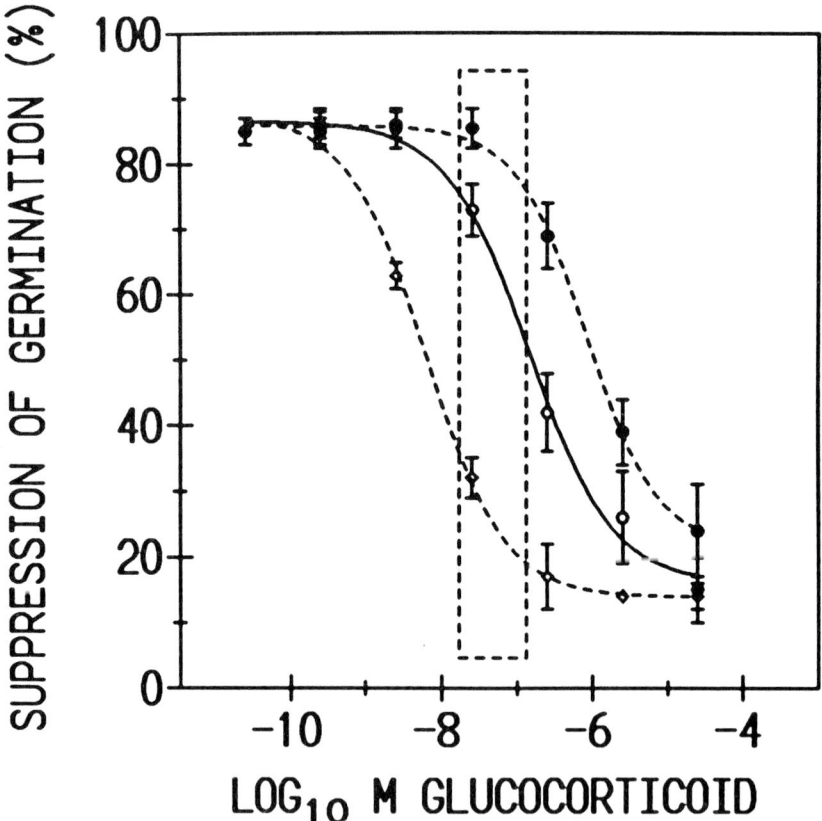

Fig. 6.3 Dose-response curve of the impairment of anti-conidial activity by glucocorticoids in human blood-derived macrophages. (○) cortisol, (◇) dexamethasone, (●) cortisol in the presence of 10^{-5} M progesterone, an antagonist of glucocorticoids at the receptor. Dashed box, normal range of diurnal peak plasma cortisol level. Adapted from Schaffner 1985.

to killing by neutrophil granulocytes (Lehrer & Jan 1970, Schaffner et al 1982). The problem of killing conidia is therefore tricky for the host. Conidia trigger the respiratory burst in neutrophils and macrophages, albeit to a lesser degree, than spores incubated to the point of germination (Levitz & Diamond 1985b), but at the time the burst is triggered, spores are not vulnerable to oxidants. Resting spores are only killed after a delay of 3 to 6 h after phagocytosis, after they have swollen, activated their metabolic machinery, and altered their cell-wall structure (Schaffner et al 1983a). Neutrophils by that time have probably exhausted their oxidative capacity, and mononuclear cells have tuned down secretion of reactive oxygen intermediates, which would serve up to that time only as a means of damaging the surrounding host tissue. By the time spores have become vulnerable to killing, only non-oxidative killing systems remain operative and apparently only macrophages but not neutrophils can therefore kill spores 6 to 24 h after phagocytosis (Schaffner et al 1982, 1983a).

The nature of this (or these) non-oxidative killing system(s) responsible for destroying resting conidia is interesting because (1) the interaction between fungal spores and phagocytes has deep evolutionary roots which may extend back to protozoa (Old & Darbyshire 1978) and the primitive coelomic phagocytes of invertebrates, (2) one effective immunosuppressive effect of cortisone appears to be the impairment of the non-oxidative anticonidial activity of macrophages, and (3) the effect of glucocorticoids on non-oxidative antimicrobial activity of macrophages is not specific for conidia but affects antimicrobial function of macrophages against a broad spectrum of pathogens such as *Listeria, Salmonella,* and *Nocardia* (Schaffner et al 1983b, Schaffner 1985, Schaffner & Rellstab 1988), pointing to the general importance of such killing mechanisms for the natural immunity of the host against many pathogens (Schaffner & Schaffner 1987).

Glucocorticoids impair antimicrobial macrophage function directly, as shown in pure cultures of macrophages. This glucocorticoid effect occurs readily at pharmacological concentrations, and the effect is receptor mediated (Fig. 6.3). Based on indirect evidence, stemming from ultrastructural studies of macrophages, which did not include specific lysosomal staining techniques, it has been proposed that by stabilizing membranes, glucocorticoids inhibit phagolysosomal fusion of macrophages from mice challenged with conidia from *A. flavus* (Merkow et al 1968). By using a lysosomal marker enzyme (Fig. 6.4) or acridine orange as a lysosomal label, we were not able to demonstrate inhibition of phagolysosomal fusion in macrophages with impaired anticonidial function (Table 6.4).

Because the ingestion rate, the triggering and magnitude of the respiratory burst, and phagolysosomal fusion are not impaired by glucocorticoids (Schaffner & Schaffner 1987, Schaffner & Rellstab 1988) it seems logical that glucocorticoids, which regulate protein synthesis, affect an antimicrobial phagolysosomal constituent of the non-oxidative antimicrobial defence. For the time being we only know that this constituent cannot be defensins, the low-molecular cationic peptides found in human neutrophils, because human macrophages (including the alveolar species), unlike macrophages from rabbits, do not produce defensins. Similarly, human mononuclear phagocytes do not contain the arginine-dependent antimicrobial system producing NO (Schaffner, unpublished).

Activation of macrophages in vitro by gamma-interferon, or lymphokines

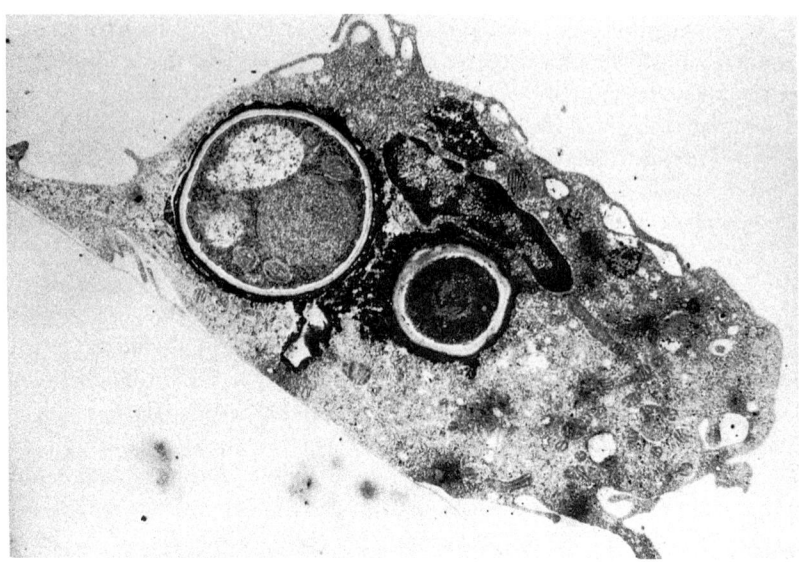

Fig. 6.4 A human-blood derived macrophage with a spore at the initiation of germination and a second, less activated, spore showing clear cut fusion of phagosomes as can be seen from the electron-dense material in the phagosome which corresponds to acid phosphatase activity (methods of Schaffner & Schaffner 1987).

Table 6.4 Effect of exposure of macrophages to 2.5×10^{-7} M of dexamethasone for 36 h prior to challenge with conidia from *A. fumigatus* on phagolysosomal fusion and suppression of germination

Macrophage type	Phagosomes fused (%) (acridin positive)	Germination rate (%) of ingested spores
Human, control	76 ± 5	18 ± 3
Human, dexamethasone	74 ± 6	86 ± 5
Mouse, control	87 ± 3	22 ± 4
Mouse, dexamethasone	91 ± 3	73 ± 2

Human blood-derived macrophages were cultured according to the method of Schaffner (1985). Mouse peritoneal macrophages were obtained 5 days after stimulation of the peritoneal cavity with 1 ml of 10% thioglycolate according to Schaffner et al (1983). Fused phagosomes = % of phagosomes with conidia with fluorescence after fusion with acridine-labelled lysosomes. Germination rates were counted 15 h (mouse) and 24 h (human) after challenge of macrophages with spores.

secreted by proliferating lymphocytes, does not improve the anticonidial activity of macrophages (Schaffner 1985, Schaffner & Rellstab 1988). Activation of macrophages also is unable to overcome the functional impairment of the non-oxidative killing system(s) caused by glucocorticoids despite an appropriate augmentation of the oxidative killing capacity by lymphokines in the presence of pharmacological concentrations of glucocorticoids (Table 6.5). Accordingly it is also not possible to enhance anticonidial activity of normal or cortisone-treated macrophages in vivo by activating macrophages during an infection with an intracellular bacterial pathogen (Fig. 6.5). There is no other convincing experimental evidence that natural immunity to *Aspergillus* can be improved significantly by antigen-dependent mechanisms of acquired immunity.

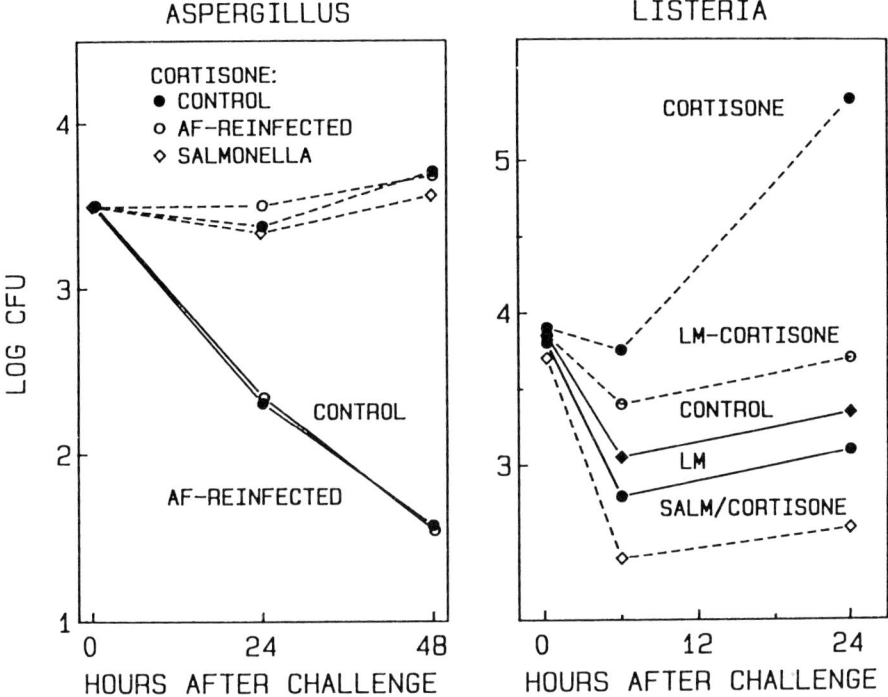

Fig. 6.5 Comparison of the effects of four injections of 2.5 mg cortisone acetate on the clearance of an i.v. challenge with *L. monocytogenes* and *A. fumigatus*. Prior infection of mice with the fungus in contrast to the bacterial infection does not enhance clearance from the liver. Similarly, heterologous infection with *Salmonella typhimurium* had no effect on clearance of conidia (omitted). Accordingly it is not possible to protect liver clearance of conidia from impairment by cortisone. In contrast, homologous and heterologous activation of macrophages enhances bacterial clearance despite immunosuppression with cortisone.

Table 6.5 Effects of dexamethasone and of gamma-interferon on the activity of human blood-derived macrophages against conidia and on secretion of H_2O_2 after a trigger by PMA

Cell type	% Spores inhibited	pmol H_2O_2 secreted per 10^5 cells
Control	83 ± 6	8550 ± 2700
Dexamethasone	11 ± 4	9600 ± 1950
Gamma-interferon	85 ± 7	$39\,150 \pm 5250$
Dexamethasone/gamma-IFN	9 ± 6	$40\,650 \pm 6150$

Adapted from Schaffner & Rellstab 1988.

CONCLUSIONS

Aspergilli are not primary pathogens and seldom establish infection in the normal host by overcoming host immune mechanisms. The host possesses two independent lines of defence, each of which on its own can protect the normal host from invasive aspergillosis. The first defence line is formed by alveolar macrophages and is directed against spores, the second by neutrophil granulocytes which attack and kill hyphae. Both phagocytic defence systems are highly efficient in the absence of specific immune mechanisms, which appear to be superfluous to the control and elimination of *Aspergillus*. Macrophages kill conidia by non-oxidative killing systems which can be impaired by pharmacological glucocorticoid concentrations. Because glucocorticoids do not interfere with phagocytosis, phagolysosomal fusion, or with oxidative killing systems, we have compared the constituents of lysosomes from glucocorticoid-treated and control macrophages in order to define these glucocorticoid-sensitive killing systems. It is interesting that aspergilli, which cannot produce extracellular elastase, are unable to germinate intracellularly even in cortisone-treated mice. This points to the possibility that elastase interferes in phagosomes with antifungal proteins which would inhibit or kill spores, even in glucocorticoid-treated macrophages.

The process of hyphal killing by neutrophils is better defined. Reactive oxygen intermediates appear to be of major importance in explaining the antimycelial activity of neutrophil granulocytes, but non-oxidative killing systems such as defensins also appear to be active. Mycelia attract neutrophils in vivo, with C5A possibly playing an important role as chemotaxin. Neutrophils can attack and kill hyphae even in the absence of opsonins, but the mechanisms by which gluco-corticoids impair the function of this defence line against hyphae have not been defined. In mice, glucocorticoids prevent mobilization of neutrophils around hyphae, but it is not known at which level of the complex process of granulocyte recruitment this impairment occurs. No studies investigating the role of cytokines in host defences against aspergillosis have been published with the exception of very recent studies in patients with chronic granulomatous disease. It is possible that experiments, such as studies with TNF-neutralizing antibodies, might provide an insight into the glucocorticoid-sensitive steps of granulocyte mobilization.

Because angiotropism of aspergilli is important in the pathogenesis of asper-gillosis, studies appear warranted which, besides defining mechanisms underlying angiotropism, investigate the role of the blood clotting system in aspergillosis. It is conceivable that platelets, which dispose of antimicrobial proteins, might affect hyphae. On the other hand, the formation of clots in response to fungi penetrating blood vessels might be counterproductive by segregating hyphae from phagocytes.

ACKNOWLEDGEMENTS

This work by the author was supported by the Swiss National Science Foundation.

REFERENCES

Bodey G P, Vartivarian S 1989 Aspergillosis. European Journal of Microbiology and Infectious Diseases 8: 413–437
Chernez-Rieux C H, Voisin C, Aerts C et al 1967 Aspergillose expérimentale du cobaye. Revue de Tuberculose et de Pneumologie 31: 705–725
Cohen B J 1977 The proteases of *Aspergilli*. In: Smith J E, Pateman (eds) Genetics and physiology of *Aspergillus*. Academic Press, London, pp 282–292
Cohen M S, Isturiz R E, Malech H L, Root R K, Wilfert C M, Gutman L, Buckley R H 1981 Fungal infection in chronic granulomatous disease. American Journal of Medicine 71: 559–566
Coonrod J D, Yoneda K 1983 Detection and partial characterization of antibacterial factor(s) in alveolar lining material of rats. Journal of Clinical Investigation 71: 129–141
Denning D W, Follansbee S E, Scolaro M, Norris S, Edelstein H, Stevens D A 1991. Pulmonary aspergillosis in the acquired immunodeficiency syndrome. New England Journal of Medicine 324: 654–662

Diamond R D, Krzesicki R, Epstein B, Jao W 1978 Damage to hyphal forms of fungi by human leukocytes in vitro. American Journal of Pathology 91: 313–328

Diamond R D, Clark R A 1982 Damage to *Aspergillus fumigatus* and *Rhizopus oryzae* hyphae by oxidative and nonoxidative microbicidal products of human neutrophils in vitro. Infection and Immunity 38: 487–495

Diamond R D, Huber E, Haudenschild C C 1983 Mechanisms of destruction of *Aspergillus fumigatus* hyphae mediated by human monocytes. Journal of Infectious Diseases 147: 474–483

Eichner R D, AlSalami M, Wood P R, Müllbacher A 1986 The effect of gliotoxin upon macrophage function. International Journal of Immunopharmacology 8: 789–797

Epstein S M, Verney E, Miale T D, Sideransky H 1967 Studies on the pathogenesis of experimental pulmonary aspergillosis. American Journal of Pathology 51: 769–788

Fauci A S, Dale D C, Balow J E 1976 Glucocorticosteroid therapy: mechanisms of action and clinical considerations. Annals of Internal Medicine 84: 304–315

Gerson S L, Talbot G H, Hurwitz S, Strom B L, Lusk E J, Cassileth P A 1984 Prolonged granulocytopenia: the major risk factor for invasive pulmonary aspergillosis in patients with acute leukemia. Annals of Internal Medicine 100: 345–351

Graham S, Tucker W S 1984 Opportunistic infections in endogenous Cushing's syndrome. Annals of Internal Medicine 101: 334–338

Gustafson T L, Schaffner W, Lavely G B, Stratton C W, Johnson H K, Hutcheson Jr R H 1983 Invasive aspergillosis in renal transplant recipients: correlation with corticosteroid therapy. Journal of Infectious Diseases 148: 230–238

Hector R F, Yee E, Collins M S 1990 Use of DBA/2N mice in models of systemic candidiasis and pulmonary and systemic aspergillosis. Infection and Immunity 58: 1476–1478

Jaffe H W, Selik R M 1984 Acquired immune deficiency syndrome: is disseminated aspergillosis predictive of underlying cellular immune deficiency? Journal of Infectious Diseases 49: 829

Kan V L, Bennett J E 1988 Lectin-like attachment sites on murine pulmonary alveolar macrophages bind *Aspergillus fumigatus* conidia. Journal of Infectious Diseases 158: 407–414

Kan VL, Benett J E 1991 Beta-1,4-oligoglucosides inhibit the binding of *Aspergillus fumigatus* conidia to human monocytes. Journal of Infectious Diseases 163: 1154–1156

Karam G H, Griffin Jr F M 1986 Invasive pulmonary aspergillosis in nonimmunocompromised, noneutropenic hosts. Reviews of Infectious Diseases 8: 357–363

Kish A L, Rosenberg P, Maydew R, Southard L 1977 Studies of the pathogenesis of immunosuppression-induced exogenous and reactivation-type murine aspergillosis. Clinical Research 25: 156A [abstract]

Kothary M H, Chase T, Macmillan J D 1984 Correlation of elastase production by some strains of *Aspergillus fumigatus* with the ability to cause pulmonary invasive aspergillosis in mice. Infection and Immunity 43: 320–325

Kozel T R, Wilson M A, Farrell T P, Levitz S M 1989 Activation of C3 and binding to *Aspergillus fumigatus* conidia and hyphae. Infection and Immunity 57: 3412–3417

Lehrer R I, Jan R G 1970 Interaction of *Aspergillus fumigatus* spores with human leukocytes and serum. Infection and Immunity 1: 345–350

Levitz S M, Diamond R D 1985a A rapid colorimetric assay of fungal viability with the tetrazolium salt MTT. Journal of Infectious Diseases 152: 938–945

Levitz S M, Diamond R D 1985b Mechanisms of resistance of *Aspergillus fumigatus* conidia to killing by neutrophils in vitro. Journal of Infectious Diseases 152: 33–42

Levitz S M, Selsted M E, Ganz T, Lehrer R I, Diamond R D 1986 In vitro killing of spores and hyphae of *Aspergillus fumigatus* and *Rhizopus oryzae* by rabbit neutrophil cationic peptides and bronchoalveolar macrophages. Journal of Infectious Diseases 154: 483–489

Mankowski Z T, Littleton B J 1954 Action of cortisone and ACTH on experimental fungus infections. Antibiotics and Chemotherapy (New York) 4: 253–258

Meeker D P, Gephardt G N, Cordasco E M, Wiedemann H P 1991 Hypersensitivity pneumonitis versus invasive pulmonary aspergillosis: two cases with unusual pathologic findings and review of the literature. American Journal of Respiratory Diseases 143: 431–436

Merkow L, Pardo M, Epstein S M, Verney E, Sideransky H 1968 Lysosomal stability during phagocytosis of *Aspergillus flavus* spores by alveolar macrophages of cortisone-treated mice. Science 160: 79–81

Merkow L P, Epstein S M, Sideransky H, Verney E, Pardo M 1971 The pathogenesis of experimental pulmonary aspergillosis: an ultrastructural study of alveolar macrophages after phagocytosis of *A. flavus* spores in vivo. American Journal of Pathology 62: 57–73

Micheli P A 1729 Nova Plantarum Genera. Florentinae

Miyaji M, Nishimura K 1977. Relationship between proteolytic activity of *Aspergillus fumigatus* and the fungus' invasiveness of mouse brain. Mycopathologia 62: 161–166

Müllbacher A, Waring P, Eichner R D 1985 Identification of an agent in cultures of *Aspergillus fumigatus* displaying antiphagocytic and immunomodulating activity in vitro. Journal of General Microbiology 131: 1251–1258

Old K M, Darbyshire J F 1978 Soil fungi as food for giant amoebae. Soil Biology and Biochemistry 10: 93–100

Rex J H, Bennett J E, Gallin J I, Malech H L, Melnick D A 1990 Normal and deficient neutrophils can cooperate to damage *Aspergillus fumigatus* hyphae. Journal of Infectious diseases 162: 523–528

Rhodes J C, Bode R B, McCuan-Kisrsch C M 1988 Elastase production in clinical isolates of *Aspergillus*. Diagnostic Microbiology and Infectious Diseases 10: 165–170

Rhodes J C, Amlung T W, Miller M S 1990 Isolation and characterization of an elastinolytic proteinase from *Aspergillus flavus*. Infection and Immunity 58: 2529–2534

Robertson M D, Seaton A, Milne L J R, Raeburn J A 1987 Suppression of host defenses by *Aspergillus fumigatus*. Thorax 42: 19–25

Roth F J, Friedman J, Syverton J T 1957 Effects of roentgen radiation and cortisone on susceptibility of mice to *Candida albicans*. Journal of Immunology 78: 122–127

Schaffner A, Douglas H, Braude A 1982 Selective protection against conidia by mononuclear and against mycelia by polymorphonuclear phagocytes in resistance to *Aspergillus*. Journal of Clinical Investigation 69: 617–631

Schaffner A, Douglas H, Braude A I, Davis C E. 1983a Killing of *Aspergillus* spores depends on the anatomical source of the macrophage. Infection and Immunity 42: 1109–1115

Schaffner A, Douglas H, Davis C E 1983b Models of T cell deficiency in listeriosis: the effects of cortisone and cyclosporin A on normal and nude BALB$_c$ mice. Journal of Immunology 131: 450–453

Schaffner A 1985 Therapeutic concentrations of glucocorticoids suppress the antimicrobial activity of human macrophages without impairing their responsiveness to gamma interferon. Journal of Clinical Investigation 76: 1755–1764

Schaffner A, Davis C E, Schaffner T, Markert M, Douglas H, Braude A I 1986 In vitro susceptibility of fungi to killing by neutrophil granulocytes discriminates between primary pathogenicity and opportunism. Journal of Clinical Investigation 78: 511–524

Schaffner A, Schaffner T 1987 Glucocorticoid-induced impairment of macrophage antimicrobial activity: mechanisms and dependence on the state of activation. Reviews of Infectious Diseases 9: S620–S629

Schaffner A, Rellstab Ph 1988 Gamma interferon restores listericidal activity and concurrently enhances release of reactive oxygen metabolites in dexamethasone-treated human monocytes. Journal of Clinical Investigation 82: 913–919

Seaton A, Robertson M D 1989 Aspergillus, asthma and amoebae. Lancet i: 893–894

Sideransky H, Friedman L 1959 The effect of cortisone and antibiotic agents on experimental pulmonary aspergillosis. American Journal of Pathology 35: 169–184

Sideransky H, Verney E 1962 Experimental aspergillosis. Laboratory Investigations 11: 1172–1183

Sideransky H, Verney E, Beede H 1965 Experimental pulmonary aspergillosis. Archives of Pathology 70: 299–309

Sideransky H, Eppstein S M, Verney E, Horowitz C 1972 Experimental visceral aspergillosis. American Journal of Pathology 69: 55–67

Syverton J T, Werder A A, Friedman J, Roth F J, Graham A B, Mira O J 1952 Cortisone and roentgen radiation in combination as synergistic agents for production of lethal infections. Proceedings of the Society for Experimental Biology and Medicine 80: 123–128

Turner K J, Hackshaw R, Papadimitriou J, Perrot J 1976 The pathogenesis of experimental pulmonary aspergillosis in normal and cortisone treated rats. Journal of Pathology 118: 65–73

Viollier A F, Peterson D E, DeJongh C A, Newman K A, Gray W C, Sutherland J C, Moody M A, Schimpf S C 1986 Aspergillus sinusitis in cancer patients. Cancer 58: 366–371

Washburn R G, Hammer C H, Bennett J E 1986 Inhibition of complement by culture supernatants of *Aspergillus fumigatus*. Journal of Infectious diseases 154: 944–951

Washburn R G, DeHart D J, Agwu D E, Bryant-Varela B J, Julian N C 1990. *Aspergillus fumigatus* complement inhibitor: production, characterization, and purification by hydrophobic interaction and thin-layer chromatography. Infection and Immunity 58: 3508–3515

Zhu W S, Wojdyla K, Donlon K, Thomas P A, Eberle H I 1990 Extracellular proteases of *Aspergillus flavus*. Fungal keratitis, proteases, and pathogenesis. Diagnostic Microbiology and Infectious Diseases 13: 491–497

112

Discussion of paper presented by A. Schaffner

Discussed by R. D. Diamond
Reported by H. C. Neu

In reviewing Dr Schaffner's presentation, Dr Diamond selected several points for discussion. He pointed out that the dimorphic pathogens and the saprophytes that cause opportunistic infection have characteristically been distinguished from each other. There clearly are differences in the transitional phases as the fungus goes through its life cycle. The resting conidia, as they evolve and swell, are subject to destruction by macrophages, but when they develop into filamentous forms they stimulate very different cellular pathways. Dr Diamond pointed out that the rodlet structures present on the conidial surface were potent surface properties in interfering with host defense mechanisms. The phagocytosed conidia which contain rodlets are poor stimulants of neutrophil and macrophage function, as demonstrated by the lack of a respiratory burst response and degranulation. Compared to conidia without the rodlets, the rodlet forms are more resistant to oxidative and non-oxidative killing mechanisms. Interestingly, even though hyphae are highly susceptible to oxidants in the test tube, hyphal organisms are killed slowly by monocytes.

It was noted that human alveolar macrophages and blood macrophages do not have arginine-mediated production of nitrous oxides so that this is not an explanation of fungal killing by these cells.

The reason why *Aspergillus fumigatus, A. flavus* and, to a much less extent, *A. niger* are the cause of infections in man when many other *Aspergillus* species can be isolated from air has not been established. However, it is possible that other species do not germinate in vivo. It was also noted that many *Aspergillus* species such as *A. terreus* have thin-walled conidia. *A. terreus,* which is very common in the environment, rarely causes disease. *A. nidulans* which is uncommon except in soil and subtropical or tropical areas is a problem in patients with chronic granulomatous disease (CGD). Thus the echinulation of conidial surfaces (cell walls) may be quite important.

The problem of aspergillosis in patients with CGD was discussed, and it was postulated that the 8–9% reported incidence probably is an underestimate since these patients are living longer. CGD patients are weakly responsive to therapy. Unfortunately, the number of CGD patients who have received gamma interferon to prevent aspergillosis is small, and the treatment success data also are based on

113

a very small number of cases. So we still do not know the ultimate role of interferon in the CGD patient.

Dr Diamond also illustrated with clinical material the problem of the host's response to fungi in terms of an excessive inflammatory reaction and cautioned that we need to learn a great deal about the use of cytokines in the infected patient.

Finally, it was generally agreed that isolation rooms with filtered air dramatically reduce the numbers of exogenous infections in leukaemia and bone marrow transplant patients. Endogenous reactivation of dormant *Aspergillus* in the lung is extremely rare, if it occurs. It was noted that although there had been some progress in the therapy of *Aspergillus* infection, if patients remained neutropenic and required continued immunosuppressive therapy they rarely if ever survived.

Session III:
Yeast genetics and morphogenesis

Chairman: M. V. Hayes

7. Novel targets for antifungal drugs

C. Nombela, J. Pla, E. Herreros, C. Gil, M. Molina, M. Sanchez

INTRODUCTION

For a number of years our group has been involved in studies of fungal cell wall functions related to the autolysis of this structure. We have addressed the question of the biological role of enzymes that degrade components of the producer's cell wall ('fungal autolysins'), by using different approaches based on biochemical and physiological aspects of the enzymes involved, as well as on the characterization of mutants altered in phenomena related to cell wall autolysis and/or morphogenesis. Our working hypothesis is that the fungal cell carries the potential for determining autolysis of its own wall. We are beginning to understand the essential aspects of the wall autolytic systems of the fungal cell and the regulation that maintains integrity of the cell under physiological conditions. Alteration of this autolytic potential eventually leads to cell death. Our interpretation of this observation is that some of the new targets that are needed for developing new antifungals might be related to this set of functions.

MAJOR COMPONENTS OF FUNGAL CELL WALLS

Fungal cell walls appear, under the electron microscope, as thick rigid structures required for maintaining cellular integrity by protecting cells against osmotic changes in the environment. The polysaccharides that form part of the wall structure differ qualitatively and quantitatively between species, and the composition of the cell wall has been tentatively used in fungal taxonomy and phylogeny. Details of the wall composition are known for many species, but aspects such as the assembly and interaction of individual components to generate the architecture of the wall are more difficult to establish.

For many years *Saccharomyces cerevisiae* has been the major experimental model for addressing the question of wall structure and organization. The picture that emerges is of a wall with two major structural crystalline polysaccharides that are responsible for rigidity and strength. One of them is a β-glucan, which consists of 1,3-β- and 1,6-β-linked homopolymers, and represents 60% of the wall material. The other homopolysaccharide is chitin which contributes only about 1% but it seems to be equally important. Other materials form the amorphous matrix that cements the structure. These are α-glucan and, mainly, mannoproteins representing 30–40% of the wall. The variety of these highly glycosylated proteins suggests an important function for them. Sentandreu and coworkers (Elorza et al 1985, 1988, Marcilla et al 1991) have recently emphasized that these proteins may play a vital role in cell wall biogenesis, on the basis of their specific interactions with structural components. Given the enzymatic activity of some of the cell wall mannoproteins (Klebl & Tanner 1989) we can also postulate that they may be important in controlling cell wall dynamics by interacting with other proteins and regulating their activity.

The studies carried out on *Candida albicans* cell walls (Shepherd 1991) are more limited, but the composition is qualitatively similar to that of *S. cerevisiae*. Glucan represents about 75% of the total wall material (Fleet & Phaff 1981, Sullivan et al 1983, Elorza et al 1983). This glucan has been fractionated into three main components, two of them being highly branched 1,3-β- and 1,6-β-linked polymers and a third linear component, chitin, which seems to be bound to the glucan. These polysaccharides are present both in blastospores and mycelia (Gopal et al 1984), although the chitin content is three to five times higher in mycelial walls (Elorza et al 1983, Sullivan et al 1983), where it might contribute additional strength to the microfibrillar network to permit the extension of the wall only by apical growth. Mannoproteins also represent the major components of the amorphous matrix of *C. albicans* wall. Up to 40 different mannoprotein components have been identified (Elorza et al 1985) and their importance for wall architecture is also emphasized by the demonstration that some of these mannoproteins are specific for either blastospore or mycelium cell walls.

THE IMPORTANCE OF CELL WALL DYNAMICS

Since the fungal wall is clearly not an inert structure, but one in a continuous state of flux, there are presumably many functions which represent possible points of interference. Thus the envelope may be relatively inert at some stages of the fungal life cycle, or in certain areas during normal vegetative growth, but it undergoes profound changes as a consequence of processes such as budding or apical extension of hyphae depending on the organism, and during dimorphic transitions and mating. The delivery of polymers to the appropriate position in the wall is also important for morphogenesis. On the other hand, the production of enzymes that hydrolyse components of the fungal wall by the growing organism suggests that cell wall hydrolases ('autolysins') must also play a physiological role based on the controlled modification of this structure.

Therefore, one can envisage cell wall dynamics are a consequence of the participation of both synthetases and hydrolases in cellular processes. In this discussion we consider the basis of both aspects in some detail, in order to substantiate our contention that interfering, or altering in some manner, fungal cell wall functions must represent the best possibility of causing a fungicidal effect. In other words, we believe that enzymes controlling cell wall dynamics must provide some of the best antifungal targets.

118

Fungal cell wall synthetases and their inhibition

The synthesis of chitin has been the most explored in most detail. It is essentially a vectorial process that leads to the polymerization of N-acetylglucosamine from its UDP-linked precursor. Two chitin synthetases were identified in membrane preparations obtained from *S. cerevisiae* (Cabib et al 1990). Both enzymes are zymogens requiring partial proteolysis for maximal in vitro activation. The structural genes for chitin synthetases I and II, namely *CHSI* (Bulawa et al 1986) and *CHS2* (Silverman et al 1988) have been cloned and sequenced, the corresponding comparison revealing a high degree of homology (42%), in a region of 660 amino acid residues.

Disruption of *CHSI* led to viable mutants, that grew and formed a normal septum, without alterations in the chitin content. Gene *CHS2* seems to be more important for chitin synthesis, since the disruption of this gene can be lethal, depending on the culture medium and the genetic background of the parental strains. After staining with Calcofluor the cells showed some fluorescence at constrictions, but no clear septa were formed. *CHS2* can be considered therefore more important for cell division than *CHSI* (Shaw et al 1991). More recently, Valdivieso et al (1991) have described a third gene involved in the formation of chitin, that was cloned by complementation of Calcofluor-resistant mutants affected in gene *CAL1*. The gene codes for what seems to be the third chitin synthetase, which is also to some extent homologous to *CHSI* and *CHS2*. This enzyme seems to play an important role in the synthesis of the chitin located in the vegetative wall, and in the synthesis of the chitosan present in the asci.

Therefore, the formation of a structural polymer such as chitin, which is present in relatively small amounts in *S. cerevisiae* walls, seems to be carried out by a complex mechanism requiring up to three different synthetases. Competitive inhibitors of chitin synthesis, such as polyoxin D and nikkomycin X and Z, are more effective against *CHSI* than against *CHS2* (Cabib 1991), an observation that could partially account for some of the differences in the in vivo and in vitro activity of these inhibitors and their derivatives. The availability of the three genes should enable efficient strategies to be implemented for the identification of targets based on inhibition of chitin synthesis. Among these are the establishment of the validity of the *S. cerevisiae* model of chitin synthesis for other fungal species of importance as pathogens. It should also be possible to compare all three enzyme sequences to carry out the molecular modelling that will establish the patterns of interaction with substrates and potential inhibitors in order to design the latter.

The counterpart of gene *CHSI* in *C. albicans* has also been cloned (Au-Young & Robbins 1990). A similar and complex system of chitin synthesis seems to operate in this yeast and it should be stressed that inhibition of chitin synthesis might also prevent the formation of hyphae, a factor that contributes to virulence, since the yeast to mycelium transition parallels an increase in the chitin content from about 1% to 5%. This is consistent with the observation that tetaine, an inhibitor of glucosamine-6-phosphate synthetase, inhibits glucose incorporation into chitin, mainly in the mycelial forms (Milewski et al 1986).

There is considerable information with regard to the biosynthesis of the structural polysaccharides 1,3-β- and 1,6-β-glucan. However, with the exception of *kre1* and *kre5* mutants concerned with β-1,6-glucan biosynthesis (Boone et al 1990, Meaden et al 1990) no data have been reported concerning the cloning of other glucan biosynthetic genes. Glucan synthetases use UDP-glucose as a precursor and are complex, consisting of soluble and membrane bound components. The former binds GTP whereas the latter carries the active centre (Kang & Cabib 1986). In any case, natural inhibitors, usually of a complex chemical structure, such as papulacandin (Kopecka 1984), aculeacin (Mizoguchi et al 1977), echinocandin (Cassone et al 1981) and cilofungin (Hall et al 1988), have been discovered. Although none of these compounds or their derivatives have so far been developed as a clinical drug, they represent a set of interesting substances for testing the possibilities of glucan synthesis as a target and deserve the attention of workers in the field of antifungals.

In summary, the synthesis of structural components of the fungal cell requires a set of enzyme systems that are being characterized in detail at the molecular and genetic level. Inhibitors that are more or less effective against the synthetic systems have been identified and are being improved by various synthetic modifications. New inhibitors of these basic processes should be discovered as a result of searches for inhibitors of specific reactions. However, studies with these inhibitors demonstrate that agents blocking specific fungal biosynthetic processes, such as formation of wall structural components that do not occur in the animal cell, will not necessarily be non-toxic. So far none of the fungal wall synthetase inhibitors have found a clear way to clinical use due to various difficulties such as toxicity, low solubility and limited penetration to the fungal target. Therefore, it is important to consider other aspects of cell wall dynamics, in particular the wall autolytic potential of the fungal cell.

Fungal cell wall lytic enzymes and their regulation
The production of enzymes capable of degrading structural components of the producer's cell wall has been documented in fungal species as well as in bacteria. Biochemical evidence of the existence of β-glucanases and chitinases produced by fungal cells have been obtained, but it has been more difficult to develop a model that would account for the role(s) and function(s) of this enzyme complement that represents a real autolytic potential. One of the major problems in drawing a clear picture of the physiological implication of fungal autolysins in morphogenesis is the diversity of these enzymes among related fungal species (Fleet 1984, Nombela et al 1988). In this respect, the situation is similar to that of bacteria.

The production and/or activation of fungal autolysins must be a regulated process. It is required by the nature of these enzymes with their potential to damage the cell wall structure were they to get out of control. In the case of glucanases, the experimental evidence shows that many fungal autolysins are specifically produced during active growth or regulated in connection with specific morphogenetic events, or alternatively a significant derepression takes place prior to situations leading to cell autolysis. In filamentous fungi that undergo autolysis when growth ceases, the production of high levels of very active 1,3-β- and 1,6-β-glucanases (Santos et al 1978) is derepressed as a consequence of the lack of a carbon source in the medium. Much lower levels of glucanase activity are observed during active growth in the presence of a readily accessible carbon source. However, in yeasts that usually do not undergo autolysis, such as *S. cerevisiae* and *C. albicans*, production of glucanases (del Rey et al 1979, Molina et al 1987) and chitinases (Barrett-Bee et al 1982, Gooday et al 1986) seems to be precisely adjusted to vegetative growth, without any derepression taking place in non-growing cells. This would suggest a role of these enzymes in morphogenesis. The observation that special differentiation processes, such as sporulation in *S. cerevisiae* (del Rey et al 1980) and germ-tube formation in *C. albicans* (Molina et al 1987), determine specific changes in glucanase production such as formation of new enzymes or the switch-off in the formation of pre-existing ones also supports the contention that the enzymes are involved in morphogenesis. Fungal autolysins are secreted enzymes but are not merely destined to be released into the extracellular medium. The secretion process sorts the enzymes for specific localizations; they might be trapped in the wall structure (Cenamor et al 1987, Klebl & Tanner 1989) or released free to the external medium (Nombela et al 1988). For this reason the use of protoplast regeneration systems to analyse protoplast secretion products has proved very useful in identifying some of the glucanases that are produced in very small amounts, but might be very important for the cell (Cenamor et al 1987), mainly because they seem to remain trapped in the wall structure.

All these studies point towards a model of fungal autolysins acting on the controlled hydrolytic modification of wall components for proper morphogenesis and development of the wall structure, their production and localization being adjusted to achieve such a role. However, genetic strategies, developed in order to obtain direct evidence regarding the role of individual fungal autolysins, reveal a more complicated picture. For example, the most abundant glucanases of *S. cerevisiae*, namely exo-1,3-β-glucanases that represent more than 60% of the glucan degrading activity in this species, are dispensable enzymes as shown by the lack of phenotypic changes in deficient mutants (Santos et al 1982) and by cloning and disruption of the corresponding gene (Nebreda et al 1986). They probably play an accessory role, and this represents a very strong indication that several of the glucanases that are produced in much smaller amounts and act as endo-hydrolases, might be critically needed. Studies ongoing in our laboratory as well as in others, aiming to clone the endo-glucanase genes, should provide evidence for this hypothesis.

LETHAL EVENTS RELATED TO CELL WALL AUTOLYSIS

Properties of lysis mutants

The existence of a wall autolytic potential in microorganisms, which is reflected by the production of enzymes that hydrolyse wall structural components, can explain the autolysis of bacteria and fungi occurring when growth ceases. However, we also find that some yeast species such as *S. cerevisiae* and *C. albicans*, do not lyse but remain stable when growth ceases. This phenomenon suggests that in these cells the autolytic potential is kept under strict control.

S. cerevisiae mutants altered in these basic functions can be isolated (Cabib & Duran 1975) and they represent the major reason for our contention that the autolytic function is controlled. Lysis mutants are thermosensitive, so that when transferred to a non-permissive temperature they cannot sustain growth and lyse rapidly. By characterizing this type of *S. cerevisiae* mutant we have identified two genes, namely *LYT1* (Nombela & Santamaria 1984) and *LYT2* (Torres et al 1991 in press), that complement with another set of lysis mutants isolated by Sansegundo & del Rey (personal communication), which defines at least three other complementation groups. Therefore, a significant number of genes may be involved in functions related to cell wall autolysis as is indicated by the number of different mutants that can be obtained.

The lytic phenotype could be essentially the result of a deficiency in wall formation or of an alteration in the control of autolysis. The impairment of membrane functions can also be envisaged as leading to a lytic phenotype. For a precise characterization of lysis mutants, we have developed a method that combines the use of 1M sorbitol as osmotic stabilizer, with the technique of flow cytometry in

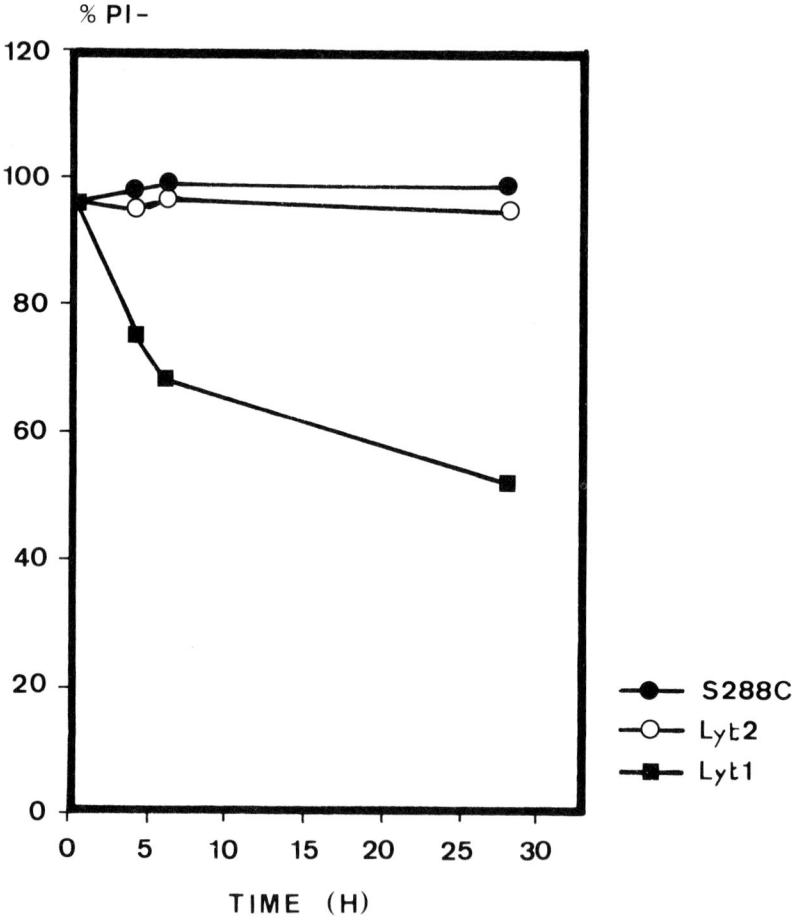

Fig. 7.1 Analysis by flow cytometry of sorbitol (1M) protection from lysis of *S. cerevisiae* strains. S288C was a wild type strain and the other two strains carried the thermosensitive lytic traits *lyt1* and *lyt2*. The percentage of propidium iodide negative (PI⁻) cells represent viable non-lysed cells in cultures grown at the non-permissive temperature of 37°C.

order to analyse large cell populations quantitatively and, even, to fractionate and sort them according to specific characteristics (de la Fuente et al 1991, in press). The method makes use of the uptake of a fluorescent dye, namely propidium iodide, that takes place in lysed cells even at initial stages of lysis. Sorbitol protection from lysis can be taken as a demonstration that it is essentially a cell wall alteration which determines the lytic phenotype, whereas mutant strains not protected by sorbitol are considered to have a membrane alteration.

This is illustrated by the results of Figure 7.1, obtained with *S. cerevisiae* lysis mutants *lyt1* and *lyt2*. Whereas the former was not protected by 1M sorbitol, the latter was rescued from lysis in the presence of the osmotic stabilizer. Lysis of the *lyt2* mutant, which could also be followed by the release of the intracellular enzyme alkaline phosphatase, took place at the non-permissive temperature and was totally dependent on active growth. It is important to emphasize at this point that alterations in cell wall development determine lethal events in growing fungal cells. Of

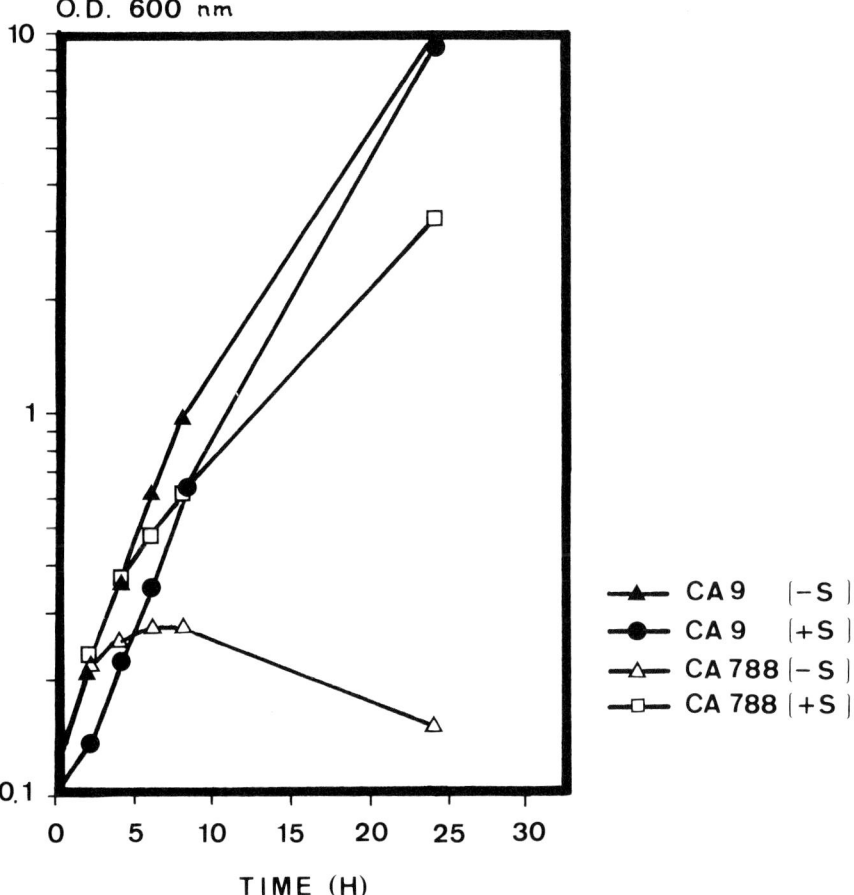

Fig. 7.2 Effect of sorbitol on growth of *C. albicans* strains at the non-permissive temperature of 42°C. Strain CA788 was lytic. Growth was measured by optical density of the cultures at 600 nm (OD 600 nm). + S, in presence of 1M sorbitol.

course, this observation does not enable one to establish the basic wall process that becomes deficient in mutant cells at the non-permissive temperature, or the regulation process related to these functions that becomes altered as a consequence of the mutation. The cloning work described later is beginning to shed some light on these 'lethal events' that we consider could be most useful in identifying novel targets for antifungals since they lead to cell death.

Lysis osmotic-remedial mutants can also be isolated from the opportunistic fungal pathogen *C. albicans* (Payton & de Tiani 1990). The number of strains that can be isolated independently is also significant, suggesting that several genes are involved in the corresponding functions. We have carried out a phenotypic characterization of several of these mutants isolated and supplied to us by M. Payton (Glaxo Institute for Molecular Biology, Geneva). As shown in Figure 7.2 the parental strain *C. albicans* CA9 (His⁻) grew at the non-permissive temperature

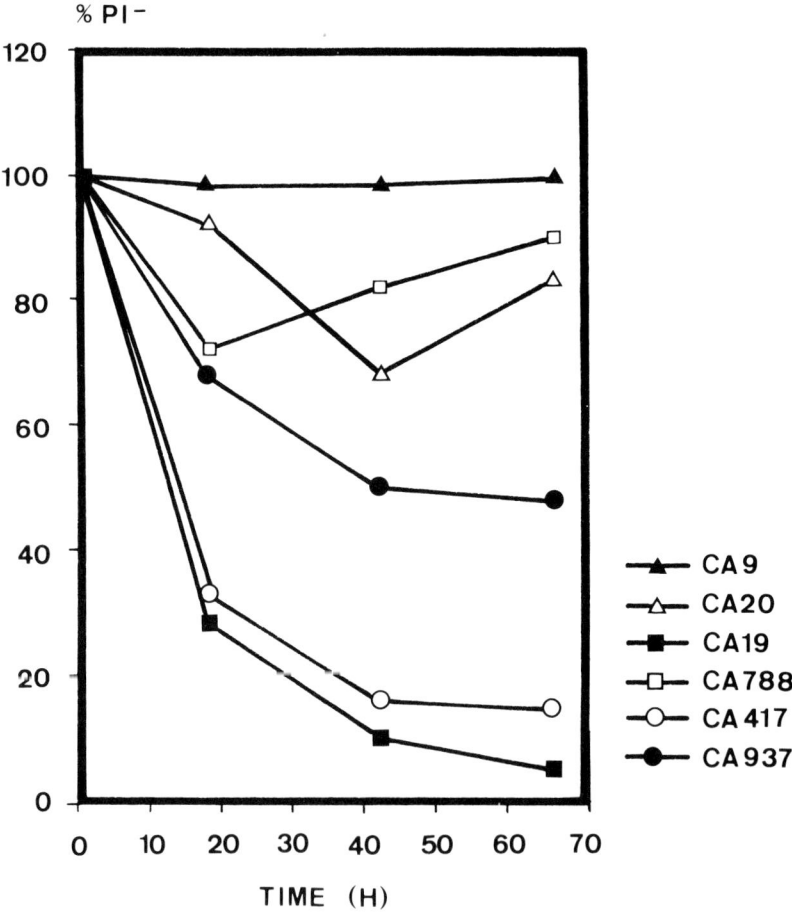

Fig. 7.3 Analysis by flow cytometry of sorbitol (1M) protection from lysis of several *C. albicans* strains. CA9 was a wild type strain and the others were thermosensitive lytic mutants. The percentage of propidium iodide negative (PI⁻) cells represent viable non-lysed cells in cultures grown at the non-permissive temperature of 42°C.

of 42°C in either the presence or absence of 1M sorbitol, whereas the lytic mutant strain CA788 could only grow under osmotically stable conditions. However, it also has to be admitted that more complex phenomena can be involved in the determination of lytic phenotypes. This is indicated by the variety of degrees of sorbitol protection that was encountered when precisely characterizing a whole set of *C. albicans* lysis mutants, isolated as osmotic remedial (Fig. 7.3). Sorbitol protection was clearly shown to occur in some strains when grown in liquid medium. But sorbitol afforded only partial protection to others and even a very limited protection to some of them.

These preliminary results enable us to propose that multiple genes are involved in *C. albicans* in the formation of a functional wall structure, so that a block in the function of these genes is lethal for growing cells.

INSIGHTS INTO THE REGULATION OF CELL WALL FORMATION

Identifying protein kinase genes involved in wall functions

Cloning of genes complementing lysis mutants should lead to the clarification of the basic functions that might represent potential antifungal targets. No cloning procedures for isolating genes using *C. albicans* as a host are yet available. Therefore, it has not been possible to undertake the cloning of the genes affected in *C. albicans* lysis mutants, although we hope to be able to carry out these cloning experiments when the development of a *C. albicans*/*S. cerevisiae* shuttle vector, that is being carried out in our laboratory, is completed. In any case, the results obtained in our laboratory on the cloning of genes complementing *S. cerevisiae* lysis mutants are very revealing. A gene was cloned on the basis of its capacity to complement the lytic phenotype of *lyt2* strains. By comparing nucleotide and amino acid sequences with the available gene banks, the cloned gene was shown to code for a putative serine/threonine protein kinase with an M_r of 55,666. This protein kinase gene, not been described previously, carries all the domains that have been shown to be specific for protein kinases, and shares a significant degree of identity with yeast protein kinases that have been implicated in the mitotic cell cycle (Reed et al 1985, Courchesne et al 1989, Elion et al 1990). Disruption of this kinase gene led to the generation of haploid disruptants that were lytic in a significant proportion of the cells when grown at 28°C and completely when grown at 37°C. The lytic phenotype of mutants with the disrupted protein kinase gene was also reversed by 1M sorbitol, indicative of a cell wall alteration caused by the lack of the protein kinase (Torres et al, in press).

Despite the similarity of phenotypes of both *lyt2* mutants and mutants with the disrupted protein kinase gene, genetic analysis shows that the cloned protein kinase gene is not the structural gene *lyt2* but a suppressor of the lytic phenotype, which we have named the *SLT2* gene. Additional evidence obtained by manipulation of the cloned gene, including site-directed mutagenesis of the putative active centre, indicated that an adequate level of expression of the protein kinase SLT2 is required for proper morphogenesis of the cell wall, both overexpression and blocking of the expression of the gene being lethal for the cells (Martin et al, unpublished data).

The implication of protein kinases in morphogenesis opens the way for understanding important aspects of the regulation of this process and its coupling to the mitotic cycle in fungal cells. Our findings with regard to gene *SLT2* can be related to other recent reports that establish implications of protein kinases in yeast morphogenesis. Protein kinase $kin1^+$ is required for morphogenesis in the fission yeast *Schizosaccharomyces pombe*, so that strains with the corresponding gene disrupted grow as spheres, with a weak cell wall that seems to be altered in composition and organization (Levin & Bishop 1990). The phenotype of Kin^- mutants is similar to the phenotype of mutants deficient in 1,3-β-glucan that display the same morphological alterations (Ribas et al 1991). Some other recent short reports indicate the involvement of novel protein kinases in yeast budding and morphogenesis (Snyder et al 1991) or in other events such as vacuolar sorting of proteins (Stack et al 1991) that might also have a relationship with morphogenesis.

PROSPECTS FOR IDENTIFICATION OF NOVEL ANTIFUNGAL TARGETS

The picture that emerges from the present discussion is not a simple one but it might reveal the way for advancement in the definition of novel targets for anti-fungals. The synthetic systems that produce and deliver structural polymers of the fungal wall, clearly represent essential functions for the formation of this envelope. But it is also shown that there are other vital functions coded by genes that are also crucial and specific in cell wall formation. These are represented by protein kinase genes that should naturally have a regulatory function. Whether that function is directly coupled to cell wall synthetases, cell wall autolysins or any other system remains to be determined. In fact, regulation by protein kinases could trigger a series of events needed for morphogenesis. It is also feasible that these events are connected to the regulation of the mitotic cycle.

Therefore, the generation of a wall structure during growth of the fungal cell requires a complex balance in the biological mechanisms whose alteration may lead to death of the fungal cell. These 'lethal points' in wall formation are not only the basic synthetic systems, but others possibly related to autolysis and the coupling of both processes. The lethality involved in the corresponding alterations may be exploited for designing new antifungals, hopefully with an efficient fungicidal effect.

The advancement in the basic knowledge of fungal wall synthesis and autolysis, specifically from the molecular biology point of view, represents the obvious way for characterizing cell wall vital functions and the extent of lethality which could be involved in the inhibition or alteration of these functions. Progress in this direction should also contribute to new antifungals development in three respects:

(i) By allowing the design of inhibitors of essential enzymes once the corresponding genes have been cloned and characterized.

(ii) By establishing a detailed comparison of proteins with similar functions in fungal and mammalian cells, in order to identify specificities of each, so that selectivity in the toxic effects for the fungal cell can be really achieved.

(ii) By contributing new, specific and simple screens for testing many molecules for their potential effects in the vital fungal functions under consideration.

SUMMARY

The growing incidence of systemic fungal infections demands the development of new drugs to overcome the difficulties and limitations of current systemic antifungal chemotherapy. These limitations are due to the reduced selectivity for the fungal parasite of antimycotics currently in use, in addition to the appearance of resistant strains. When considering fungal functions that are really specific to the fungal cell, it becomes clear that the processes leading to the biogenesis of the cell wall do not occur in the mammalian host.

The isolation and characterization of lysis mutants from *S. cerevisiae* and *C. albicans* that are affected in different cell wall functions indicates that several events in cell wall formation can be altered with a lethal effect. A detailed study of these 'lethal points' at the molecular level may lead to the identification of novel antifungal targets whose inhibition may lead to the desired fungicidal effects. Cloning work related to the aforementioned mutants is beginning to reveal the participation of protein kinases in the regulation of events leading to cell wall autolysis. The protein kinases must play a regulatory role in key events in wall formation. Work in progress is expected to lead to a more complete understanding of cell wall autolysis and its regulation as a means to design and/or discover new inhibitors to act on those targets crucial for fungal cell viability.

ACKNOWLEDGEMENTS

Work in the authors laboratory was supported in part by a grant from Glaxo Spain. Support was also obtained from Comision Interministerial de Ciencia y Tecnologia (BI089-0387-C02-01).

REFERENCES

Au-Young J, Robbins P W 1990 Isolation of a chitin synthase gene (*CHS1*) from *Candida albicans* by expression in *Saccharomyces cerevisiae*. Molecular Microbiology 4: 197–207

Barrett-Bee K J, Lees J, Henderson W 1982 Variation in the activities of enzymes associated with cell wall metabolism during a growth cycle of *Candida albicans*. FEMS Microbiology Letters 15: 275–278

Boone C, Sommer S S, Hensel A, and Bussey H, 1990 Yeast kre genes provide evidence for a pathway of cell wall β-glucan assembly. Journal of Cell Biology 110: 1833–1843

Bulawa C E, Slater M, Cabib E, Au-Young J, Sburlati A, Adair W L, Robbins P W 1986 The *Saccharomyces cerevisiae* structural gene for chitin synthase is not required for chitin synthesis in vivo. Cell 46: 213–225

Cabib E, Duran A 1975 Simple and sensitive procedure for screening yeast mutants that lyse at non-permissive temperatures. Journal of Bacteriology 124: 1604–1606

Cabib E, Silverman S J, Sburlati A, Slater M L 1990 Chitin synthesis in yeast (*Saccharomyces cerevisiae*). In: Kuhn P J, Trinci A P J, Jung M J, Goosey M W, Copping L G (eds) Biochemistry of cell walls and membranes in fungi. Springer-Verlag, Berlin, pp 31–41

Cabib E 1991 Differential inhibition of chitin synthetases 1 and 2 from *Saccharomyces cerevisiae* by polyoxin D and nikkomycins. Antimicrobial Agents and Chemotherapy 35: 170–173

Cassone A, Mason R E, Kerridge D 1981 Lysis of growing yeast-form cells of *Candida albicans* by echinocandin: a cytological study. Sabouraudia 19: 97–110

Cenamor R, Molina M, Galdona J, Sanchez M, Nombela C 1987 Production and secretion of *Saccharomyces cerevisiae* β-glucanases: differences between protoplast and periplasmic enzymes. Journal of General Microbiology 133: 619–628

127

Courchesne W E, Kunisawa R, Thorner J 1989 A putative protein kinase overcomes pheromone-induced arrest of cell cycling in *Saccharomyces cerevisiae*. Cell 58: 1107–1119

de la Fuente J M, Alvarez A, Nombela C, Sanchez M 1991 Flow cytometric analysis of *Saccharomyces cerevisiae* autolytic mutants and protoplast. Yeast (in press)

del Rey F, Garcia-Acha I, Nombela C 1979 The regulation of β-glucanase synthesis in fungi and yeast. Journal of General Microbiology 110: 83–89

del Rey F, Santos T, Garcia-Acha I, Nombela C 1980 Synthesis of β-glucanases during sporulation in *Saccharomyces cerevisiae*: formation of a new sporulation-specific 1,3-β-glucanase. Journal of Bacteriology 143: 621–627

Elion E A, Grisafi P L, Fink G R 1990 *FUS3* encodes a cdc2 + /CDC28 related kinase required for the transition from mitosis into conjugation. Cell 60: 649–664

Elorza M V, Rico H, Sentandreu R 1983 Calcofluor white alters the assembly of chitin fibrils in *Saccharomyces cerevisiae* and *Candida albicans* cells. Journal of General Microbiology 129: 1577–1582

Elorza M V, Murgui A, Sentandreu R 1985 Dimorphism in *Candida albicans*: contribution of mannoproteins to the architecture of yeast and mycelial cell walls. Journal of General Microbiology 131: 2209–2216

Elorza M V, Marcilla A, Sentandreu R 1988 Wall mannoproteins of the yeast and mycelial cells of *Candida albicans*: nature of the glycosidic bonds and polydispersity of their mannan moieties. Journal of General Microbiology 134: 2393–2403

Fleet G H, Phaff H J 1981 Fungal glucans. Structure and metabolism. In: Tanner W, Loewus F A (eds) Plant carbohydrates II. Extracellular carbohydrates. Encyclopedia of plant physiology: new series. Springer-Verlag, Berlin, pp 516–440

Fleet G H 1984 The occurrence and function of endogenous wall-degrading enzymes in yeasts. In: Nombela C (ed) Microbial cell wall synthesis and autolysis. Elsevier, Amsterdam, pp 227–238

Gooday G W, Humphreys A M, McIntosh W H 1986 Roles of chitinases in fungal growth. In: Muzzarelli R A A, Jeuniaux C, Gooday G W (eds) Chitin in nature and technology. Plenum Press, New York, pp 83–91

Gopal P K, Shepherd M G, Sullivan P A 1984 Analysis of wall glucans from yeast, hyphal and germ tube forming cells of *Candida albicans*. Journal of General Microbiology 130: 3295–3301

Hall G S, Myles C, Pratt K J, Washington J A 1988 Cilofungin (LY121019), an antifungal agent with specific activity against *Candida albicans* and *Candida tropicalis*. Antimicrobial Agents and Chemotherapy 32: 1331–1335

Kang M S, Cabib E 1986 Regulation of fungal cell wall growth: a guanine nucleotide-binding, proteinaceous component required for activity of (1–3)-β-D-glucan synthase. Proceedings of the National Academy of Sciences of USA 83: 5808–5812

Klebl F, Tanner W 1989 Molecular cloning of a cell wall exo-β-1,3-glucanase from *Saccharomyces cerevisiae*. Journal of Bacteriology 171: 6259–6264

Kopecka M 1984 Lysis of growing cells of *Saccharomyces cerevisiae* induced by papulacandin B. Folia Microbiologica 29: 115–119

Levin D E, Bishop J M 1990 A putative protein kinase gene (*kin1+*) is important for growth polarity in *Schizosaccharomyces pombe*. Proceedings of the National Academy of Sciences of USA 87: 8272–8276

Marcilla A, Elorza M V, Mormeneo S, Rico H, Sentandreu R 1991 *Candida albicans* mycelial wall structure: supramolecular complexes released by zymolyase, chitinase and β-mercaptoethanol. Archives of Microbiology 155: 312–319

Martin H, Arroyo J, Molina M, Sanchez M, Nombela C 1991 (Unpublished)

Meaden P, Hill K, Wagner J, Slipetz D, Sommer S A, Bussey H 1990 The yeast kre5 gene encodes a probable endoplasmic reticulum protein required for (1–6)-β-D-glucan synthesis and normal cell growth. Molecular Cell Biology 10: 3013–3019

Milewski S, Chmara H, Borowski E 1986 Antibiotic tetaine: a selective inhibitor of chitin and mannoprotein biosynthesis in *Candida albicans*. Archives of Microbiology 145: 234–240

Mizoguchi J, Saito T, Mizuno K, Hayano K 1977. On the mode of action of a new antifungal antibiotic, aculeacin A: inhibition of cell wall synthesis in *Saccharomyces cerevisiae*. Journal of Antibiotics 30: 308–313

Molina M, Cenamor R, Nombela C 1987 Exo-1,3-β-glucanase activity in *Candida albicans*: effect of the yeast-to-mycelium transition. Journal of General Microbiology 133: 609–617

Nebreda A R, Villa T G, Villanueva J R, del Rey F 1986 Cloning of genes related to exo-β-glucanase production in *Saccharomyces cerevisiae*: characterization of an exo-β-glucanase structural gene. Gene 47: 245–259

Nombela C, Santamaria C 1984 Genetics of yeast cell wall autolysis. In: Nombela C (ed) Microbial cell wall synthesis and autolysis. Elsevier, Amsterdam, pp 249–260

128

Nombela C, Molina M, Cenamor R, Sanchez M 1988 Yeast β-glucanases: a complex system of secreted enzymes. Microbiological Sciences 5: 328–332

Payton M A, de Tiani M 1990 The isolation of osmotic-remedial conditional lethal mutants of *Candida albicans*. Current Genetics 17: 293–296

Reed S I, Hadwiger J A, Lörincz A T 1985 Protein kinase activity associated with the product of the yeast cell division cycle gene *CDC28*. Proceedings of the National Academy of Sciences of USA 82: 4055–4059

Ribas J C, Roncero C, Rico H, Duran A 1991 Characterization of a *Schizosaccharomyces pombe* morphological mutant altered in the galactomannan content. FEMS Microbiology Letters 79: 263–268

Sansegundo P, del Rey F 1991 Personal communication

Santos T, Sanchez M, Villanueva J R, Nombela C 1978 Regulation of the β-1,3-glucanase system in *Penicillium italicum*: glucose repression of the various enzymes. Journal of Bacteriology 133: 465–471

Santos T, del Rey F, Villanueva J R, Nombela C 1982 A mutation (*exb1-1*) that abolishes exo-1,3-β-glucanase production does not affect cell-wall dynamics in *Saccharomyces cerevisiae*. FEMS Microbiology Letters 13: 259–263

Shaw J A, Mol P C, Bowers B, Silverman S J, Valdivieso M H, Duran A, Cabib E 1991 The function of chitin synthetase 2 and chitin synthetase 3 in *Saccharomyces cerevisiae* cell cycle. Journal of Cell Biology (in press)

Shepherd M G 1991 Function and architecture of *Candida albicans* cell wall. In: XI Congress of the International Society for Human and Animal Mycology. Program and abstracts volume. Canada, p 44

Silverman S J, Sburlati A, Slater M L, Cabib E 1988 Chitin synthase 2 is essential for septum formation and cell division in *Saccharomyces cerevisiae*. Proceedings of the National Academy of Sciences of USA 85: 4735–4739

Snyder M, Gehrung S, Page B, Madden K, Costigan C 1991 Analysis of cell polarity and cell morphogenesis in *Saccharomyces cerevisiae*. In: Yeast genetics and molecular biology meeting. Program and abstract volume. San Francisco, p 63

Stack J, Herman P, Emr S 1991 Protein kinase complex required for vacuolar protein sorting in yeast. In: Yeast genetics and molecular biology meeting. Program and abstract volume. San Francisco, p 60

Sullivan P A, Yin C Y, Molloy C, Templeton M D, Shepherd M G 1983 An analysis of the metabolism and cell wall composition of *Candida albicans* during germ tube formation. Canadian Journal of Microbiology 29: 1514–1525

Torres L, Martin H, Garcia-Sez M I, Arroyo A, Molina M, Sanchez M, Nombela C 1991 A protein kinase gene complements the lytic phenotype of *Saccharomyces cerevisiae lyt2* mutants. Journal of Molecular Microbiology (in press)

Valdivieso M H, Mol P C, Shaw A, Cabib E, Duran A 1991 *CAL1* a gene required for activity of chitin synthetase 3 in *Saccharomyces cerevisiae*. Journal of Cell Biology (in press)

Discussion of paper presented by C. Nombela

Discussed by M. G. Shepherd
Reported by M. V. Hayes

In his discussion of Dr Nombela's paper, Dr Shepherd re-emphasized the importance of fungal walls as potential sites for new antifungals. He highlighted two
obvious advantages of these target sites. Firstly, antifungals may not have to
transverse the plasma membrane to reach their target and secondly, many of the
wall components are not found in mammalian cells. Therefore, these components,
and indeed the enzymes associated with their synthesis and turnover, are favoured
targets for new antifungals.

Nombela stressed the dynamic nature of the cell wall and Dr Shepherd reinforced
this view with data from his own laboratory. Thus, using streptococci that had
been labelled with tritiated methyl thymidine, he measured the effects of various
growth conditions on the ability of *Candida albicans* to adhere to and coaggregate
with the streptococci. There was a small amount of coaggregation of cells when
grown in a defined (phosphate buffered glucose) or a more enriched (yeast nitrogen
base) media at 28° or 37°C. However, starving those *C. albicans* cells for a period
of 30 min allowed almost all of the cells to coaggregate with the streptococci.
Hence, very dynamic changes in adherence properties were seen to occur in the wall
over a very short period. These changes were not associated with the morphogenesis
event (i.e. hyphal formations), but occurred before that event took place. Indeed,
if a protein synthesis inhibitor such as trichodermin was added to the culture, it
abolished the emergence of the coaggregation effectors resulting from the starvation – hence, giving some putative evidence for the occurrence of de novo protein
synthesis during the starvation period. The coaggregation results from a lectin-
type interaction involving a carbohydrate on the cell surface of the streptococci.
Dr Shepherd's group has isolated the carbohydrate which comprises a repeating
sequence of oligosaccharides containing fucose and galactose with phospho-
diester linkages. Dr Shepherd suggested that colonization may represent an
alternative point of intervention for novel antifungals. The targets could be the
molecules necessary for the dynamic change of the wall that is associated with
adherence.

In reviewing the architecture of the fungal cell wall, Dr Shepherd noted that the
mannoproteins on the outer surface of the wall are likely to be associated with
receptors and the molecules for cellular adhesion. Mannoproteins on the outer

130

surface may be some of the molecules that alter during changes on the dynamics of the wall.

Dr Shepherd stressed some of the differences between *Candida* and *Saccharomyces* cell walls, one of the major differences being the amount of β-1,6 glucan. In *C. albicans*, β-1,6 glucan is the major structural component making up 30 or 40% of the components in the wall, whereas in *S. cerevisiae* the β-1,6 glucan is responsible for only 5 or 6% of the glucan. There are also considerable differences in the linkages of the O-linked oligosaccharides for the mannoproteins. However, the greatest differences are in the outer chain, where two examples were given. Firstly, there was more phosphate in the mannoprotein of *C. albicans* and secondly, but more importantly, considerable branching of the *C. albicans* outer chain was observed. Dr Shepherd's group is currently carrying out acetolysis of the *C. albicans* mannoproteins followed by nuclear magnetic resonance analysis to give a greater insight into these structural differences.

In his concluding remarks, Dr Shepherd turned his attention to the linkage of wall polymers. His group has recently confirmed an association between glucan and mannoprotein. Unfortunately, he could not comment on the nature of that linkage. A model for the rearrangement and cross-linking of β-1,3 and β-1,6 glucans was presented. Dr Shepherd made the point that all the rearrangements involving linkages of glucan have to be carried out in the wall in order to give the finished product. He showed evidence for a potential cross-linking enzyme. Pat Sullivan and his colleagues have investigated the *Candida* exoglucanase under various assay conditions using G3 oligosaccharide as a substrate, and were able to demonstrate some glucose transhydrolase activity. The G4 and greater oligosaccharides made up the bulk of the products. Therefore, the enzyme had cross-linking activity although, unfortunately, all of that activity was β-1,3. This still leaves the question of how the β-1,6 glucan is produced in the wall. The enzymes involved in the cross-linking of polymers required for the structural integrity of the wall conceivably represent additional antifungal targets to the wall synthetases.

Several speakers mentioned the difficulty of obtaining vectors that are useful for studying genes from *C. albicans* and *C. cerevisiae*. Dr Shepherd finished his discussion by bringing to the attention of the audience a useful vector that is available from his group. The essential elements of the vector are the *C. albicans* ARS which will function in both *Candida* and *Saccharomyces*, the LEU2 gene from *C. albicans* and the URA3. The LEU2 is useful for selection in *Saccharomyces* AH22 and the URA3 for selection in *C. albicans* SG243. The vector also has ampicillin resistance, an *Escherichia coli* origin of replication, multiple cloning sites and a *lac* gene for selection of inserted DNA.

In general discussion, Dr Nombela responded to a question from Dr Verhoef relating to protein kinase inhibitors as fungicidal agents, by suggesting that the proteins regulated by the kinases may represent better targets than the kinases. Clearly, protein kinases are present in mammalian systems and it would be essential to demonstrate high specificity for an inhibitor before it could be considered as an antifungal agent. The protein kinase described by Dr Nombela differed substantially from other yeast and mammalian protein kinases and may represent a selective target.

Dr Nombela has not investigated the autophosphorylation properties of the

SLT2 protein kinase; however, he did mention that site directed mutagenesis of the active site but not the phosphorylation site abolished the kinase activity. Furthermore, he added that he was planning to attempt to identify similar kinases in *Candida* by complementation studies.

Dr Odds pointed out that with the few substances that do inhibit cell wall synthesis (e.g. nikkomycin, echinocandins), their spectrum of activity is rather limited; however, their enzyme specificity is considerable. He asked whether it is likely that the inhibition of precisely the same enzyme function will have precisely the same effect across a wide range of fungi, or whether it will be necessary to develop variant drugs to deal with a wide range of species. Dr Shepherd responded by providing evidence that in the nikkomycins, the poor activity is a reflection of the inability of the antibiotic to effectively penetrate the cell wall rather than lack of activity against the target enzyme(s). He stressed the importance of access to the drug target.

Dr Nombela commented that it was important to carry out both biochemical and genetic studies of enzymes from different species in order to answer the question of broad spectrum activity. As an example, he cited the exoglucanase of *Saccharomyces* which is not necessary for growth; the counterpart in *Candida* has been cloned by a New Zealand group and once it has been established whether or not it is essential for growth, a clearer view will emerge of its potential as a target for inhibitors.

Dr Cole raised an interesting issue of access when targetting an autolysin with an inhibitor, given that the autolysin is located in a rapidly growing, dynamic wall that is undergoing crystallization. He also suggested that once the nascent polymers were converted to a crystallized form, particularly involving cross-linking of glucans, the target may be lost. Dr Shepherd did not necessarily agree with this view, suggesting that the ease with which he can make protoplasts would indicate that it is possible to gain access to targets and make them susceptible. He commented that perhaps as an alternative approach to inhibition of autolysins we perhaps should consider the activation of them. He added that his group has cloned a chitobiase and he was looking at a strategy for activation of this hydrolase.

8. Molecular genetics of dimorphism in *Candida albicans*

C. Birse, W. A. Fonzi, S. Saporito, M. Irwin, P. S. Sypherd

INTRODUCTION

The difficulty of pursuing the dimorphism of *Candida albicans* at the genetic level would be all too daunting, were it not for the imperatives of human disease. On the one hand *C. albicans* has no sexual cycle to facilitate the experimental recombination of genes, and it is permanently diploid, reducing the convenience of mutations in studying aspects of its biology. The rise in systemic candidosis associated with the increase in AIDS and in the use of cytotoxic drugs in the treatment of cancers, gives urgency to studies aimed at understanding features of the organism that make it pathogenic. Our interest has been in understanding, at the molecular level, control of the events that lead to morphogenetic transition from yeasts to hyphae, events that undoubtedly lead to invasiveness and pathology.

From a theoretical perspective, the morphogenetic events in *C. albicans* can be viewed within the context of developmental systems that involve an extrinsic signal, including environmental stress, and morphological change in response to that signal. Although this context can be made very complex to accommodate a vast array of systems, it can also be generalized to include the following events: (1) generation of an environmental signal; (2) signal perception and processing; (3) development of appropriate intracellular biochemistry, including the movement and/or activation of enzyme packets (vesicles); and finally (4) the synthesis of new cellular structures from new or redesigned macromolecules. Biological models abound for attacking each of these and related events, from the signalling by a hormone (i.e. pheromone), and secondary messengers for signal transduction, to the intracellular transport of organelles by processes that involve cytoskeletal elements. Thus, the problems are beautifully poised for genetic approaches, but ironically in an organism seemingly designed by nature to thwart their implementation.

The gloom surrounding mounting a genetic attack on dimorphism in *C. albicans* was only partially dispelled by the heroic efforts of Sarachek & Bish (1976), Kwon-Chung & Hill (1970) and Poulter et al (1981) to develop mutants and 'parasexual' analyses, since these approaches were both tortuous (to the investigators) and labour intensive. For the molecular biologist, the development of molecular genetics, using transformation and recombinant DNA techniques (Kurtz et al 1986,

1987), literally forged a new frontier of research for understanding the molecular nature and the control of dimorphism in *C. albicans*.

The role played by hyphal formation in the pathogenesis of *C. albicans* has been investigated extensively and recently reviewed (Odds 1985, 1988), with the weight of the evidence confirming the relationship. Our own emphasis on the events of hyphal formation rests on two hypotheses: that hyphal formation results from the activation of gene products not expressed in yeasts, and that these gene products will be potentially useful as the targets for new and potent antifungals.

Since the focus of our efforts is on *genes*, we have taken two approaches using the new molecular genetic tools. The first of these was to use heterologous gene probes in an attempt literally to guess if the analogous genes in *C. albicans* would show changes in levels of expression during the yeast–hyphal transition. The second approach, which has a similar degree of uncertainty to the first, has been to clone genes that are differentially expressed during hyphal formation, and then attempt to determine the functions of these genes.

HETEROLOGOUS GENE PROBES

In our earlier work on dimorphism in *Mucor racemosus*, we found that the gene for the protein synthesis factor EF-1α, was represented by three unlinked copies that yielded identical proteins when translated. Knowing of the differential expression of the actin gene family during development in *Drosophila* (Fyrberg et al 1983), we used oligonucleotide probes specific for each EF-1α gene, and found that there was a bias in the transcription of these three genes during morphogenesis.

Attempting to transfer these findings to *C. albicans*, we used a *M. racemosus* EF-1α gene probe to identify two genes for EF-1α in *C. albicans*. Each gene from *C. albicans*, while yielding identical proteins, had sufficient heterogeneity in the 3′ untranslated region of the mRNA to allow us to prepare gene specific oligo-nucleotide probes. Using these probes we found that both genes were transcribed (Sundstrom et al 1990), and appeared to be translated (Sundstrom et al 1991), but neither appeared to be expressed differentially between yeast and hyphal forms (Sundstrom et al 1990).

Pursuing elongation factors further, we focused attention on EF-3, a factor believed to be specific to fungi (Kamath & Chakraburtty 1989, Qin et al 1987, Skogerson & Wakatama 1976) By using a probe from the EF-3 gene of *Saccharomyces cerevisiae* (provided by Calvin McLaughlin) we examined the DNA of *C. albicans* and *Pneumocystis carinii*. The latter organism was examined because although its phylogeny is in doubt, recent evidence suggests that it is a fungus (Edman et al 1988). We have cloned the genes for EF-3 from both *C. albicans* and *P. carinii* and shown them to be highly homologous to the EF-3 of *S. cerevisiae*. These data add support to both the notion that EF-3 could be a useful antifungal target, and to the fungal nature of *P. carinii*.

Our next choice of heterologous probes was based upon some evidence of the biochemistry of the process. For example, it has been suggested that calcium and calmodulin (Paranjape et al 1990, Sabie & Gadd 1989, Roy & Datta 1987) play a role in promoting hyphal growth in dimorphic fungi. We regarded these clues as

134

important ones, since they fit into our model mentioned above, that involved signal processing and cytoskeletal movement of vesicles in order to bring about the change in morphology. Calcium and its carrier, calmodulin, are of course involved in many physiological processes, but there did not seem to be a great intellectual leap to imagine a role for calmodulin in either a signal process involving triphosphoinositol (Berridge et al 1984) or in the control of cytoskeletal assembly and activity (Greer & Schekman 1982).

Cloning and characterization of the calmodulin gene

Using a probe containing the calmodulin gene of *Saccharomyces cerevisiae* (provided by Jeremy Thorner), the *C. albicans* calmodulin gene was isolated from a genomic lambda library containing *C. albicans* SC5314 DNA completely digested with *Hind*III (provided by Myra Kurtz & Donald Kirsch; Squibb Pharmaceuticals). A 3.8 kb *Hind*III insert was subcloned in M13mp18 and designated pSMS11. The calmodulin gene was localized within the insert of pSMS11. Southern blots of total SC5314 DNA digested with one of several restriction endonucleases were probed with a subfragment of the calmodulin gene. In each digest, a single hybridizing band was detected, suggesting that calmodulin is encoded by a single gene in *C. albicans* (Fig. 8.1). Multiple calmodulin genes have been characterized in several organisms including man (Fischer et al 1988), frog (Chien & Dawid 1984) and a trypanosome (Tschudi et al 1985), while unique genes have been identified in *Drosophila* (Smith et al 1987), *Dictyostelium* (Goldhagen & Clarke 1986) and yeast (Davis et al 1986, Takeda & Yamamoto 1987). The genomic sequence, along with

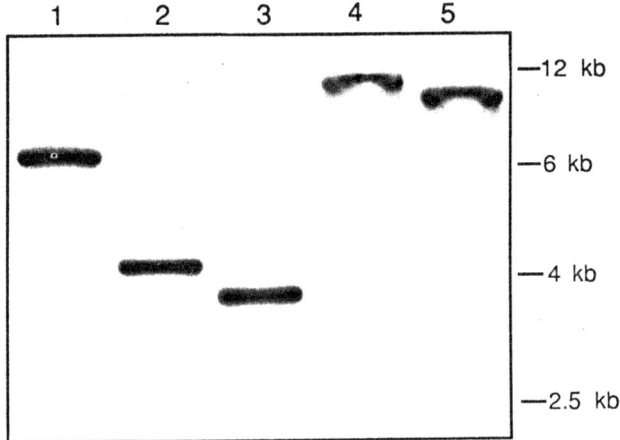

Fig. 8.1 Southern blot analysis of *C. albicans* genomic DNA. Approximately 10 µg genomic SC5314 DNA was cut with several restriction endonucleases; *Bgl*II (lane 1), *Eco*RI (lane 2), *Hind*III (lane 3), *Pst*I (lane 5), and *Xho*I (lane 6). DNA fragments were separated on a 1% agarose gel in 1 × TBE and transferred to nylon membrane. The probe consisted of a 300 bp *Hind*II genomic DNA fragment identified in a genomic library of *Candida* DNA by hybridization to the *CMD1* gene of *S. cerevisiae*. pSMS11 was ^{32}P-labelled using the random primer method (Feinberg & Vogelstein 1984) and used as a probe. The hybridization buffer consisted of 5 × SSPRE (0.75 M NaCl, 0.005 M EDTA, 0.05M sodium phosphate, pH 7.4), 50% formamide 5 × Denhardts (0.1% Ficoll, 0.1% polyvinylpyrrolidone, 0.1% BSA), 0.1% SDS and 200 µg/ml denatured salmon sperm DNA. Hybridizations and washes were carried out under relatively low stringency conditions (25°C).

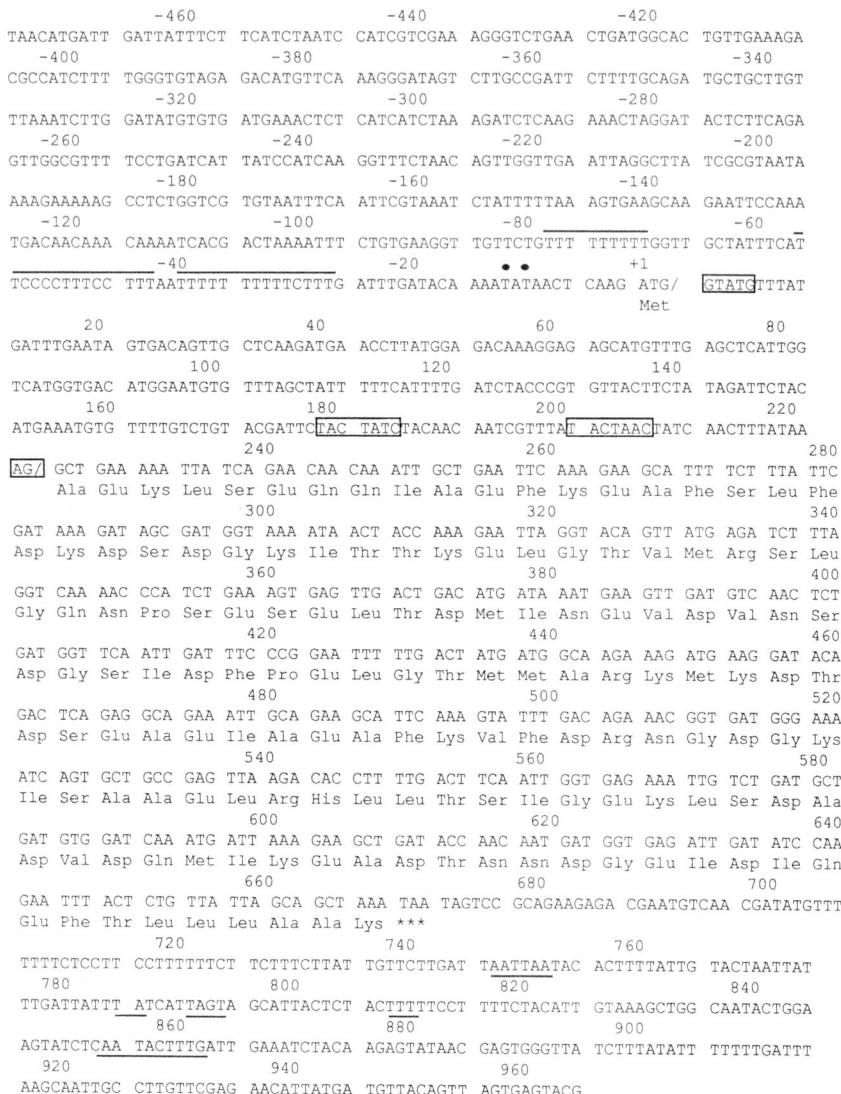

Fig. 8.2 The nucleotide and deduced amino acid sequence of the *CMD1* gene. The numbering indicates the distance, in nt, from the start of the first exon. The arrows indicate the 5′ termini of two cDNA clones examined. Pyrimidine tracts are overlined. The 5′/GTATGT, internal TACTAAC and TACTATC, and 3′ AG/splice signals are boxed. The stop codon is denoted by***. Possible termination and polyadenylation signals are underlined. The nucleotide sequence data reported in this paper have been submitted to GenBank and assigned the accession number M61128. The nucleotide sequence was determined by the dideoxy chain termination method (Sanger et al 1977, Tabor & Richardson 1987) with M13 universal sequencing primers or prepared oligonucleotide primers (Operon) and the Sequenase kit (US Biochemical Corp.).

the deduced amino acid sequence for the *C. albicans CMD1* gene is shown in Figure 8.2. Comparison of a cDNA sequence to the genomic sequences identified a putative intron of 222 bp immediately following the initiating ATG codon. An intron positioned immediately following the start codon has been conserved in the cal-

SEQUENCE COMPARISONS BETWEEN CALMODULIN OF CANDIDA ALBICANS AND OTHER ORGANISMS

```
C. albicans    MAEKLSEQQI AEFKEAFSLF DKDSDGKITT KELGTVMRSL GQNPSESELT DMINEVDVNS
S. cerevisiae  -SSN-T-E-- ------A--- ---NN-S-SS S--A------ -LS---A-VN -LM--I--DG
S. pombe       TTRN-TDE-- ---R------ -R-Q--N--S N---V----- --S-TAA--Q ------ADG
A. nidulans    --DS-T-E-V S-Y------- --G--Q---- ---------- ---------Q ----EADN
A. klebsiana   --DQ-T---- ----G----- --G--T---- --V------- ----T-A--Q -----ADG
Tetrahymena    --DQ-T-E-- ---------- --G--T---- ---------- ----T-A--Q -----ADG
Bovine brain   --DQ-T-E-- ---------- --G--T---- ---------- ----T-A--Q -----ADG

C. albicans    DGSTDFPEFL TMMARKMKDT DSEAEIA#AF KVFDRNGDGK ISAAELRHLL TSIGEKLSDA
S. cerevisiae  NHQ-E-S--- AL-S-QL-SN ---Q-LLE-- ----K----L ----K-V--- -----T---
S. pombe       N-T---T--- ---------- -N-E-VRE-- ----K---Y -TVE--T-V- --L--R--QE
A. nidulans    N-T------- ---------- ---E--RE-- -----DNN-F --------VM -----T-D
A. klebsiana   N-[------- ---------- ---E--LE-- QG--KD-N-F --------MM -NL----T-E
Tetrahymena    --T------- SL-------- ---E-LIE-- ---D--L- -T-----VM -NL----T-E
Bovine brain   N-T------- ---------- ---E--RE-- R---KD-N-Y --------VM -NL----T-E

C. albicans    DVDQMIKEAD TNNDGEIDIQ EFTLLLAAK    149
S. cerevisiae  F--D-LR-VS #DGS---N-- Q-AA--SK     147   60%
S. pombe       E-AD--R--- -DG--V-NYE --SRVISS-    149   61%
A. nidulans    E--E--R--- QDG--R--VN --VQ-MMQK    149   69%
A. klebsiana   E--E--R--- IDG--Q-NTE --VRMMMSK    149   70%
Tetrahymena    E--E--R--- IDG--H-NYE --VRMM-      147   71%
Bovine brain   E--E--R--- IDG--QV-YE --VQMMTAK    148   71%
```

Fig. 8.3 Alignment of the amino acid sequences from the calmodulin genes from *C. albicans*, *S. cerevisiae* (Davis et al 1986), *S. pombe* (Takeda & Yamamoto 1987), *A. nidulans* (Rasmussen et al 1990), *A. klebsiana* (LeJohn 1989) and bovine brain (Watterson et al 1980). Identical residues are represented as a dash (–). The # symbol indicates a one residue gap introduced into the *S. cerevisiae* and *C. albicans* sequence to give maximal alignment with the other proteins. Putative calcium binding domains are overlined. The number of total amino acid residues of each protein is given. The degree of identity is calculated in per cent identical residues.

137

modulin genes of *C. albicans, Schizosaccharomyces pombe* (Takeda & Yamamoto 1987) and *Aspergillus nidulans* (Rassmussen et al 1990).

Both the 5' splice junction ARTG/GTATGT and the 3' splice junction AG/GCT of the intron match the consensus splice site sequences identified in other eukaryotes (Mount 1982). In addition to the splice site sequence homology, the calmodulin intron contains a short internal sequence identified in fungal introns. In *S. cerevisiae*, the TACTAAC box has been shown to be essential for efficient splicing (Langford et al 1984). In the *C. albicans* calmodulin intron, an exact match of the TACTAAC box is located 15 bp upstream from the 3' splice junction and a slightly degenerate second box, TACTATC is found 14 bp upstream from the first. Such internal sequences have been found in all of the *C. albicans* introns examined thus far (Smith et al 1988, Losberge & Ernst 1989a). Although the role of such boxes in *C. albicans* has yet to be examined, it may be assumed that they also function as internal guides for the splicing machinery (Langford & Gallwitz 1983, Langford et al 1984).

By comparison to the consensus polyadenylation sequences identified by Proudfoot & Brownlee (1976), a potential polyadenylation signal AATTAA, was found in the 3' flanking squences centred at nucleotide +753. The tripartite termination sequence (TAG ... TAGT ... TTT) of *S. cerevisiae* has been found in the downstream regions of several *C. albicans* genes (Au-Young & Robbins 1990, Sundstrom et al 1990) but not all (Koser et al 1990). The sequences in Figure 8.2 show that this termination consensus sequence is absent in the *CMD1* gene, although related sequences can be found. The sequence CAATACTTTG at position 856–865 may also be important in transcriptional termination of the *CMD1* gene. The similar sequence CAATATTTG has been shown to be the site of transcription termination in some yeast genes (Henikoff et al 1983, Henikoff & Cohen 1984).

Alignment of the deduced amino acid sequence of *C. albicans* calmodulin with the calmodulins of other organisms is shown in Figure 8.3. When compared to analogous genes of other species, the *Candida* gene usually shows the highest degree of amino acid similarity with *S. cerevisiae*; such as elongation factor EF-1α (90%, Sundstrom et al 1990), tubulin (82%, Smith et al 1988) and actin (94%, Losberger & Ernst 1989b). However, only 60% of the amino acid residues of *C. albicans* calmodulin are identical to those of *S. cerevisiae* and *S. pombe*. A higher degree of identity, 70%, is shared with filamentous fungi and the vertebrates. Although the degree of similarity between *C. albicans* calmodulin and the other calmodulins increases when conservative amino acid substitutions are considered, the overall relationship remains the same, with *C. albicans* calmodulin showing a closer relationship to the calmodulins of vertebrates and filamentous fungi than to those of yeast.

Calmodulin mRNA levels in yeast and hyphal cell forms

Increased calmodulin activity has recently been detected during hyphal development (Paranjape et al 1990). Northern analysis was employed to determine if calmodulin gene expression levels also varied during the yeast to hyphal transition. Total RNA was isolated from SC5314 cells grown in non-inducing and hyphal inducing medium (see legend to Fig. 8.4). Steady state RNA levels were measured

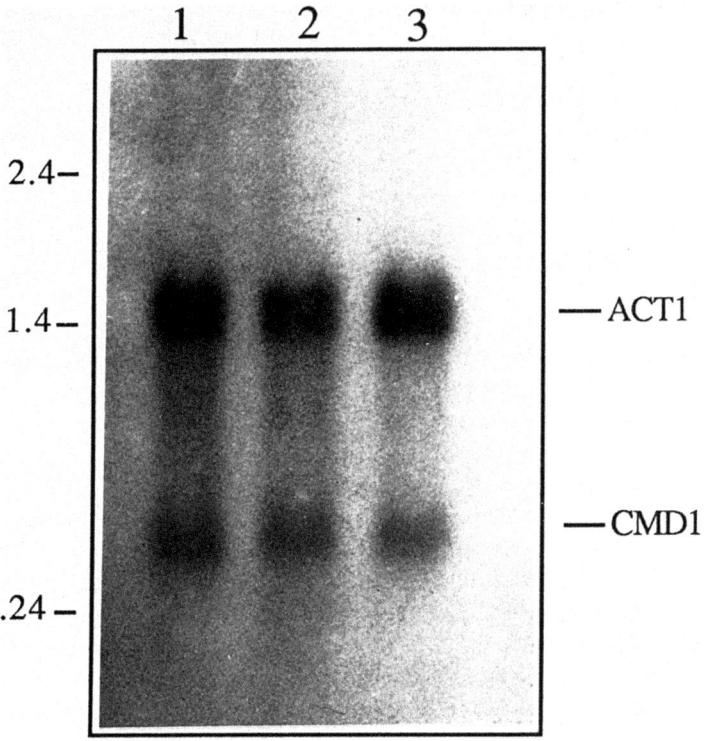

Fig. 8.4 *CMD1* mRNA analysis. The pH mediated hyphal induction method (Brummel & Soll 1982) was used to prepare yeast and hyphal cells. SC5314 cells were grown overnight at 25°C in Lee's medium, pH 4.5 (Lee et al 1975) to stationary phase. The cells were washed in distilled water and suspended to a cell density of 10^7 cells/ml in fresh Lee's medium (pH 4.5, 25°C) to prepare yeast cells or in Lee's medium (pH 6.5, 37°C) to prepare germ tube-forming cells. Cultures were incubated for 2 and 5 h for hyphae induction or for 5 h for yeast growth. Under these conditions, none of the cells grown at pH 4.5 (25°C) had initiated germ tube formation while greater than 98% of the cells grown at pH 6.5 (37°C) had germ tubes. Cells were harvested at appropriate times by adding cycloheximide to a final concentration of 150 μg/ml followed by centrifugation for 10 min at 7 K. The washed cells were suspended in lysis buffer (50 mmol Tris, pH 8.0; 1 mmol EDTA; 200 μg/ml heparin; 0.5% SDS). An equal volume of equilibrated phenol was added and RNA was isolated by vortexing with glass beads at 4°C. The aqueous phase was further extracted with phenol:chloroform (1:1) and chloroform prior to precipitation with ethanol. Total RNA (25 μg per lane) was separated on a 1.2% agarose/1.1% formaldehyde gel in 1 × MOPS buffer (20 mmol MOPS, 5 mmol NaOAc, 0.25 mmol EDTA, pH 7.0), transferred to nitrocellulose and hybridized with a *CMD1* gene specific probe as described in Figure 8.1 and subjected to autoradiography. Steady state RNA levels were detected in yeast cells (lane 1) and in cells pH-induced for hyphal formation for 2 h (lane 2) and 5 h (lane 3). The detection of actin mRNA levels was used as an internal control by rehybridizing the filter with the *C. albicans* actin gene (a gift from Stuart Riggsby, University of Tennessee). Sizes of the RNA species were determined using RNA molecular weight size markers (Bethesda Research Laboratory).

in yeast cells and cells induced for germ tube formation for 2 and 5 h as shown in Figure 8.4. A single 650 nucleotide transcript was detected in both cell types. The level of transcription did not vary significantly in the different morphological forms when normalized to actin mRNA, an internal control. The increased calmodulin activity reported by Paranjape and coworkers (1990) may therefore be due to post-transcriptional regulation of calmodulin rather than mRNA accumulation. Furthermore, specific calmodulin binding proteins, such as kinases, may be activated by the calcium–calmodulin complex in response to morphogenic signals. Paranjape and coworkers (1990) have measured an increase in protein phosphorylation in hyphal cells.

CLONED GENES DIFFERENTIALLY EXPRESS DURING HYPHAL DEVELOPMENT

One of the most intriguing aspects of dimorphism is the possibility that the morphogenesis is accompanied by changes in gene expression. This question has been approached indirectly by several investigators who have analysed the distribution of polypeptides in the two forms using either one- or two-dimensional electrophoresis. In one thorough study, using 2D-PAGE, and pH-induced morphogenesis, Finney et al (1985) identified only two proteins that appeared unique to yeasts and two proteins unique to hyphae, out of a total of over 300 reproducible spots. Similar studies, using alternative means of hyphal induction, have yielded differing results, but when found, there were never more than a few changes between the forms (cf. Soll et al 1990).

The question of differential gene expression has also been studied indirectly by examining potential antigenic differences between yeasts and hyphae (Syverson et al 1975, Brawner & Cutler 1986, Sundstrom et al 1987). Such differences, however, do not distinguish the molecular basis of change, and could be attributed to post-translational modifications involving carbohydrates. Antigenic differences, where found, are usually not unambiguously related to *form* as opposed to the conditions which were used to induce the transition. Our approach, then, was to use differential cDNA hybridization to screen for genes that were developmentally regulated.

Isolation of genes differentially expressed during dimorphism

The experimental design of the screen was to prepare a λ phage cDNA library from cells in the process of hyphae formation and to hybridize plaques of the plated library with labelled first-strand cDNAs prepared from either blastospores (yeast) or hyphae. The first-strand cDNA probes were prepared from cells grown in Lee's medium (Lee et al 1975), pH 4.5, at 25°C, or cells grown in Lee's medium, pH 6.5, at 37°C. The cells grow with a yeast morphology under the former conditions and grow with a hyphal morphology under the latter. These two probes were anticipated to be sensitive to differences due either to morphology or to the environmental conditions of temperature and pH. Temperature and pH are critical environmental parameters; a neutral pH and temperature of approximately 37°C are required for hyphal induction by all of the in vitro regimes.

The experiment was conducted using a *C. albicans* clinical isolate designated SC5314 (Gillum et al 1984). The cDNA library was prepared in the phage vector λ ZAPII (Stratagene) using polyA$^+$ RNA derived from cells induced to form hyphae by incubation for 60 min in tissue culture medium 199 (TC199) (Landau et al 1965). Duplicate plaque lifts of the library were hybridized under standard conditions with one or the other of the first strand cDNA probes (Sambrook et al 1989). Approximately 2000 plaques were screened and 65 plaques which hybridized with the hyphae-derived probe, but not the yeast-derived probe, were identified.

The differentially hybridizing plaques could have been derived from several differentially expressed genes or from a single, highly expressed one. To differentiate which plaques were derived from unique genes, a random primer labelled probe was prepared from a randomly chosen clone and hybridized with a panel containing all 65 isolates. A second clone, which did not hybridize with the first one, was selected, labelled, and hybridized with the same panel of clones. In this manner 21 unique clones were identified. One gene was represented by 27 clones, a second by 20 cDNA clones, and a third by eight cDNA clones. The remainder were represented by one or a few clones.

Genes whose expression correlates with cell length

ECE1, ECE2 and ECE3 (Extent of Cell Elongation) define a particularly intriguing class of genes identified by the differential screen. There appears to be a direct correlation between the level of expression of these genes (i.e. amount of transcript) and the degree of cell elongation. The Northern blot shown in Figure 8.5 illustrates the characteristics of ECE gene expression and the photomicrographs in Figure 8.6 illustrate the corresponding morphology. No expression of ECE1 can be

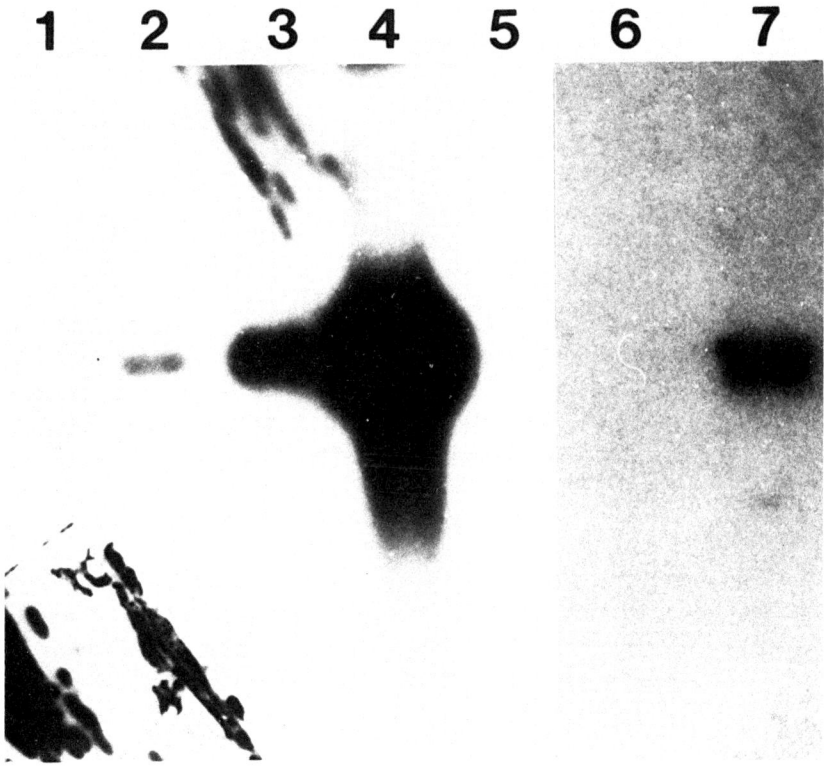

Fig. 8.5 Northern blot analysis of ECE1 expression. Each lane was loaded with 20 μg of RNA from strain SC5314 grown in Lee's medium, pH 4.5, 25°C (lane 1), pH 6.5, 25°C (lane 2), pH 4.5, 37°C (lane 3), pH 6.5, 37°C (lane 4) or from strain SGY 243 grown in Lee's medium, pH 6.5, 37°C (lane 5) or from strain SGY 243 grown in TC199 at 25°C (lane 6) or 37°C (lane 7). The blot was hybridized with the ECE1 cDNA.

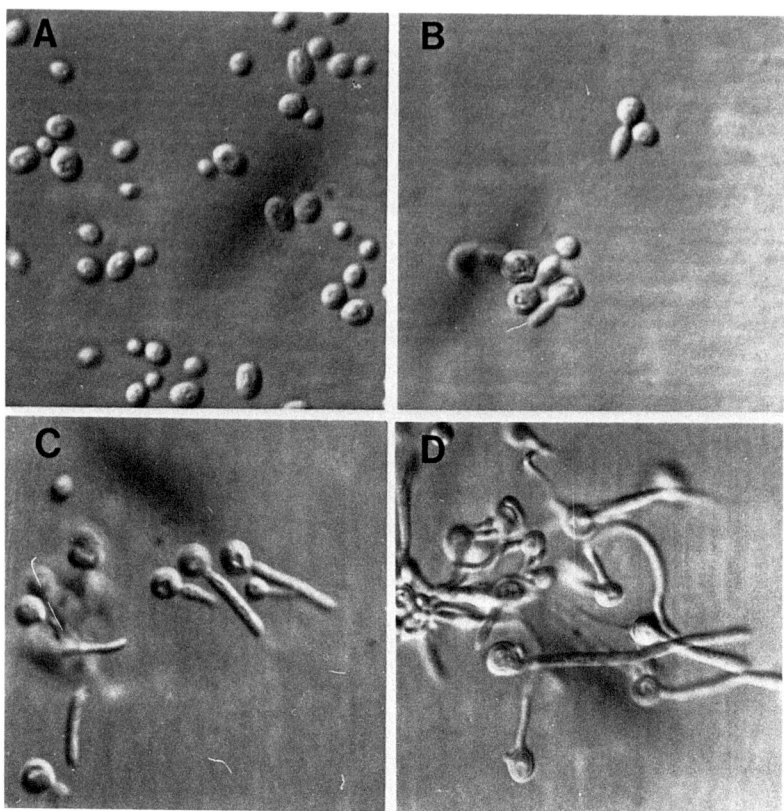

Fig. 8.6 Morphology of strain SC5314 grown in Lee's medium, pH 4.5, 25°C (A), pH 6.5, 25°C (B), pH 4.5, 37°C (C), or pH 6.5, 37°C (D).

detected in cells of strain SC5314 when they are grown as yeast at 25°C in Lee's medium adjusted to pH 4.5 (Fig. 8.5, lane 1), even after 5 days of exposure of the blot shown. These cells exhibit the typical ovoid yeast morphology (Fig. 8.6, panel A). Adjusting the pH of the medium to 6.5 results in an easily detectable, but low, amount of ECE1 expression (Fig. 8.5, lane 2) and results in cells which are still yeast-like, but are distinctly more elongated than the cells cultured at pH 4.5 (Fig. 8.6, panel B). Maintaining the pH at 4.5, but shifting the temperature to 37°C results in a substantial accumulation of ECE1 mRNA (Fig. 8.5, lane 3) and the morphology of the cells is substantially elongated (Fig. 8.6, panel C). Maximal expression of ECE1 is observed when the medium is at pH 6.5 and the cultures are incubated at 37°C (Fig. 8.5, lane 4). Under these culture conditions the most highly elongated cell form, true hyphae, are observed (Fig. 8.6, panel D). The level of ECE expression does not appear to reflect a subpopulation of true hyphae as determined by microscopic examination of the cultures. Expression of ECE2 and ECE3 are qualitatively similar to ECE1 expression (data not shown). ECE1 is rapidly induced upon introduction of stationary phase cells into the culture medium with maximal levels of mRNA accumulating by the time of germ tube emergence (data not shown). Expression is sustained with no evidence of fluctuations during the cell cycle.

142

Additional evidence of the correlation between ECE1 expression and cell elongation was obtained by examining strain SGY243 (Kelly et al 1987). SGY243 (ade2/ade2 Δura3::ADE2ura) is a transformable *C. albicans* strain developed by Kelly et al (1987). This strain is unusual in that growth in Lee's medium, even at a pH of 6.5 and temperature of 37°C, is always in the yeast form. However, it will form hyphae when inoculated into Tissue Culture Medium 199 (TC199) at 37°C. SGY243 is auxotrophic only for uridine and the basis of this media-conditional response is unclear. However, it should be noted that this strain has been heavily mutagenized in the course of its construction and likely bears a number of mutations that may affect its dimorphic response. When strain SGY243 is cultured in Lee's medium at pH 6.5, there is no detectable mRNA for ECE1 at 37°C in accordance with its yeast morphology (Fig. 8.5, lane 5). Similarly, when inoculated into TC199 at 25°C, SGY243 grows as yeast and no ECE1 mRNA is detected (Fig. 8.5, lane 6). However, when inoculated into TC199 at 37°C, hyphae are formed and, correspondingly, ECE1 mRNA is expressed (Fig. 8.5, lane 7). Interestingly, expression of ECE1 in SGY243 does not respond to pH or temperature in Lee's medium as was observed for strain SC5314. This may suggest that these response pathways have been altered in SGY243 and this alteration directly affects its ability to form hyphae.

Consideration of the foregoing data highlights an interesting aspect of dimorphism in *Candida* and the particular significance of these ECE genes. *C. albicans* is generally regarded as having three vegetative morphologies, yeast, pseudohyphae, and hyphae (Odds 1988). Pseudohyphae are distinguished from 'true hyphae' by their budding mode of reproduction, as evidenced by visible constrictions between cells. Individual pseudohyphal cells can vary greatly in length and, in extreme forms, can approximate the appearance of true hyphae. The developmental relationship, if any, between pseudohyphae and true hyphae is unknown. The expression pattern of the ECE genes is the first data to suggest that pseudohyphae result from the *incremental expression* of the constituents of 'true hyphae'. This observation may account, in part, for the inability of previous investigations to detect distinguishing characteristics of hyphae (Soll 1990). The significance of these genes goes beyond an insight into 'dimorphism'. Obviously, the correlation between ECE expression and cell elongation is suggestive of a causal relationship, although this need not be so. But regardless of whether a causal relationship exists or not, expression of the ECE genes is responsive to both temperature and pH, two significant environmental parameters controlling dimorphism. Dissecting the control of ECE gene expression could provide significant insight into the nature of *Candida* dimorphism.

Deletion of the ECE1 gene
To determine if a causal relationship exists between ECE1 gene expression and hyphal development, we have initiated efforts to construct a strain containing homozygous null alleles of this gene. The methods of *C. albicans* gene deletion directly parallel those developed for *S. cerevisiae* (Kelly et al 1987). A DNA fragment containing a selectable marker substituted for the deleted gene sequences is constructed in vitro and used to replace the endogenous genomic region by transformation and homologous integration (Kelly et al 1987). However, since

Candida is a diploid organism (Olaiya & Sogin 1979, Whelan et al 1980), both wild type alleles must be replaced to detect recessive mutations. Constructing homozygous gene deletions is essentially the same as constructing the single allele deletion except that two in vitro constructs must be made containing different selectable markers and the corresponding double mutant strain must be available. The only published account of constructing double deletions via sequential transformation has employed strain SGY484 (Kelly et al 1988), a *ura3 leu2* derivative of strain SGY243, with the URA3 and LEU2 genes used as selectable markers (Kurtz & Marrinan 1989). The disadvantages of this approach are that two in vitro constructs must be made, the *leu2* mutation in SGY484 is unstable (Kurtz & Marrinan 1989), and this strain has been further mutagenized beyond that of SGY243 (Kelly et al 1988). As discussed earlier, SGY243 is already altered in its dimorphic response. In light of these concerns, we have tested an alternate means of constructing the double mutants in *C. albicans* by adapting the method of Alani et al (1987) which utilizes a construct consisting of the *S. cerevisiae* URA3 gene flanked by direct repeats of the *E. coli hisG* gene. An analogous construct for use in *C. albicans* was prepared from plasmid pNK51 (Alani et al 1987). The *S. cerevisiae* URA3 was removed by digestion with *Hind*III and replaced by blunt-end ligation with a 1.36 kb ScaI-XbaI fragment containing the *C. albicans* URA3 gene (Losberger & Ernst 1989a). This construct was used to replace the gene to be deleted. The deleted construct was transformed into *Candida* and *ura*⁺ transformants were selected. The unique advantage of the construct is that subsequent homologous recombination between the direct repeats of the *hisG* sequences results in excision of the URA3 gene. These excision events, which occur at frequencies of 10^{-5} to 10^{-4} (Alani et al 1987), can be selected by plating the cells in the presence of 5-fluoro-orotic acid (5FOA). Only *ura*⁻ cells grow in the presence of 5FOA (Boeke et al 1984). After excision of URA3, the target gene is now deleted and replaced with the *hisG* sequences and the cell is returned to a *ura*⁻ phenotype. A second round of transformation with the same construct should allow the second homologue to be deleted. Thus only a single selectable marker is necessary and only a single in vitro construct need be made. In the case of *S. cerevisiae* the authors reported that this technique could be used to disrupt as many as four genes within

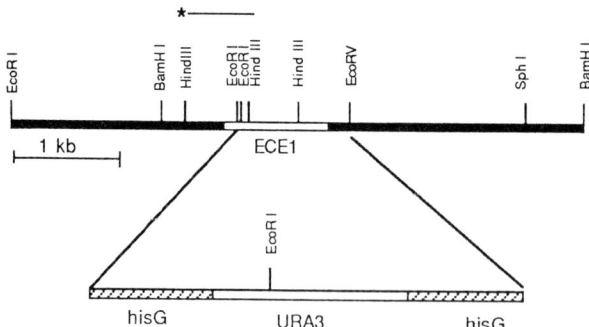

Fig. 8.7 Restriction map of ECE1 gene and construction of deleted construct. The open bar indicates the ECE1 coding region. The bar above the graph indicates the *Hind*III fragment hybridized to the Southern blot in Figure 8.8.

144

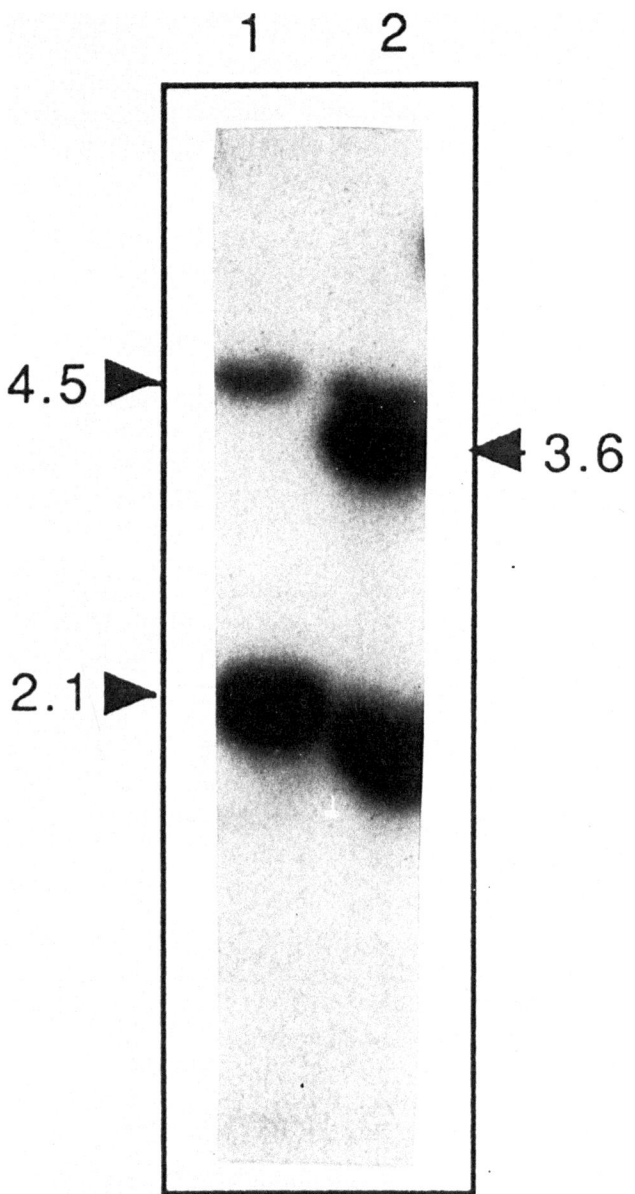

Fig. 8.8 Southern blot analysis of genomic DNA from SGY243 (lane 1) and *his*G-URA3-*his*G transformant (lane 2). The DNA was digested with *Eco*RI and the blot was probed with the ECE1 DNA fragment indicated in Figure 8.7. The size of the hybridizing bands, in kb, are indicated.

one strain without any apparent negative effects. The authors also report that the nature of the flanking sequences is not critical and sequences other than *his*G may be used to further extend the use of the method (Alani et al 1987). The primary requirements of this approach, homologous recombination, URA3 as a selectable marker, and 5FOA selection of *ura⁻* cells, have all been demonstrated for *Candida*

145

(Scherer & Magee 1990, Kelly et al 1987). Consequently, the technique should be directly applicable to *Candida*.

To prepare a null strain deleted of the ECE1 gene, a genomic clone of the gene was isolated from a genomic library in phage lambda using the cDNA as a hybridization probe. The library was prepared by ligation of a partial Sau3A digestion of SC5314 genomic DNA into λ-GEM12 (Promega) (unpublished results). A restriction map of the ECE1 genomic clone and the design of the deletion construct are shown in Figure 8.7. The region between the first *Eco*RI site and the *Eco*RV site, which contains nearly the entire open reading frame of the ECE1 gene, was removed and blunt-end ligated with the 4.0 kb *Bam*HI-*Bgl*II fragment containing the *his*G-URA3-*his*G construct. Following digestion with *Hin*dIII and *Sph*I, which recognize 5′ and 3′ flanking restriction sites respectively, the deleted construct was transformed into strain SGY243 as described in Kurtz et al (1986). A Southern blot of one of the transformants is shown in Figure 8.8. The presence of an additional 3.6 kb hybridizing band in the transformant indicated that the correct integration event occurred. This additional band also hybridized with *his*G DNA as expected (data not shown). Thus, this strain contains a heterozygous deletion of the ECE1 gene.

The transformant shown above was inoculated into defined medium (2% glucose and Difco yeast nitrogen base) and grown to stationary phase. The stationary phase cells were spread on 5FOA plates to select *ura*⁻ cells which would occur by an intragenic recombination between flanking *his*G sequences. The *ura*⁻ derivatives were obtained at a variable frequency of 0.3 to 10×10^{-5}. Twenty six *ura*⁻ colonies were picked and screened by Southern blot hybridization. Of the 26 isolates, three retained *his*G sequences, suggesting that approximately one in eight *ura*⁻ clones were derived from intragenic recombination events between the *his*G sequences flanking the URA3 marker gene.

Nucleotide sequence of ECE1
The nucleotide sequence and the predicted translation product of the ECE1 gene are shown in Figure 8.9. A 675 bp open reading frame was present which was somewhat shorter than the approximately 1 kb mRNA observed in Northern blots. The open reading frame could encode a protein 225 amino acids in length. Neither the nucleotide sequence or the presumptive polypeptide contained discernible homology with any of the sequences present in the Genbank computer files. The protein contains two interesting features including three tandem repeats of the sequence Ala-Pro-Ala and multiple dispersed repeats of the sequence Lys-Arg-Asp. The functional significance, if any, of these features is not yet clear.

Hyphal-specific genes
Two differentially expressed genes, HSG1 and HSG2 (Hyphal-Specific Gene), appear to be expressed only in hyphae. As seen in the Northern blot in Figure 8.10, HSG1 mRNA is observed only in SC5314 cells incubated in Lee's medium at pH 6.5 and 37°C (lane 4) where true hyphae form, but not when the cells are incubated at lower pH or lower temperature (lanes 1, 2 and 3). HSG1 is also expressed in SC5314 cells induced to form hyphae by serum, proline, or N-acetylglucosamine (data not shown). Since all of these inducing conditions have in

AGAATTGAAGATATAAATACATCAAATAACCCACCTATTTC

AAAATTGTTTTATTTTTGTTTATCTCTACAACAAACAACTTTCCTTTATTTTTACTACCAACTATTTTCCATTCGTTAAA

```
121/1                                151/11
ATG AAA TTC TCC AAA ATT GCC TGT GCT ACT GTT TTT GCT TTA TCT TCT CAA GCT GCC ATC
Met lys phe ser lys ile ala cys ala thr val phe ala leu ser ser gln ala ala ile
181/21                               211/31
ATC CAC CAT GCT CCA GAA TTC AAC ATG AAG AGA GAT GTT GCT CCA GCT GCC CCA GCT GCT
ile his his ala pro glu phe asn met lys arg asp val ala pro ala ala pro ala ala
241/41                               271/51
CCA GCT GAC CAA GCA CCT ACT GTT CCT GCA CCT CAA GAA TTC AAT ACT GCT ATT ACC AAA
pro ala asp gln ala pro thr val pro ala pro gln glu phe asn thr ala ile thr lys
301/61                               331/71
AGA AGT ATT ATT GGA ATT ATT ATG GGT ATT CTT GGC AAC ATT CCA CAA GTA ATC CAA ATC
arg ser ile ile gly ile ile met gly ile leu gly asn ile pro gln val ile gln ile
361/81                               391/91
ATC ATG AGT ATT GTC AAA GCT TTC AAA GGT AAC AAG AGA GAA GAT ATT GAT TCT GTT GTT
ile met ser ile val lys ala phe lys gly asn lys arg glu asp ile asp ser val val
421/101                              451/111
GCT GGT ATC ATT GCT GAT ATG CCA TTT GTT GTC AGA GCT GTT GAC ACA GCC ATG ACT TCT
ala gly ile ile ala asp met pro phe val val arg ala val asp thr ala met thr ser
481/121                              511/131
GTT GCT TCT ACC AAG AGA GAT GGA GCT AAT GAT GAC.GTT GCT AAT GCC GTC GTC AGA TTG
val ala ser thr lys arg asp gly ala asn asp asp val ala asn ala val val arg leu
541/141                              571/151
CCA GAA ATT GTT GCT CGT GTT GCC ACT GGT GTT CAA CAA TCC ATC GAA AAT GCC AAG AGA
pro glu ile val ala arg val ala thr gly val gln gln ser ile glu asn ala lys arg
601/161                              631/171
GAT GGC GTT CCA GAT GTT GGC CTT AAT CTT GTT GCT AAT GCT CCA AGA CTT ATC TCT AAC
asp gly val pro asp val gly leu asn leu val ala asn ala pro arg leu ile ser asn
661/181                              691/191
GTT TTT TTA TCT CTA ACG TTT TTG ATG GCG TCC TGG AAA CTG TTC AAC AAG CTA AGA GAG
val phe leu ser leu thr phe leu met ala ser trp lys leu phe asn lys leu arg glu
721/201                              751/211
ATG GTC TTG AAG ATT TTC TTG ATG AAC TTC TTC AAA GAC TCC CAC AAC TCA TTA CTA GAT
met val leu lys ile phe leu met asn phe phe lys asp ser his asn ser leu leu asp
781/221
CAG CTG AAT CTG CTT TGA AAGACAGTCAACCAGTTAAAAGAGATGCCGGCTCAGTAGCACTTAGCAATTTAAT
gln leu asn leu leu OPA
```

Fig. 8.9 Nucleotide sequence and predicted protein of the ECE1 gene.

common a near neutral pH and a temperature of 37°C, it is not possible to determine whether HSG expression is specific to morphology or specific to the environmental conditions. Nonetheless, HSG expression is more tightly controlled and does not exhibit the incremental expression apparent with the ECE genes. It

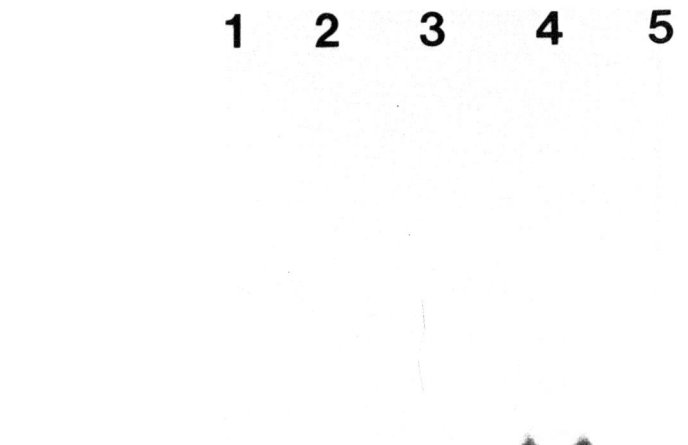

Fig. 8.10 Northern blot analysis of HSG1 expression. Each lane was loaded with 20 μg of RNA from strain SC5314 grown in Lee's medium, pH 4.5, 25°C (lane 2), pH 4.5, 37°C (lane 3), pH 6.5, 37°C (lane 4), or from strain SGY243 grown in Lee's medium, pH 6.5, 37°C (lane 5). The blot was hybridized with HSG1 cDNA.

might be noted that HSG1 is not expressed in strain SGY243 incubated in Lee's medium, pH 6.5, at 37°C (lane 5), conditions which do not elicit hyphae formation in this strain.

pH-responsive genes

The pH of the external environment appears to be an important parameter monitored by *C. albicans* in its morphological decision making (Odds 1988). In more general terms, the ability to respond and adapt to changes in the pH of the external environment would seem to be of particular significance to organisms, such as *Candida*, that inhabit the vertebrate gut and must cope with extreme variations in external pH. Thus, it is not surprising that differential expression in response to external pH has been demonstrated for several intestinal inhabitants including *Escherichia coli* (Bingham et al 1990, Heyde & Portalier 1987, Slonczewski et al 1987), *Shigella flexneri* (Headley & Payne 1990), and *Salmonella typhimurium* (Aliabadi et al 1988). Not only can such responses affect growth and survivability, they can directly affect expression of virulence determinants (Headley & Payne 1990, Miller et al 1989). Similarly, the response of *C. albicans* to changes in external pH may be essential to morphogenesis. There are examples in other cells of the role that pH changes play in regulating intracellular events that have morphogenetic consequences. Increases in both intracellular Ca^{2+} and pH are implicated in the control of protein kinase C, an essential element in signal transduction, in HeLa

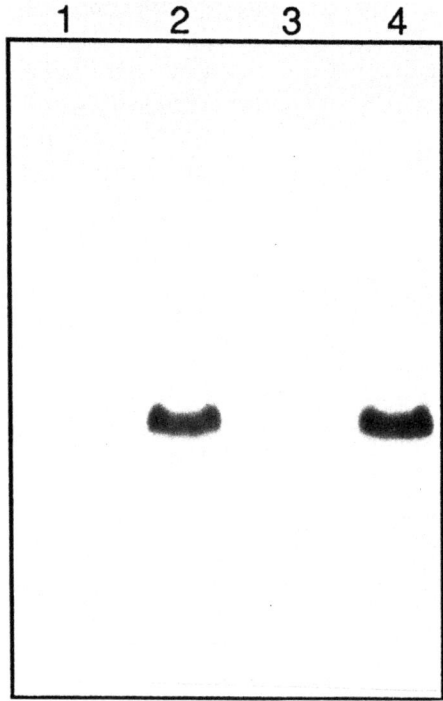

Fig. 8.11 Northern blot analysis of PHR1 expression. Each lane was loaded with 20 μg of RNA from strain SC5314 grown in Lee's medium, pH 4.5, 25°C (lane 1), pH 6.5, 25°C (lane 2), pH 4.5, 37°C (lane 3), pH 6.5, 37°C (lane 4). The blot was hybridized with the PHR cDNA.

cells (Tilly et al 1990). In addition, increases in intracellular pH positively affect the Ca^{2+} activation of chemo-mechanical forces in mammalian cardiac cells (Solaro et al 1989). Furthermore, changes in intracellular pH are correlated with developmental changes in *Dictyostelium* (Inouye 1989, Furukawa et al 1990, Iijima & Maeda 1990).

The expression of the pH-responsive genes was highly induced at near neutral pH and significantly diminished at low pH. A Northern blot analysis of the expression of one of these genes, tentatively designated PHR1 (pH responsive), is shown in Figure 8.11. PHR1 is highly expressed in strain SC5314 grown in Lee's medium, pH 6.5, (lanes 2 and 4) but barely detectable in cells grown in the same medium at pH 4.5 (lanes 1 and 3). Expression is independent of temperature since the same response is seen with cells incubated at 25°C or incubated at 37°C. Expression is also independent of the morphology of the cells since comparable levels of expression are seen in yeast cells (25°C, pH 6.5, lane 2) and hyphal cells (37°C, pH 6.5, lane 4). The response was not specific to strain SC5314 or the growth medium. Similar levels of expression were seen with strains SGY243, 3153a, and ATCC38696 and in serum, N-acetylgucosamine, and proline induction media (data not shown). These results demonstrate that *C. albicans* responds to the pH of its environment with specific changes in gene expression, and may indicate that the pH constraints of morphological development reflect a requirement for the products of these genes rather than, or in conjunction with, a requirement for general metabolic changes that might accompany alterations in the pH of the growth media.

CONCLUSION

Comparing yeast-hyphal morphogenesis in *C. albicans* to other morphogenetic and developmental systems has an inherent risk, but on the whole seems appropriate. The proof that new gene expression is involved, as it is in development in higher organisms, has been difficult to obtain, owing largely to the difficulty of obtaining and analyzing mutations. Molecular gene cloning offers the possibility of identifying such genes, if they are involved. Our finding of several genes that are specifically transcribed in hyphal cells or in response to the signals that lead to hypha formation, is a significant new avenue for analysis. One such gene, which responds to the higher pH required to initiate hyphal formation, bears a striking sequence similarity to a protein found in *S. cerevisiae* and which contains glycosylphosphatidylinositol (GPI), a plasma membrane anchoring structure (Vai et al 1991). This protein in *S. cerevisiae* is found in the cytoplasmic membrane and is highly regulated in a cell cycle specific manner. Interestingly, a protein with similar properties, SERA, is found in the blood stage of *Plasmodium falciparum* (Li et al 1989). These relationships, however tenuous, will undoubtedly be strong factors in determining our future lines of research.

REFERENCES

Alani E, Cao L, Kleckmer N 1987 A method for gene disruption that allows repeated use of URA3 selection in the construction of multiply disrupted yeast strains. Genetics 116: 541–545

Aliabadi Z, Park Y K, Slonczewski J L, Foster J W 1988 Novel regulatory loci oxygen- and pH-regulated gene expression in *Salmonella typhimurium*. Journal of Bacteriology 170: 842–851

Au-Young J, Robbins P W 1990 Isolation of a chitin synthase gene (*CHS1*) from *Candida albicans* by expression in *Saccharomyces cerevisiae*. Molecular Microbiology 4: 197–207

Berridge M J, Heslop J P, Irvine R F, Brown K D 1984 Inositol triphosphate formation and calcium mobilization in Swiss 3T3 cells in response to platelet-derived growth factor. Journal of Biochemistry 222: 195–201

Bingham R J, Hall K S, Slonczewski J L 1990 Alkaline induction of a novel gene locus, alx, in *Escherichia coli*. Journal of Bacteriology 172: 2184–2186

Boeke J D, LaCroute F, Fink G R 1984 A positive selection for mutants lacking orotidine-5′-phosphate decarboxylase activity in yeast: 5-fluoro-orotic acid resistance. Molecular and General Genetics 197: 345–346

Brawner D L, Cutler J G 1986 Variability in expression of cell surface antigens of *Candida albicans* during morphogenesis. Infection and Immunity 51: 337–343

Brummell M, Soll D R 1982 The temporal regulation of protein synthesis during synchronous bud or mycelial formation in the dimorphic fungus *Candida albicans*. Developmental Biology 89: 211–217

Chien J-H, Dawid I B 1984 Isolation and characterization of calmodulin genes from *Xenopus laevis*. Molecular and Cellular Biology 4: 507–513

Davis T N, Urdea M S, Masiarz F R, Thorner J 1986 Isolation of the yeast calmodulin gene: calmodulin is an essential protein. Cell 47: 423–431

Edman J C, Kovacs J A, Masur H, Santi D V, Elwood H J, Sogin ML 1988. Nature 334: 519–522

Feinberg A P, Vogelstein B 1984 A technique for radio-labelling DNA restriction endonuclease fragments to high specific activity. Analytical Biochemistry 132: 6–13

Finney R, Langtimm C J, Soll D R 1985 The programs of protein synthesis accompanying the establishment of alternative phenotypes in *Candida albicans*. Mycopathologia 91: 3–15

Fischer R, Koller M, Flura M et al 1988 Multiple divergent mRNAs code for a single human calmodulin. Journal of Biological Chemistry 263: 17055–17062

Furukawa R, Wampler J E, Fechheimer M 1990 Cytoplasmic pH of *Dictyostelium discoideum* amebae during early development: identification of two cell subpopulations before the aggregation stage. Journal of Cell Biology 110: 1947–1954

Fyrberg E E, Mahaffery J W, Bond B J, Davidson 1983 Transcripts of the six *Drosophila* actin genes accumulate in a stage- and tissue-specific manner. Cell 33: 115–123

Gillum A M, Tsay E J H, Hirsch D R 1984 Isolation of the *Candida albicans* gene for orotidine-5′-phosphate decarboxylase by complementation of *S. cerevisiae, ura*3 and *E. coli pyr*F mutations. Molecular and General Genetics 198: 179–182

Goldhagen H, Clarke M 1986 Identification of the single gene for calmodulin in *Dictyostelium discoideum*. Molecular and Cellular Biology 6: 1851–1854

Greer C, Schekman R 1982 Calcium control of *Saccharomyces cerevisiae* actin assembly. Molecular and Cellular Biology 2: 1279–1286

Headley V L, Payne S M 1900 Differential protein expression by *Shigella flexneri* in intracellular and extracellular environments. Proceedings of the National Academy of Sciences, USA 87: 4179–4183

Henikoff S, Kelly J D, Cohen E H 1983 Transcription terminates in yeast distal to a control sequence. Cell 33: 607–614

Henikoff S, Cohen E H 1984 Sequences responsible for transcription termination of a gene segment in *Saccharomyces cerevisiae*. Molecular and Cellular Biology 4: 1515–1520

Heyde M, Portalier R 1987 Regulation of major outer membrane porin proteins of *Escherichia coli* K12 by pH. Molecular and General Genetics 208: 511–517

Iijima N, Maeda Y 1990 The influence of pH on the choice between sexual and asexual development in *Dictyostelium mucoroides*. Journal of General Microbiology 136: 1739–1745

Inouye K 1989 Regulation of cytoplasmic pH in the differentiating cell types of the cellular slime mold *Dictyostelium discoideum*. Biochimica et Biophysica Acta 1012: 64–68

Kamath A, Chakraburtty K 1989 Role of yeast elongation factor 3 in the elongation cycle. Journal of Biological Chemistry 264: 15423–15428

Kelly R, Miller S M, Kurtz M B, Kirsch D R 1987 Directed mutagenesis in *Candida albicans*: One-step gene disruption to isolate *ura*3 mutants. Molecular and Cellular Biology 7: 199–207

Kelly R, Miller S M, Kirtz, M B 1988 One-step gene disruption by cotransformation to isolate double auxotrophs in *Candida albicans*. Molecular and General Genetics 214: 24–31

Koser P L, Livi G P, Levy M A, Rosenberg M, Bergsma D J 1990 A *Candida albicans* homolog of a human cyclophilin gene encodes a peptidyl-prolyl *cis-trans* isomerase. Gene 96: 189–195

Kurtz M B, Cortelyou M W, Kirsch D R 1986 Integrative transformation of *Candida albicans*, using a cloned *Candida* ADE2 gene. Molecular and Cellular Biology 6: 142–149

150

Kurtz M B, Cortelyou M, Miller S, Lai M, Kirsch D 1987 Development of autonomously replicating plasmids for *Candida albicans*. Molecular and Cellular Biology 7: 209–217

Kurtz M B, Marrinan J 1989 Isolation of Hem3 mutants from *Candida albicans* by sequential gene disruption. Molecular and General Genetics 217: 47–52

Kwon-Chung K J, Hill W B 1970 Studies on pink adenine deficient strains of *Candida albicans*. I. Cultural and morphological characteristics. Sabouraudia 8: 48–61

Landau J W, Dabrowa N, Newcomer V D 1965 The rapid formation in serum of filaments by *Candida albicans*. Journal of Investigative Dermatology 44: 171–179

Langford C J, Gallwitz D 1983 Evidence for an intron-contained sequence required for the splicing for yeast RNA polymerase II transcripts. Cell 33: 519–527

Langford C J, Klinz F-J, Donath C, Gallwitz D 1984 Point mutations identify the conserved, intron-containing TACTAAC box as an essential splicing signal sequence in yeast. Cell 36: 645–653

Lee K L, Buckley H R, Campbell C C 1975 An amino acid liquid synthetic medium for the development of mycelial and yeast forms of *Candida albicans*. Sabouraudia 13: 273–277

LeJohn H B 1989 Structure and expression of fungal calmodulin gene. Journal of Biological Chemistry 264: 19366–19472

Li W B, Bzik D J, Horii T, Inselberg J 1989 Structure and expression of *Plasmodium falciparum* SERA gene. Molecular and Biochemical Parasitology 33: 13–25

Losberger C, Ernst J F 1989a Sequence and transcription analysis of the *C. albicans* URA3 gene encoding orotidine-5′-phosphate decarboxylase. Current Genetics 16: 153–157

Losberger C, Ernst J F 1989b Sequence of the *Candida albicans* gene encoding actin. Nucleic Acids Research 17: 9488

Miller S L, Kukral A M, Mekalanos J J 1989 A two-component regulatory system (*pho*P *pho*Q) controls *Salmonella typhimurium* virulence. Proceedings of the National Academy of Sciences, USA 86: 5054–5058

Mount S M 1982 A catalogue of splice junction sequences. Nucleic Acids Research 10: 459–472

Odds F C 1985 Morphogenesis in *Candida albicans*. CRC Critical Review Microbiology 12: 45–93

Odds F C 1988 *Candida* and candidosis. A review and bibliography, 2nd edn. Bailliere Tindall, London

Olaiya A F, Sogin S J 1979 Ploidy determination of *Candida albicans*. Journal of Bacteriology 140: 1043–1049

Paranjape V, Roy B G, Datta A 1990 Involvement of calcium, calmodulin and protein phosphorylation in morphogenesis of *Candida albicans*. Journal of General Microbiology 136: 2149–2154

Poulter R, Jeffery K, Hubbard M J, Shepherd M G, Sullivan P A 1981 Parasexual genetic analysis of *Candida albicans* by spheroplast fusions. Journal of Bacteriology 146: 833–840

Proudfoot N J, Brownlee G G 1976 3′ non-coding region sequences in eukaryotic mRNA. Nature 263: 211–214

Qin S, Moldave K, McLaughlin C S 1987 Isolation of the yeast gene encoding elongation factor 3 for protein synthesis. Journal of Biological Chemistry 262: 7802–7807

Rasmussen C D, Means R L, Lu K P, May G S, Means A R 1990 Characterization and expression of the unique calmodulin gene of *Aspergillus nidulans*. Journal of Biological Chemistry 265: 13767–13775

Roy B G, Datta A 1987 A calmodulin inhibitor blocks morphogenesis in *Candida albicans*. FEMS Microbiology Letters 41: 327–329

Sabie F T, Gadd G M 1989 Involvement of a Ca^{2+}-calmodulin interaction in the yeast-mycelial (Y-M) transition of *Candida albicans*. Mycopathologia 108: 47–54

Sambrook J, Frisch E F, Maniatis T 1989 Molecular cloning. A laboratory manual, 2nd edn. Cold Spring Harbor Press, Cold Spring Harbor, New York, Vol 1, pp 2.14–2.17

Sanger F, Nicklen S, Coulson A R 1977 DNA sequencing with chain-terminating inhibitors. Proceedings of the National Academy of Sciences, USA 74: 5463–5467

Sarachek A, Bish J T 1976 Effects of growth temperature and caffeine on genetic responses of *Candida albicans* to ethyl methane-sulfonate, nitrous acid and ultraviolet irradiation. Mycopathologia 60: 51–56

Scherer S, Magee P T 1990 Genetics of *Candida albicans*. Microbiological Review 54: 226–241

Skogerson L, Wakatama E 1976 A ribosome-dependent GTPase from yeast distinct from elongation factor 2. Proceedings of the National Academy of Sciences, USA 73: 73–76

Slonczewski J L, Gonzalez T N, Bartholomew F M, Holt N J 1987 Mu d-directed lacZ fusions regulated by low pH in *Escherichia coli*. Journal of Bacteriology 169: 3001–3006

Smith R A, Allaudeen H S, Whitman M H, Koltin Y, Gorman J A 1988 Isolation and characterization of a β-tubulin gene from *Candida albicans*. Gene 63: 53–63

Smith V L, Doyle K E, Maune J F, Munjaal R P, Beckingham K 1987 Structure and sequence of the *Drosophila melanogaster* calmodulin gene. Journal of Molecular Biology 196: 471–485

151

Solaro R J, El-Saleh S C, Kentish J C 1989 Ca^{2+}, pH and the regulation of cardiac myofilament force and ATPase activity. Molecular and Cellular Biochemistry 89: 163–167

Soll D R 1990 Dimorphism and high frequency switching in *Candida albicans* In: Kirsch D, Kelly R, Kurtz M (eds). The genetics of *Candida*. CRC Press, Boca Raton, Florida, pp 147–176

Sundstrom P M, Nichols E J, Kenny G G 1987 Antigenic differences between mannoproteins of germ tubes and blastospores of *Candida albicans*. Infection and Immunity 55: 616–620

Sundstrom P, Smith D, Sypherd P S 1990 Sequence analysis and expression of the two genes for elongation factor 1α from the dimorphic yeast *Candida albicans*. Journal of Bacteriology 172: 2036–2045

Sundstrom P, Irwin M, Smith D, Sypherd P S 1991 Both genes for EF-1α in *Candida albicans* are translated. Molecular Microbiology, in press.

Syverson R G, Buckley H R, Campbell C C 1975 Cytoplasmic antigens unique to the mycelial or yeast phase of *Candida albicans*. Infection and Immunity 12: 1184–1188

Tabor S, Richardson C C 1987 DNA sequence analysis with a modified bacteriophage T7 RNA polymerase. Proceedings of the National Academy of Sciences, USA 84: 4767–4771

Takeda T, Yamamoto M 1987 Analysis and in vivo distruption of the gene coding for calmodulin in *Schizosaccharomyces pombe*. Proceedings of the National Academy of Sciences, USA 84: 3580–3584

Tilly B C, Lambrechts A C, Tertoolen L G J, de Laat S W, Moolenaar W H 1990 Regulation of phosphoinositide hydrolysis induced by histamine and guanine nucleotides in human HeLa carcinoma cells. Federation of European Biochemical Societies 265: 80–84

Tschudi C, Young A S, Ruben L, Patton C L, Richards F F 1985 Calmodulin genes in trypanosomes are tandemly repeated and produce multiple mRNAs with a common 5′ leader sequence. Proceedings of the National Academy of Sciences, USA 82: 3998–4002

Vai M, Gatti E, Lacana E, Popolo L, Alberghina 1991 Isolation and deduced amino acid sequence of the gene encoding gp115, a yeast glycophospholipid-anchored protein containing a serine-rich region. Journal of Biological Chemistry 266: 12242–12248.

Watterson D M, Shanef F, Vanaman T C 1980 The complete amino acid sequence of the Ca^{2+}-dependent modulator protein (calmodulin) of bovine brain. Journal of Biological Chemistry 255: 962–975

Whelan W L, Partridge R M, Magee P T 1980 Heterozygosity and segregation in *Candida albicans*. Molecular and General Genetics 180: 107–113

Discussion of paper presented by P. S. Sypherd

Discussed by M. F. Tuite
Reported by M. V. Hayes

Dr Tuite started his discussion by defining the stages of dimorphism from the cell biological, biochemical and genetic point of view. He commented that dimorphism should be viewed as a gradual change in cell morphology through basically four cell types (yeast, 'pseudo-yeast', pseudohyphae and hyphae) and not as a sequential step-by-step process. Clearly, there is an obvious need for accurate identification of morphological forms to allow for the correct interpretation of data relating to studies of dimorphism. In developing Dr Sypherd's theoretical perspective of the morphogenetic events in *Candida albicans*, Dr Tuite described dimorphism as a process similar to protein synthesis with distinct initiation, elongation and termination events associated with the yeast–hyphal transition.

A diverse collection of signals (e.g. pH, temperature, nutritional factors) can act as initiators or effectors of hyphal formation. Dr Tuite highlighted that these signals do not appear to have any common physical or chemical properties. He raised the question of whether they all act on the yeast cell in the same way. He argued that because certain strains of *C. albicans* respond to some but not all known effectors, there are probably different pathways involved in the initial detection of the primary signal for the morphological change.

In common with Dr Sypherd's view, Dr Tuite proposed that the way that the signal is received and transmitted to its intracellular targets could be analogous to the process of signal transduction in mammalian cells and perhaps to the pheromone response in *Saccharomyces*. The signal transduction process may be mediated by one or more second messengers and, as mentioned by Dr Sypherd, calmodulin may be one of the prime candidates. Dr Tuite suggested that cellular pH and cyclic AMP may also act as second messengers for dimorphism.

Dr Sypherd presented some convincing data that new gene expression occurs and is probably required to initiate cell elongation. Dr Tuite pointed out that previous attempts to demonstrate the occurrence of new proteins or changes in the levels of certain proteins associated with the dimorphic switch were largely unsuccessful. He highlighted the limitations of 2D gel electrophoretic techniques which can only give information on a small subset of proteins (i.e. 10–20%) from the yeast and hyphal forms of *Candida*.

Dr Sypherd has started a detailed genetic analysis of dimorphism which is likely to yield an important insight into this complex morphogenic process. Dr Tuite pointed out that there are some encouraging new developments in the classical genetic analysis of *Candida*, that will benefit such studies. For example, Mark Payton's laboratory (Glaxo Institute of Molecular Biology, Geneva) has now constructed a collection of temperature-sensitive mutants of *C. albicans*, and Richard Barton (University of Minnesota) has shown that by a combination of inducing aneuploidy in *C. albicans* with an antimycotic agent followed by a round of mutagenesis, it is possible to uncover a large number of recessive mutations.

Dr Sypherd's working hypothesis that new gene expression is required for dimorphism is based on his discovery of a series of genes whose transcription levels change during dimorphism. Dr Tuite made the point that changes in RNA levels do not necessarily result in changes in the level of encoded protein. There are significant levels of post-transcriptional control of gene expression in *S. cerevisiae* and in other eukaryotes and it is likely that *Candida* will also exhibit a degree of post-transcriptional control. A good example in support of this notion may be calmodulin, where Dr Sypherd's data showed that the calmodulin gene transcriptional levels are approximately the same throughout dimorphism, whereas the data from the group of Datta suggest that the levels of calmodulin activity change significantly during the yeast–hyphal transition. However, nobody has actually determined the concentration of the calmodulin protein directly.

In concluding his discussion, Dr Tuite raised an issue that was also mentioned by Dr Sypherd; namely, how to determine from a DNA sequence the structure and function of the encoded polypeptide. The basic assumption is that the DNA sequence allows for a prediction of the protein sequence. Dr Tuite stated that this concept may have to be reconsidered for *C. albicans*, because his group has recently discovered the existence of an unusual transfer RNA in this organism which suggests that the decoding of messenger RNA by *C. albicans* may not be typical. This leucyl-tRNA has many unique features including a primary sequence that is highly homologous to seryl-tRNAs and a G-residue in position 33 with the tRNA which is almost universally a U-residue in other tRNAs. The unusual G^{33} residue apparently will induce significant conformational changes in the anticodon stem-loop region. Dr Tuite showed in vitro translation data that demonstrated that this 'novel' tRNA causes significant mistranslation on non-*C. albicans* messenger RNAs. His working hypothesis is that it frameshifts at certain leucine codons, possibly in the region of the termination codon, resulting in an elongated polypeptide. The discovery of this tRNA would suggest that there may be something very unusual about the *C. albicans* translational machinery and may explain the difficulty in expressing non-*Candida* genes in *C. albicans*. To date, the *S. cerevisiae* *LEU2* gene is the only reported heterologous gene to be expressed in *Candida albicans* (M Kurtz, Merck, USA).

In the course of general discussion, Dr Hobden challenged the idea that in protein synthesis the elongation factor EF-3 was unique to fungi and wondered if it actually depends on the definition of a ribosome versus an elongation factor. Dr Sypherd commented that there was evidence from anti-EF-3 antibody studies to support an EF-3 function that is indeed built into the mammalian ribosome. He stated that he remained enthusiastic about EF-3 as an antifungal target because of the possibility that the contact between EF-3 and the ribosome could actually be the site for the rational development of a broad spectrum antifungal agent. Dr

Tuite added that he believed one of the functions of EF-3 is to supply ATPase activity essential for ribosome function.

The question of multiple pathways to control yeast–hyphal morphogenesis was also discussed. Dr Sypherd expressed the view that if hyphal formation is really essential for invasion in an organism that has lived in association with higher mammals for several million years or so, it might well have developed some back-up systems. The existence of these multiple pathways that can induce morphological change may well complicate 'knock-out' mutant studies for some of the genes involved, because in such mutants new genes may now turn on alternative pathways to give hyphae.

9. Switching and its possible role in *Candida* pathogenesis

D. R. Soll

INTRODUCTION

Candida albicans is highly adapted to the human body. As a commensal, it can be carried in the oral cavity, gastrointestinal tract, anus and genital regions of healthy individuals (Odds 1988, Soll et al 1991b), and it is assumed that commensal strains are the source of subsequent infections. As a pathogen, *C. albicans* is capable of invading virtually every tissue and cavity of the human body, and in the case of systemic infections, which occur primarily in immunocompromised hosts, it can readily cause death. The reasons for the success of *C. albicans* as a pathogen still elude us, and although several phenotypic traits have been implicated as virulence factors (e.g. hypha formation, selective adhesion, and acid protease secretion), we still do not know the magic combination of traits which provide the species with an advantage over other related fungi for commensalism and subsequent pathogenesis in the human body.

The success of *C. albicans* may in part be based on its capacity to thrive in a variety of ecologically distinct environments. This capacity could be achieved in a number of ways. First, within the species, there may exist a variety of strains, each adapted to a different environmental circumstance. In this case, each environmental niche or physiological state of the host would select the most highly adapted strain available. Second, each individual cell may have in its developmental repertoire a variety of phenotypes in addition to the basic bud and hyphal form, and the expression of each phenotype would be cued by a different environmental circumstance. Third, each individual organism may contain a spontaneous, high-frequency switching system which continually generates variability in a population, and each environmental circumstance would select the most adapted phenotype from this repertoire. Finally, most strains of *C. albicans* may share one general, basic phenotype capable of effectively handling every niche in the human body and every physiological state of the host. In the discussion which follows, I will make the case that almost all of these possibilities combine to provide *C. albicans* with adaptive advantages for both commensalism and pathogenesis, and that high-frequency, reversable phenotypic switching may play a role in rapid adaptation.

156

THE ABSENCE OF MEIOTIC RECOMBINATION AS A VARIABILITY SYSTEM

Candida albicans has been demonstrated to be diploid, and there has been no indication of any sexual cycle (Whelan 1987, Scherer & Magee 1990). In one study, balanced lethals were demonstrated in a single strain, suggesting that, at least in this strain, haploidization would lead to death (Whelan & Soll 1982). Therefore, the variability which normally results from meiotic recombination and segregation is not available to *C. albicans*. Heterozygosity and mitotic recombination have been demonstrated (Whelan & Magee 1981, Whelan & Soll 1982), but the latter does not represent a reasonable source of rapid and reversible variability since it results in homozygosity. Reversibility in this case would be achieved primarily through low frequency mutation.

STRAIN VARIABILITY

A diploid organism such as *C. albicans* does not need a sexual cycle to generate strain variability. Through mutation, translocation, and recombination between repetitive sequences, genetically diverse strains can be rapidly generated. In the case of the moderately repetitive sequence Ca7, located at the ends of chromosomes, rearrangements have been demonstrated to occur in select strains at extraordinarily high frequencies (Soll et al 1987, Sadhu et al 1991), and in the case of the moderately repetitive sequence Ca3 (also 27A), rearrangements are frequent enough to generate diversity between Southern blot hybridization patterns of over 99% of independently isolated strains (Soll et al 1987, Scherer & Stephens, 1988 Schmid et al 1990). Reorganization of ribosomal cistrons also occurs at extraordinarily high frequencies (Iwaguchi et al 1990), and chromosomal rearrangements identifiable by chromosome separation gels seem to occur quite frequently (Magee & Magee 1987, Merz, 1990).

The phenotypic diversity of strains has long been a subject of investigation, primarily because it was assumed that it would facilitate the identification of virulence traits. There is a voluminous literature, reviewed in detail by Odds (1988), demonstrating differences between strains in (1) antigenicity, (2) secretion of acid protease, (3) environmental constraints on hypha formation, (4) sensitivity to antifungal agents, (5) adhesion to different epithelia and plastic, (6) sugar assimilation, and (7) a number of other parameters. There is little argument that strains of *C. albicans* differ to varying degrees in every aspect of cell physiology, and that this variability may be related to adaptation. However, there has been little firm evidence that manipulation of any single phenotypic variable provides a set of strains with an advantage for a particular body location, a particular disease, or a particular immunological or physiological state.

Although there is no clear view of the particular sets of phenotypic traits which provide strains with selective advantage, two recent studies have established that there is both strain adaptation, and environmental selection. First, using biotyping methods to discriminate between strains, Odds and co-workers (1989) demonstrated that in 58% of cases in which vaginal and oral isolates of *Candida* spp.

were obtained simultaneously from the same asymptomatic patient, the pair of isolates exhibited different biotypes. These results suggested that different strains can be carried in different anatomical locations of the same individual and, therefore, that different strains are more highly adapted to different locations, in this case the oral cavity and the vaginal canal. Unfortunately, discrimination by biotyping runs the risk of grouping genetically unrelated strains with similar biotypes, and separating genetically related strains with different biotypes. This risk has been underscored by the demonstration that reversible phenotypic switching can impact on biotype parameters (Soll et al 1991a). However, the biotyping results of Odds and co-workers were confirmed in a genetic analysis of strain relatedness performed in our laboratory (Soll et al 1991b). Both the intensity of carriage and strain relatedness were assessed in 52 healthy women each sampled at 17 anatomical locations using an isolation procedure which facilitates cloning from the site of carriage (Soll 1991), and a computer assisted DNA fingerprinting system which computes genetic similarity between strains and generates dendrograms on the basis of the patterns of Southern blots probed with the moderately repetitive

Table 9.1 The unrelatedness of *C. albicans* strains simultaneously isolated from the oral cavity and vaginal canal of the same individuals[a]

Locations	Individual[b]	Strains[c]	S_{AB}[d]	Mean $S_{AB}(+SD)$
Vaginal canal–oral[f]	hp2	vw[e],bt	0.00	0.62±0.34
	hp13	vw,bt[e]	0.00	
	hp22	vw,bt	0.67	
	hp27	vw,ch	0.91	
	hp28	vw,bt	0.67	
	hp29	vw,ch	0.65	
	hp31	vw,bt	0.96	
	hp33	vw,bt	0.63	
	hp36	vw,bt	0.96	
	hp37	vw,bt	0.90	
	hp39	vw,bt	0.50	
Vulva–vaginal canal[f]	hp11	vu,vw	0.98	0.99±0.01
	hp13	vu,vw	1.00	
	hp22	vu,vw	1.00	
	hp27	vu,vw	1.00	
	hp29	vu,vw	0.96	
	hp31	vu,vp	1.00	
	hp33	vu,vw	1.00	
	hp36	vu,vw	1.00	
	hp49	vu,vw	1.00	

[a] For details of this study, see Soll et al 1991b.
[b] hp, healthy patients.
[c] vw, vaginal wall; vp, vaginal pool; bt, back of tongue; ch, cheek.
[d] S_{AB} values represent the similarity coefficient calculated through the comparison of Southern blot hybridization blots probed with the moderately repetitive sequence Ca3 according to the methods of Schmid et al 1990. An S_{AB} of 1.00 represents identicalness and 0.00 complete unrelatedness.
[e] In these cases, little or no hybridization was observed with the species-specific probe Ca3 demonstrating that the isolate was not of the species *C. albicans*
[f] In all cases of simultaneous vulva and vaginal canal isolates, the patterns were identical. In the cases of simultaneous vaginal and oral isolates, seven pairs were unrelated (S_{AB} of 0.00 to 0.67) and four pairs were similar but nonidentical (S_{AB} of 0.90 to 0.96).

158

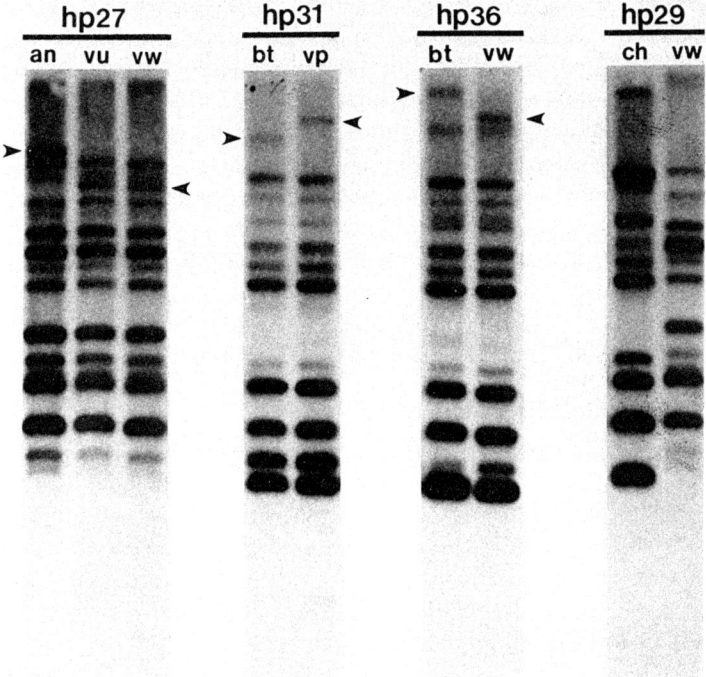

Fig. 9.1 Southern blot hybridization patterns of EcoRI-digested DNA probed with the moderately repetitive sequence Ca3. For each healthy patient (hp) commensal strains of *C. albicans* were simultaneously isolated from different anatomical locations and fingerprinted. For hp27, the anal (an) isolate differs from the vulval (vu) and vaginal wall (vw) isolates by the position of one high molecular weight fragment containing a Ca3 sequence; for hp31 and hp36, the back of tongue (bt) isolates differ from the vaginal pool (vp) isolate, in the former case, and the vaginal wall isolate, in the latter case, by the location of one band; for hp29, the cheek (ch) and vaginal wall isolate are completely unrelated.

sequence Ca3 (Schmid et al 1990). 73% of test individuals carried *Candida*, and at least half of these individuals did so in more than one of three major body locations (oral, vulvovaginal, anorectal). Isolates from different body locations of the same individual were either (1) completely unrelated, (2) similar but non-identical, or (3) identical. In the 11 cases in which *Candida* spp. were simultaneously isolated from the oral cavity and vulvovaginal region, seven pairs were genetically unrelated, and four pairs were genetically similar but nonidentical (Table 9.1). Therefore, in 11 cases of simultaneous carriage in the oral and vaginal regions, no pairs were identical. Scherer & Stevens (1988) also observed that in two of three pairs of isolates from the same patients probed with the moderately repetitive sequence 27a, the isolates were genetically similar but non-identical. The fact that genetically non-identical strains simultaneously inhabit different anatomical locations of the same individual suggests that there is strain adaptation to different environmental niches, and that there is little mixing. In the case of strains which are genetically similar but non-identical (Fig. 9.1), it is likely that they have evolved from a single strain, a point which will be returned to in a later section of this essay. Results are therefore beginning to accumulate which indicate that there is very refined strain adaptation for different anatomical locations, and that phenotypic variation between strains plays a major role in both carriage and pathogenesis. Strain selection was also demonstrated at the genetic level in analysis of colonization during three sequential episodes of recurrent vaginitis in a single patient (Soll et al 1989). During the three episodes, separated by periods of imidazole treatment (the first infection was treated with clotrimazole and the second with butoconazole), a single strain persisted in the vulvovaginal region and was the cause of each successive infection, and a completely unrelated strain persisted in the oral cavity. The phenotypic traits which make one strain more adapted to the vulvovaginal region, and another more adapted to the oral cavity have not been elucidated.

MULTIPLE PHENOTYPES IN A BASIC DEVELOPMENTAL REPERTOIRE

Candida albicans and related species are dimorphic, capable of growing in the primary budding form, and in the elongate hyphal form (Soll 1986). It has been assumed that the hyphal form has evolved as a mechanism for tissue penetration and that the developmental capacity to form a hypha represents a major virulence factor for *Candida* pathogenicity. There is little doubt that hypha formation is important for *Candida* pathogenesis, and hypha-minus mutants are, as one would expect, less virulent when injected into a mouse (Sobel et al 1984). However, one cannot discriminate strains from different body locations or different disease states based simply on the capacity to form hyphae since, in all such studies, the majority of pathogens and commensals possess this capacity. In addition, one cannot assign selective advantages to the bud or hypha form for carriage in the oral cavity versus vaginal canal, since in the commensal state, the bud form usually predominates in all body locations (Soll & Galask, unpublished observations). One could hypothesize that each strain of *C. albicans* possesses in its phenotypic repertoire a far greater number of basic phenotypes, each adapted to a particular set of environmental conditions, but if these phenotypes are not as blatantly identifiable as the bud or hypha morphology, they would not be readily identifiable in wet mounts. *C. albicans* is capable of graded morphologies between the bud and hyphal phenotypes (Merson-Davies & Odds 1989), and it has been proposed that the major differences between bud and hypha formation involve temporal, spatial and quantitative changes, as well as qualitative ones (for review, see Soll 1986). If such phenotypic differences are involved in adaptation, then one would expect particular graded phenotypes to prevail in different anatomical locations, or in different types of infections. Although there is a propensity for hyphal formation at sites of infection, the hyphal phenotype alone cannot be considered diagnostic of an infection (Odds 1988), and no evidence that I am aware of has demonstrated the specificity of graded phenotypes for particular environmental niches or different types of infection. There has also been no demonstration that environmentally induced phenotypic transitions other than the basic bud-hypha transition are included in the basic developmental repertoire of *C. albicans*. However, that does not mean they do not exist.

A SINGLE GENERAL PHENOTYPE

Although there are well over 200 *Candida* species, *C. albicans* is the most pervasive fungal commensal and pathogen in man (for review, see Odds 1988). This suggests that most strains of the species *C. albicans* share a basic general phenotype which provides them with common commensal and pathogenic advantages over other species. Several studies have uncovered very interesting phenotypic differences between *C. albicans* and other pathogenic species (e.g. Barrett-Bee et al 1985, MacDonald 1984). However, as reviewed in an earlier section of this essay, not all *C. albicans* strains are equal in their capacity to colonize different body locations, suggesting that superimposed upon a general *C. albicans* phenotype, there are subtle variations which result in strain adaptation.

HIGH FREQUENCY PHENOTYPIC SWITCHING

Many pathogens have developed quite sophisticated mechanisms for spontaneously generating variability within a population through high-frequency switching. In several bacteria, including *Escherichia coli* and *Salmonella typhimurium*, phase transitions are effected by the conserved inversion of DNA sequences leading to changes in the expression of genes involved in cell surface morphology and antigenicity (Glasgow et al 1989). These phase transitions are spontaneous and reversible. In *E. coli*, spontaneous inversion controls expression of the fimA gene that encodes the type 1 fimbrial protein, which is necessary for attachment to host cells and virulence (Dorman & Higgins 1987, Eisenstein et al 1987). In *Salmonella typhimurium*, inversion controls expression of the alternative flagellin genes, H1 and H2, leading to alternative antigenic states (Silverman & Simon 1980, Zieg & Simon 1980). In *Borrelia hermsii*, nonreciprocal recombination occurs between silent and expressed loci of the variable outer membrane protein genes on linear plasmids, leading to antigenic variation (Barbour 1989). In *Neisseria gonorrhoea*, a number of partial unexpressed pilin genes are clustered around an expressed gene, and variation is generated by gene conversion of the variable stretches of the partial genes (Swanson & Koomey 1989). Switching mechanisms have also been demonstrated in eucaryotic pathogens. In the African trypanosomes, up to 1000 genes for variant surface glycoproteins are dispersed throughout the genome, and through rearrangement, are moved into and out of expression sites (Donelson 1989). In all of these systems, DNA reorganization occurs spontaneously, generating variants within the infecting population. Variants enrich in a changed environment in which they now have selective advantage over the previously dominating phenotype. In the majority of cases, the environmental change involves the genesis by the host of antibodies to the surface antigen(s) of the originally dominating strain.

Candida spp. are also capable of high-frequency, reversible phenotypic switching, but the molecular mechanism of switching has not been elucidated (Soll 1992). In the majority of strains of *Candida* spp. so far tested, switching can be demonstrated by high-frequency, reversible changes in colony phenotype. For example, in the common laboratory strain 3153A, cells are capable of switching between roughly seven general phenotypes (Slutsky et al 1985), each characterized by a very specific colony phenotype, resulting from the spatial, temporal and quantitative dynamics of bud, pseudohyphal and hyphal phenotypes in the developing colony dome (Soll 1988, 1990). Switching in strain 3153A must be distinguished from the bud–hypha transition. In a switch, cells change colony phenotype, but cells in the different switch phenotypes are all capable of generating hyphae. Therefore, the switch causes a change in the environmental constraints on the bud–hypha transition, and spontaneous switching provides the cell with a number of general phenotypes superimposed upon the basic bud–hypha transition.

In subsequent analyses of switching in other strains, it was determined that several different switching systems, distinguishable by the different colony morphologies in their switching repertoires, existed in *C. albicans* and *C. tropicalis* (Soll et al 1988), but switching in each system appeared to follow the same general rules as strain 3153A. These rules included (1) a limited number of switch phenotypes, (2) the capacity for extremely high frequencies of switching, (3) reversibility and interconvertibility, (4) high- and low-frequency modes of switching usually correlating with the different switch phenotypes, and (5) inducibility of switching by UV-irradiation (Soll 1990).

High frequency switching in *C. albicans* provides us, at least in theory, with a mechanism for rapid variation in a commensal or pathogenic population. However, if switching plays a role in the pathogenic success of *Candida albicans*, we would expect it (1) to affect one or more putative virulence traits, (2) to occur at the site of carriage or infection, and (3) to generate strains adapted to different environmental circumstances.

THE EFFECTS OF SWITCHING ON CELLULAR PHENOTYPE

Although switching has been primarily studied through its impact upon colony morphology, colony formation is not an attribute of an infecting population of *C. albicans* in situ. Rather, variation in colony morphology reflects physiological changes which can affect rates of growth and hypha formation on agar. An example of this can be seen in the 'smooth-heavy myceliated' switching system common in isolates from vaginal infections (Soll et al 1987b), in which a reversible transition occurs between a colony morphology with minimal hypha formation under the dome, and one with a dense hyphal perimeter and bumps in the colony dome (Fig. 9.1).

Perhaps the most severe effect of switching on cellular phenotype has been demonstrated for the white–opaque transition in strain WO-1 (Slutsky et al 1987, Rikkerink et al 1988, Bergen et al 1990, Soll et al 1991a). In the white–opaque transition, cells switch at relatively high frequencies between a white and an opaque colony-forming unit, distinguishable by colour, size and height of the dome. The differences in cellular phenotype between white and opaque are dramatic (Anderson & Soll 1987, Anderson et al 1989, 1990, Soll et al 1991a). First, opaque cells are twice as large and exhibit twice the mass of white cells, but approximately the same amount of total cellular DNA. Opaque cells also exhibit alterations in cellular architecture. A large vacuole containing vesicular material is positioned in the cell centre, squeezing the remaining cytoplasm with nucleus and mitochondria against the plasma membrane–cell wall periphery. Cell wall architecture is also altered, with pimples containing channels and, in some cases, exhibiting membrane bound vesicles at the pimple apices. In addition to cellular architecture, the white–opaque transition has a dramatic effect upon lipid and sterol contents both quantitatively and qualitatively (Ghannoum et al 1990). More importantly, the WO-1 transition has been demonstrated to affect a number of putative virulence traits (Table 9.2).

Table 9.2 Phenotypic traits affected by switching between the white and opaque phenotypes of strain WO-1

Trait	Reference
1. Colony morphology	Slutsky et al 1987
2. Lipid and sterol content	Ghannoum et al 1990
3. Susceptibility to antifungal agents	Soll et al 1989, Ghannoum et al 1990, Soll et al 1991
4. Cell morphology and wall architecture	Slutsky et al 1987, Anderson & Soll 1987, Anderson et al 1989, 1990
5. F-actin localization	Anderson et al 1987
6. Dynamics of wall expansion	Staebell & Soll unpublished observation
7. Gene expression	Soll et al 1991, Thyagarajan, Morrow & Soll unpublished observation
8. Adhesion to buccal epithelium and cohesion	Kennedy et al 1988
9. Sensitivity to PMNs and oxidants	Kolatila & Diamond 1990
10. Accessibility of vital dyes	Rikkerink et al 1988, Anderson & Soll 1987
11. Antigenicity	Anderson & Soll 1987, Anderson et al 1989, 1990
12. Acid protease secretion	Ray et al 1988
13. Sugar assimilation patterns	Soll 1990
14. Enviromental induction of switch to opposite phenotype	Rikkerink et al 1988, Slutsky et al 1987, Morrow et al 1989
15. Virulence in a mouse model	Ray & Payne 1990, Morron et al, in preparation

Hypha formation
Hypha formation has been considered a paramount virulence trait for *C. albicans*, and, as previously stated, hypha-defective mutants are less virulent in mouse models (Sobel et al 1984). Although both white and opaque cells are capable of generating morphologically indistinguishable hyphae (Anderson et al 1989), the environmental constraints on the bud–hypha transition differ. Budding opaque cells are less prone to pH-stimulation of hypha formation than budding white cells (Slutsky et al 1987), but do form hyphae en masse when dispersed on buccal epithelium (Anderson et al 1989). Changes in the environmental constraints on the bud–hypha transition have also been demonstrated for the star phenotype (originally referred to as M10) in the switching repertoire of strain 3153A (Bedell & Soll 1979). The parental strain, in this case, forms hyphae readily when released from stationary phase into amino acid-rich defined medium at 37°C, pH 6.7, but accumulates in the budding phase as singlets in G1 when entering stationary phase in the same medium at 25°C. In contrast, cells in the star colony phenotype (M10) form hyphae not only when leaving the stationary phase at high temperature and pH, but also when entering stationary phase as 25°C. Hypha formation under these latter conditions is inhibited by micromolar concentrations of zinc. In contrast, hypha formation after release from stationary phase at 37°C, pH 6.7, is zinc-insensitive.

Adhesion

Adhesion appears to play a major role in pathogenesis in bacteria and we have assumed that the same is true for *C. albicans* (Calderone & Braun 1991). As noted, switching in *E. coli* regulates an adherence system which is basic to epithelial invasion (Eisenstein 1987). Switching in strain WO-1 also affects adherence (Kennedy et al 1988). White budding cells are significantly more adhesive to buccal epithelial cells than opaque ones, but opaque budding cells are more cohesive than white budding cells. However, white budding cells are less hydrophobic.

Secretion of acid protease

The secretion of both acid protease and phospholipase have been considered to be potential virulence traits (Ruchel 1981, Pugh & Cawson 1977), and mutants defective in protease secretion have been found to be less virulent (MacDonald & Odds 1980, Kwon-Chung et al 1985). It has been assumed that the secretion of these enzymes facilitates tissue penetration. Opaque cells secrete far more acid protease into their environment than do white cells, and this can be readily demonstrated by clearing activity on agar plates containing albumin (Ray et al 1988).

Antigenicity

In most of the switching systems which have been characterized in both prokaryotic and eukaryotic pathogens, the major result of the switching process is a change in antigenicity, providing a mechanism for evading the immune system. Two studies suggest that switching in *C. albicans* also results in antigenic variability. First, we demonstrated that opaque cells express opaque-specific wall antigens (Anderson & Soll 1987, Anderson et al 1988, 1989). Second, Poulain and co-workers (personal communication) demonstrated that a serotype-specific antiserum to cell surface polysaccharides stained sectors in colonies of the opposite serotype, suggesting that switching resulted in antigenic variability. These results should in no way be interpreted as demonstrating that *C. albicans* switches between antigenic states to escape the immune system as in the case of other switching pathogens. In systems like *S. typhimurium, Borrelia* and the trypanosomes, variable antigenic states represent replacement systems in which multiple genes code for alternative antigens. In both the WO-1 system and Poulain et al's results, antigens have been demonstrated to be present or absent, but no evidence has been presented for a replacement system.

Resistance to antifungal agents

The capacity to survive or elude drug therapy may play a major role in the persistence or recurrence of a *C. albicans* infection. Several observations demonstrate that switching in *C. albicans* affects susceptibility to a number of antifungal agents. In strain WO-1, it has been demonstrated that white and opaque cells differ in susceptibility to a number of antifungal agents. However, a more interesting study demonstrated that changes in drug susceptibility could accompany switching at the site of infection (Soll et al 1989). In a recurrent vaginitis patient, followed through three successive infections separated by two periods of imidazole treatment, the same infecting strain, determined by DNA fingerprinting, changed colony morphology in each successive episode. The switch phenotype in the second episode

164

exhibited an increased sensitivity to clotrimazole and a decreased sensitivity to butoconazole. In the third episode, the strain switched back to the original colony morphology expressed by the strain in the first episode, and returned to the original sensitivities to clotrimazole and butoconazole. Therefore, switching in this case affected the repertoire of drug sensitivities, changing it in a reversible fashion in successive infections.

INTERACTIONS WITH THE IMMUNE SYSTEM

As in the case of other pathogens, *C. albicans* is vulnerable to polymorphonuclear leukocytes (PMNs), and any form of resistance to PMN candidacidal activity or phagocytosis would facilitate infectivity. Kolotila & Diamond (1990) demonstrated that although white and opaque cells of strain WO-1 were equally phagocytosed, white cells were more resistant to the candidacidal activity of intact PMNs, as well as to cell-free oxidants. More surprisingly, they demonstrated that both intact PMNs and oxidants stimulated switching from white to opaque.

SWITCHING AT THE SITE OF INFECTION

It is therefore clear that switching can affect in a reversible fashion a number of phenotypic characteristics, including putative virulence traits (Table 9.2), but if switching is involved in commensalism and/or pathogenesis, it must occur in situ. In three studies, evidence has been presented that switching occurs at the sight of carriage and infection. In the first study (Soll et al 1987b), cells were clonally plated directly from the vaginal canals of single episode yeast vaginitis patients, and colony morphologies assessed. In four of the 11 sets of isolates from vaginal wall and pool, multiple colony phenotypes were observed in the primary plating. Cells from multiple phenotypes were subsequently demonstrated to represent the same strain by DNA fingerprinting with the moderately repetitive probe Ca3 (referred to in the original paper by Soll et al in 1987 as JH3). Interconvertibility in vitro of the mixed phenotypes was demonstrated by subsequent plating experiments. The results of this study suggested that switching does occur in at least some strains at the site of infection. In a second study already discussed (Soll et al 1989), the morphology of the infecting strain changed with each successive episode of vaginitis following imidazole therapy. In a third study of vaginal carriage in healthy women, it was demonstrated that switching can occur in the commensal population, and an example of multiple phenotypes of the same strain in a primary plating of a commensal isolate from the vagina is shown in Figure 9.2. These results strongly suggest that switching occurs spontaneously in both commensal and infecting populations in situ. However, the extent of switching observed in these studies must be an underestimate since the frequency of variant cells in a population can be as low as 10^{-4} (Soll et al 1987b, 1988, 1989, Rikkerink et al 1988, Bergen et al 1990, Soll et al 1991a), and in primary cultures of cells isolated from sites of low level carriage or colonization, the number of clonal colonies is usually too low to observe variants. This may further be prejudiced by enrichment of a dominant primary phenotype more highly adapted to the particular niche sampled.

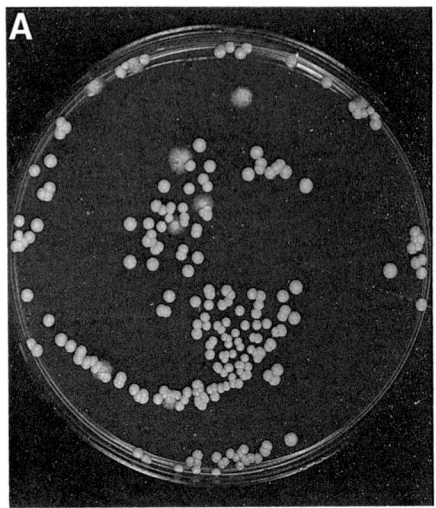
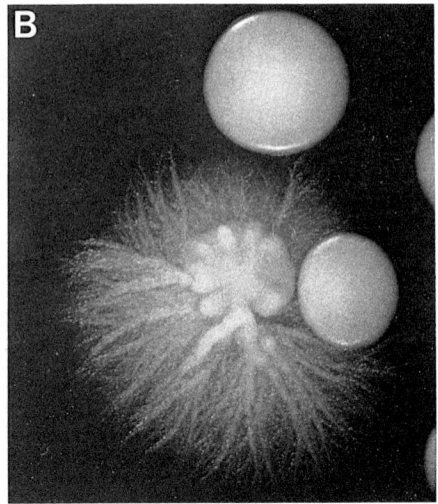

Fig. 9.2 Example of phenotypic variability in a primary sample from the vaginal wall of an asymptomatic patient. The two phenotypes fingerprinted as the same strain and subsequent plating experiments demonstrated a high level of interconvertibility.

ADAPTATION TO DIFFERENT HOST CIRCUMSTANCES

The most convincing demonstration that switching in *C. albicans* plays a role in commensalism and pathogenesis would be to isolate different switch phenotypes of the same strain from different body locations of the same host, from the same host before and after a physiological change resulting in an infection, or from different hosts in different physiological states. This has not yet been accomplished, but it is not clear if a study to test this possibility has ever been correctly performed. In an early comparison of commensal and pathogenic strains isolated from the oral cavity, pathogenic strains appeared to switch on average more frequently than commensal strains (Soll et al 1987a). In a more detailed repeat of this study, it was found that in pathogenic strains, variant phenotypes other than smooth white predominated in one-third of 30 isolates from oral lesions, while smooth white was dominant in all 30 commensal isolates (Helstein, Fotos, Schmid & Soll, in preparation). These results suggest that pathogenic strains switch at higher frequencies, on average, than commensal strains, but unfortunately they do not demonstrate that particular switch phenotypes of a single strain are more highly adapted to different environmental niches.

In the recurrence study (Soll et al 1989) which has been referred to several times in this discussion, switching occurred in sequential episodes of vaginitis separated by imidazole therapy. This result may actually be interpreted as contradicting the notion that switch phenotypes are selectively adapted to different anatomical locations, since one would expect the same switch phenotype to predominate in each recurrent infection even if drug therapy initially selected a different switch phenotype. The strain should have been continually capable of generating the most adapted phenotype by switching, and this one phenotype should have rapidly enriched in the population in each recurrent episode. However, we may be demanding a bit too much within the time frame of the study. If the rate of reversion from the switch phenotype which escaped drug therapy to the original switch phenotype was low, and selection for the original phenotype not very strong, the time of sampling may have been too early to observe dominance by the original phenotype. The patient was treated with an antifungal agent immediately after presenting with the second infection, so time was not at our disposal for determining such an outcome. Interestingly, in two subsequent studies of recurrence, a single strain with a constant colony phenotype prevailed in successive episodes (Soll, Rotman, Galask & Schmid, in preparation).

It is therefore too early to assess whether different switch phenotypes predominate in different host circumstances, primarily because the proper studies have not been performed. However, what form would such a study take? First, if one could identify the same strain in disparate anatomical locations (e.g. the vulvovaginal region and the oral cavity) of the same individual by DNA fingerprinting, one could then clone from the sites of carriage and test for different switch phenotypes. If different switch phenotypes prevailed, then interconvertibility would have to be demonstrated in vitro. As far as I know, this type of study has not been reported. Second, if one demonstrated by DNA fingerprinting that an original commensal strain was responsible for a subsequent infection in an individual, one could then compare clonal phenotypes of the commensal and pathogenic states for differences. Again, such a study has not yet been reported.

Although the studies proposed to test whether different switch phenotypes are better adapted to different host circumstances appear to be straightforward, negative data may not be so easily interpretable. Interpretation in this case is based upon our ability to identify switch phenotypes, and that is based solely upon colony morphology. However, there are reasons to believe that switching in many cases may not impart variant colony morphologies, and that this form of switching may be more pervasive than that identified through colony morphology. Anderson et al (1989) demonstrated that different clones of opaque cells exhibited extreme variability in hypha formation, and that variability within a clone was far less than between clones. These results suggested that heritable and reversible changes affecting hypha formation occurred at high frequency which could be dissociated from the white–opaque transition. We may therefore be faced with the problem of not being readily able to discriminate switch phenotypes other than those which manifest themselves in variant colony morphology.

SWITCHING AND RAPID ADAPTATION

The DNA fingerprinting study of commensal strains in different anatomical locations of healthy individuals described in a preceding section lends support to the notion that adaptation between strains and substrains is involved in commensalism (Soll et al 1991b). In this study, it was demonstrated that in 11 cases in which *Candida* was isolated simultaneously from both the oral cavity and vulvovaginal region, each of seven pairs of isolates were completely unrelated, while each of the remaining four pairs were similar but non-identical (Table 9.1, Fig. 9.1). These results suggested that the oral cavity and vulvovaginal region represent very distinct environmental niches with very different selective pressures. However, the most interesting result in this study was identification of highly similar but non-identical strains simultaneously isolated from the oral cavity and vulvovaginal region. The minor differences between the fingerprint patterns of these strains (Fig. 9.1) probably reflects divergence at the sites of carriage since simultaneous isolates from the vulva and vaginal canal, tested in the same manner as the oral–vaginal pairs from the time of isolation, were in all nine cases identical. Therefore similar but non-identical vaginal–oral pairs most probably evolved from the same progenitor strain, and are in the process of genetic divergence. Genetic divergence in two body locations by a single strain suggests that the geographically separated substrains have adapted to the alternative niches. Otherwise, one would expect one substrain to dominate in all body locations given the likely acessibility. It is not unreasonable to propose that the rapid phenotypic variability basic to this apparently rapid adaptation could be accomplished through high-frequency phenotypic switching.

THE LEVELS OF PHENOTYPIC VARIABILITY REVISITED

I have attempted in this essay to assess the role of phenotypic variability in *Candida albicans* pathogenesis. In Table 9.3, I have outlined the potential levels of phenotypic variability in the developmental repertoire of the species, and it is hard not to conclude that variability relevant to pathogenic success occurs at every level. At the species level, most strains of *C. albicans* must share a combination of phenotypic traits which provide this species with an advantage over the other species for human commensalism and pathogenesis, and I have referred to this combination as the 'general phenotype' of the species. However, within the context of this general species phenotype, there is indeed strain variability which must be the basis for the anatomical adaptation we have uncovered in the human commensal flora of healthy patients (Soll et al 1991b) and in the flora of one recurrent patient (Soll et al 1989). If one strain can exist in the oral cavity at the same time that another, unrelated strain exists in the vaginal canal of the same individual, then the former must be more highly adapted to the oral cavity, and the latter more highly adapted to the vaginal region. We can now begin to consider whether orotropic and vaginotropic strains, first suggested by Sobel (1985), indeed exist. However, we, as well as Scherer & Stevens (1988), have also demonstrated by DNA fingerprinting that different anatomical locations of the same individual can be colonized by genetically similar but non-identical strains (Soll et al 1991b), and we have suggested that these represent genetically diverging substrains of a single progenitor strain. I have proposed that the evolution of this incipient diversity may result from selective adaptation, and that the basis for the alternative phenotypes is high-frequency, reversible phenotype switching. I have argued that several observations support a role for switching in pathogenesis, but the most definitive evidence has not been reported, primarily because the correct studies have never been performed. The format for such studies has been outlined in this essay, but they may be hard to interpret since we are limited in our capacity to assess switching by our dependence upon colony morphology, which may not be expressed by the

Table 9.3 The levels of phenotypic variability in *C. albicans*

Level of regulation	Phenotype
Species	The general phenotype of *Candida albicans* provides most strains in the species with an advantage over other species for commensalism and pathogenesis in the human body.
Strains	Strain variability leads to subtle changes in phenotype which provide adaptive advantages in different environmental circumstances.
Populations	Spontaneous and reversible high frequency switching generates variants in both commensal and colonizing populations which can enrich in a changed environment for which they are more adapted.
Cells	Dimorphism and perhaps other phenotypic transitions built into the developmental repertoire of each cell and responsive to environmental cues at the cellular level provide specialized cell types for different commensal and pathogenic functions.

majority of switch phenotypes. Finally, I have relegated the variability obtained from the bud–hypha transition as a virulence trait included in the general phenotype of the species, manipulated both by switching and strain variation. I have suggested that cells may possess far more phenotypic variability within their developmental repertoire which is responsible immediately to environmental cues, but that we are again limited by our capacity to assess only the phenotypic changes in the bud–hypha transition.

Most importantly, I have tried to place in context the levels of variability (Table 9.3) at the disposal of a colonizing population of *C. albicans*, so that we can begin to consider what role may be played by high frequency phenotypic switching. Without real evidence, and with the licence presented to us in this symposium for speculation, I have proposed that the real role of switching is to provide the organism with rapid phenotypic variability for adaptation. Experiments must now be performed to test this hypothesis.

SUMMARY

The success of *Candida albicans* is reflected in its capacity to live as a commensal in a number of diverse anatomical locations and to infect most tissues as a pathogen. In a recent analysis of commensalism in healthy individuals, it was demonstrated that different strains of *C. albicans* were simultaneously carried in the oral cavity and vaginal canal. These results were interpreted to mean that different strains of *C. albicans* were more highly adapted than others for either the vaginal canal or oral cavity. However, in four of the 11 cases in which *C. albicans* was simultaneously isolated from the oral cavity and vaginal canal, the strains were genetically highly similar but nonidentical, suggesting that they evolved from the same progenitor. It is suggested that high frequency switching provided the original phenotypic variability for rapid adaptation. In order to consider the relationship of strain adaptation and the role of switching, most of this discussion explores the potential levels of phenotypic variability which may contribute to the commensal and pathogenic success of *C. albicans*.

ACKNOWLEDGEMENTS

The author is indebted to Dr R. Galask for collaborative efforts, and to Dr J. Schmid, Dr J. Anderson and B. Morrow for research interactions. This research was supported by Public Health Service grant AI23922.

REFERENCES

Anderson J M, Soll D R 1987 Unique phenotype of opaque cells in the white–opaque transition of *Candida albicans*. Journal of Bacteriology 169: 5579–5588

Anderson J, Cundiff L. Schnars B, Gao M, Mackenzie I, Soll D R 1989 Hypha formation in the white–opaque transition of *Candida albicans*. Infection and Immunity 57: 458–467

Anderson J, Mihalik R, Soll D R 1990 Ultrastructure and antigenicity of the unique cell wall pimple of the *Candida* opaque phenotype. Journal of Bacteriology 172: 224–235

Barbour A 1989 Antigenic variation in relapsing fever *Borrelia* species: genetic aspects. In: Berg D E, Howe M M (eds) Mobile DNA. ASM Press, Washington, DC, pp 783–797

Barrett-Bee K, Hayes Y, Wilson R G, Ryley J F 1985 A comparison of phospholipase activity, cellular adherence, and pathogenicity of yeasts. Journal of General Microbiology 131: 1217–1221

Bedell G W, Soll D R 1979 Effects of low concentrations of zinc on the growth and dimorphism of *Candida albicans*: Evidence for zinc-resistant and -sensitive pathways for mycelium formation. Infection and Immunity 26: 348–354

Bergen M, Voss E, Soll D R 1990 Switching at the cellular level in the white–opaque transition of *Candida albicans*. Journal of General Microbiology 136: 1925–1936.

Calderone R A, Braun P C 1991 Adherence and receptor relationships of *Candida albicans*. Microbiological Reviews 55: 1–20

Donelson J E 1989 DNA rearrangements and antigenic variation in African trypanosomes. In: Berg D E, Howe M M (eds) Mobile DNA. ASM Press, Washington, DC, pp 763–781

Dorman C J, Higgins C F 1987 Fimbrial phase variation in *Escherichia coli*: dependence on integration host factor and homologies with other site-specific recombinases. Journal of Bacteriology 169: 3840–3843

Eisenstein B I 1987 Pathogenic mechanisms of *Legionelle pneumophila* and *Escherichia coli*. ASM News 53: 621–622

Eisenstein B I, Sweet D, Vaughn V, Friedman D I 1987 Integration host factor is required for the DNA inversion that controls phase variation in *Escherichia coli*. Proceedings of the National Academy of Sciences, USA 84: 6506–6510

Ghannoum M A, Swairjo I, Soll D R 1990 Variation in lipid and sterol contents in *Candida albicans* white and opaque phenotypes. Journal of Medical and Veterinary Mycology 28: 103–115

Glasgow A C, Hughes K T, Simon M I 1989 Bacterial DNA inversion systems. In: Berg D E, Howe M M (eds), Mobile DNA. ASM Press, Washington, DC, pp 637–659

Iwaguchi S, Homma M, Tanaka K 1990 Variation in the electrophoretic karyotype analyzed by the assignment of DNA probes in *Candida albicans*. Journal of General Microbiology 136: 2433–2442

Kennedy M J, Rogers A L, Hanselman L R, Soll D R, Yancey R J 1988 Variation in adhesion and cell surface hydrophobicity in *Candida albicans* white and opaque phenotypes. Mycopathologia 102: 149–156

Kolotila M P, Diamond R D 1990 Effect of neutrophils and in vitro oxidants on survival and phenotypic switching of *Candida albicans* WO-1. Infection and Immunity 58: 1174–1179

Kwon-Chung K J, Lehman D, Good C, Magee P T 1985 Genetic evidence for the role of extracellular proteinase in virulence of *Candida albicans*. Infection and Immunity 49: 571–575

MacDonald F, Odds F C 1980 Inducible proteinase of *Candida albicans* in diagnostic serology and in the pathogenesis of systemic candidiasis. Journal of Medical Microbiology 13: 423–436

MacDonald F 1984 Secretion of inducible proteinase by pathogenic *Candida* species. Sabouraudia 22: 79–82

170

Magee, B B, Magee P T 1987 Electrophoretic karyotypes and chromosome numbers in *Candida* species. Journal of General Microbiology 133: 425–430

Merson-Davies L A, Odds F C 1989 A morphology index for characterization of cell shape in *Candida albicans*. Journal of General Microbiology 135: 3143–3152

Merz W G 1990 *Candida albicans* strain delineation. Clinical Microbiology Reviews 3: 321–334

Morrow B, Anderson J, Wilson E, Soll D R 1989 Bidirectional stimulation of the white–opaque transition of *Candida albicans* by ultraviolet irradiation. Journal of General Microbiology 135: 1201–1208

Odds F C 1988 Candida and candidosis: a review and bibliography. Baillière Tindall, London

Odds F C, Webster C E, Fisk P G, Riley V C, Mayuranathan P, Simmons P D 1989 *Candida albicans* biotypes in women attending clinics in genitourinary medicine. Journal of Medical Microbiology 29: 51–54

Pugh D, Cawson R A 1977 The cytochemical localization of phospholipase in *Candida albicans* infecting the chick chorio-allantoic membrane. Sabouraudia 15: 29–35

Ray T L, Payne C D, Soll D R 1988 Variable expression of *Candida* acid proteinase by 'switch phenotypes' of individual *Candida albicans* strain. Clinical Research 36: 687A

Ray T L, Payne C D 1990 *Candida albicans* acid protease: a role in virulence. In: Ayaib E M, Cassell G H, Branche W C Jnr, Henry T J (eds) Microbial determinants of virulence and host response. American Society for Microbiology, Washington, DC, pp 163–178

Rikkerink E H A, Magee B B, Magee P T 1988 Opaque–white phenotype transition: a programmed morphological transition in *Candida albicans*. Journal of Bacteriology 170: 895–899

Rüchel R 1981 Properties of purified proteinase from the yeast *Candida albicans*. Biochimicha et Biophysica Acta 659: 99–113

Sadhu C, McEachern M J, Rustchenko-Bulgac E P, Schmid J, Soll D R, Hicks J B 1991 Telomeric and dispersed repeat sequences in *Candida* yeasts and their use in strain identification. Journal of Bacteriology 173: 842–850

Scherer S, Stevens D A 1988 A *Candida albicans* dispersed, repeated gene family and its epidemiologic applications. Proceeding of the National Academy of Sciences USA 85: 1452–1456

Scherer S, Magee P T 1990 Genetics of *Candida albicans*. Microbiological Reviews 54: 226–241

Schmid J, Voss E, Soll D R 1990 Computer-assisted methods for assessing *Candida albicans* strain relatedness by Southern blot hybridization with repetitive sequence Ca3. Journal of Clinical Microbiology 28: 1236–1243

Silverman M, Simon M I 1980 Phase variation: genetic analysis of switching mutants. Cell 19: 845–854

Slutsky B, Buffo J, Soll D R 1985 High frequency switching of colony morphology in *Candida albicans*. Science 230: 666–669

Slutsky B, Staebell M, Anderson J, Risen L, Pfaller M, Soll D R 1987 'White–opaque transition': a second high-frequency switching system in *Candida albicans*. Journal of Bacteriology 169: 189–197

Sobel J D, Muller G, Buckley H R 1984 Critical role of germ tube formation in the pathogenesis of candidal vaginitis. Infection and Immunity 44: 576–580

Sobel J D 1985 Epidemiology and pathogenesis of recurrent vulvovaginal candidiasis. American Journal of Obstetrics and Gynaecology 152: 924–935

Soll D R 1986 The regulation of cellular differentiation in the dimorphic yeast *Candida albicans*. Bioessays 5: 5–11

Soll D R, Slutsky B, Mackenzie S, Langtimm C, Staebell M 1987a Switching systems in *Candida albicans* and their possible roles in oral candidiasis. In: Mackenzie J, Squier C, Dabelsteen E (eds) Oral mucosa diseases: biology, etiology and therapy. Laegeforeningens Folarg, Denmark, pp 52–59

Soll D R, Langtimm C J, McDowell J J, Hick, Galask R 1987b High frequency switching in *Candida* strains isolated from vaginitis patients. Journal of Clinical Microbiology 25: 1611–1622

Soll D R 1988 High frequency switching in *Candida albicans*. In: Berg D E, Howe M M (eds), Mobile DNA. ASM Press, Washington, DC, pp 791–789

Soll D R, Staebell M, Langtimm C, Pfaller M, Hicks J, Rao T V G 1988 Multiple *Candida* strains in the course of a single systemic infection. Journal of Clinical Microbiology 26: 1448–1459

Soll D R, Galask R, Isley S et al 1989, switching of *Candida albicans* during successive episodes of recurrent vaginitis. Journal of Clinical Microbiology 27: 681–690

Soll D R 1990 Dimorphism and high frequency switching in *Candida albicans*. In: Kirsch D R, Kelly R, Kurtz M B (eds) The genetics of *Candida*. CRC Press, Boca Raton, pp 147–176

Soll D R 1991 Current status of the molecular basis of *Candida* pathogenicity. In: Cole G, Hoch H (eds) The fungal spore and disease initiation in plants and animals. Plenum Inc., New York, pp 503–540

Soll D R, Anderson J, Bergen M, 1991a The developmental biology of the white–opaque transition in *Candida albicans*. In: Prasad R (ed) The molecular biology of *Candida albicans*. Springer-Verlag, Berlin, pp 20–45

Soll D R, Galask R, Schmid J, Hanna C, Mac K, Morrow B 1991b Genetic dissimilarity of commensal strains of *Candida* spp. carried in different anatomical locations of the same healthy women. Journal of Clinical Microbiology 29: 1702–1710

Soll D R 1992 High frequency switching in *Candida*. Clinical Microbiological Reviews, (submitted)

Swanson J, Koomey J M 1989 Mechanisms for variation of pili and outer membrane protein II in *Neisseria gonorrhoeae*. In: Berg D E, Howe M M (eds). Mobile DNA, ASM Press, Washington, DC, pp 743–761

Whelan W L 1987 The genetics of medically important fungi. CRC Critical Reviews in Microbiology 21: 99–170

Whelan W L, Magee P T 1981 Natural heterozygosity in *Candida albicans*. Journal of Bacteriology 145: 896–903

Whelan W L, Soll D R 1982 Mitotic recombination in *Candida albicans*: recessive lethal alleles linked to a gene required for methionine biosynthesis. Molecular and General Genetics 187: 477–485

Zieg J, Simon M I 1980 Analysis of the nucleotide sequence of an invertible controlling element. Proceedings of the National Academy of Sciences USA 77: 4196–4200

Discussion of paper presented by D. R. Soll

Discussed by P. T. Magee
Reported by M. V. Hayes

In reviewing the possible roles for the plasticity of the *Candida albicans* genotype required for switching, Dr Magee commented that he particularly liked Dr Soll's idea of rapid adaptation to various host circumstances being based on a variety of properties of *C. albicans*. These properties range from the general phenotype of the strain to the specific phenomenon of switching. However, he pointed out that there are alternative ways for generating reversible phenotypes that may not be related to switching. Because *C. albicans* is diploid, it may have a way of generating heterozygosity that can remain recessive and not be selected against. Later, mitotic crossing-over can render these recessive mutations homozygous and therefore expressed. While it is not possible to ever go back to the pre-existing condition, it is possible for the organism to become heterozygous again through a reversion or a new mutation.

One possible hypothesis proposed by Dr Soll is that *Candida* strains are found in particular niches because they are capable of adapting to that environment and therefore are best suited for that site. An alternative view expressed by Dr Magee is that strains may be in a particular niche because that happens to be where they started; for example, inoculation can lead to a population of some cells in a particular niche where other cells could equally well have survived. For example, a vulvo-vaginal strain could equally well survive in the mouth.

Dr Magee's experimental approach to decide between the two hypotheses would be to carry out multiple sampling from any orifice over a relatively short period of time and comprehensively analyse every strain on the isolation plate. He stressed the need to analyse every colony to avoid self-selection. He argued that the advantage of this approach over the characterization of a small number of isolates is that a whole population can be studied, rather than a few isolates that may not necessarily be typical of the resident population.

An interesting issue raised by Dr Magee for which there does not appear to be any data, is whether there is sufficient time for adaptation during colonization by *Candida*. He suggested it would be interesting to determine how rapidly cells divide when they are in a carrier state as distinct from an infectious state. This information would be useful because if there is to be adaptation there clearly has to be reproduction and the ability for selection of variants.

In further considering variability in *C. albicans*, Dr Magee pointed out the difficulty in defining a single strain, particularly when this organism appears to lack genetic exchange. Thus, the characters that are used for identification are necessarily those characters which have a certain amount of stability, but we do not know what characters there are that vary in a very short span of generations. Those would be the characters that without single cell analysis, as suggested above, probably would not be identified because they would be rapidly homogenized in any kind of colony. In summarizing this part of his discussion, Dr Magee re-emphasized the need to be careful about the interpretation of data used in generating ideas relating to strain adoption, particularly taking note of the caveats described above.

Finally, Dr Magee turned his attention to the key issue of strain identification. He showed a restriction fragment length polymorphism (RFLP) picture from a Scherer and Stevens publication of two strains that had been probed using the 27A probe. The strains appeared identical from the point of view of RFLPs for this probe. As Dr Soll pointed out, this technique is a remarkably subtle way of differentiating between strains and provides greater discrimination than the use of RFLP alone. However, in this case the probe technique did not differentiate between the two strains. Dr Magee determined the karotype of the whole group of strains described by Scherer and demonstrated an extra chromosome band in one of the strains showing that these strains were not precisely identical as indicated by the 27A analysis. Therefore, strains may differ in their karyotype but appear identical by RFLP using 27A. Hence, they have undergone translocations or possibly deletions to change the migration rate of their chromosomes. Finally, Dr Magee re-emphasized three key points to be considered in the interpretation of data on switching and its role in commensalism and pathogenesis. These were making sure that the entire population is sampled, that the kind of selection that is proposed to take place has time to proceed in certain niches, and that it is essential to define very carefully what is meant by similarity and differences between strains. From the work of Dr Soll and others it is anticipated that information will become available that will give us a better understanding of exactly how infections establish themselves and how carrier status is maintained.

In general discussion, Dr Shepherd returned to the question of switching occurring at the infection site and mentioned Dr Magee's point about the rate of division that must occur between the commensal and the infected tissue. Dr Shepherd suggested that the infected tissue contains cells in a whole range of polymorphic states, and asked Dr Soll if he was seeing an increase in switching as a consequence of the cells now being pathogenic rather than anything to do with the switching phenomenon being involved in their pathogenic phenotype.

Dr Soll responded to this question by giving details of a study he performed with his colleagues in Iowa. Hence, isolates in the first plating of commensals from healthy mouths were almost all in 'original' smooth states, and most of the strains could switch at moderate to high frequency, or switching could be initiated with UV. However, in leukoplakial lesion isolates, in about 30% of the cases unusual phenotypes were found which are in switching repertoires; they were not in the O-smooth phenotype. Genetic analysis of this with CA3, followed by dendrogram analysis, shows that the strains mix. There were no genetically distinct hypervirulent strains and there was convergence, not divergence, for phenotype. So in terms of cell division, he concluded that it does not seem to be important whether cells are dividing slow or fast, when considering the main switch phenotype. So, even if there is enrichment, slow dividing strains would have a chance to express a specific switch phenotype and enrich. Therefore, there must be some advantage in that situation, that results in selection. Dr Magee argued that there could be something like a 'founder's effect'. For example, a strain that became pathogenic could switch early and, because of its pathogenicity, outgrow the strains which were normal. One possible interpretation of such an observation could be that switching was associated with the emergence of the major population in that particular niche. However, in fact switching was a fortuitous event early in the infection and not the cause of pathogenicity.

Dr Soll added that he has seen strain replacement. In his study with Dr Odds of strains from Leicester AIDS patients they found a remarkable decrease in diversity in the strains in this group compared with commensals isolated in the same hospital in the same period. They thought at first it was a single strain infecting most of the AIDS patients and that patients had acquired it from other patients and undergone strain replacement that way. However, the minor differences between the strains DNA fingerprinting patterns remained intact throughout a year, suggesting that the differences probably reflect the selection from the environment of similar strains but not the same strain diverging in different individuals. Their interpretation is that these AIDS patients actually had replacement at an early stage in AIDS because of the commensal diversity, and that these strains held true.

The concept of patients keeping the same strains over long periods of infection was highlighted by Dr Hicks. In a study with oral isolates in San Francisco AIDS patients through several remissions in drug treatments, the same patients kept the same strains over 3 years, with one case of transfer between partners. Dr Hicks suggested that it would be worth comparing the dendrograms of the strains from his study with those from the Leicester study to look for similar patterns.

Session IV:
Cryptococcus

Chairman: J. Verhoef

10. Capsule synthesis and immunity to *Cryptococcus neoformans*

G. J. Bancroft, E. R. Rockett, H. L. Collins

INTRODUCTION

Cryptococcus neoformans (*C. neoformans*) is an encapsulated, basidiomycetous yeast capable of causing life-threatening human disease. Two varieties of the organism have been described, *C. neoformans* var. *neoformans* and *C. neoformans* var. *gattii,* which differ in their geographic distribution, antigenicity and epidemiology (Ellis & Pfeiffer 1990). Exposure to *C. neoformans* occurs via inhalation of the yeast from the environment, but in the majority of cases this is not associated with symptomatic disease. Clinical infection can occur in apparently healthy individuals, but most cases are associated with conditions of impaired cell-mediated immunity and, in particular, defects in macrophage and T-cell function. *C neoformans* is a significant opportunistic pathogen in haematological malignances such as Hodgkin's lymphoma, or in renal transplant recipients. However, most significantly, with the global emergence of AIDS, the incidence of cryptococcosis is increasing and *C. neoformans* represents the major life-threatening fungal infection in these patients (Diamond 1991). The incidence of infection with *C. neoformans* in AIDS patients varies from approximately 3–15% although it has been said to approach 30% in some regions of Africa (Holmberg & Meyer 1986). HIV-positive individuals may develop infection either as the initial AIDS-defining illness or later in the progression of immunodeficiency. The majority of patients present with meningitis and/or disseminated infection which may involve many different organ systems. In this setting, cryptococcal meningitis is invariably lethal without treatment, and life-long maintenance therapy is required to prevent relapse (Diamond 1991).

Cryptococcus is unique among the pathogenic fungi in expressing an extensive polysaccharide capsule which is the primary determinant of virulence in vivo. The capsular polysaccharides possess important immunomodulatory properties including a potent anti-phagocytic action and the capacity to induce immunological suppression (Deepe & Bullock 1990). Thus, defining the interaction between encapsulated yeasts and the immune system is essential in understanding the mechanisms of host resistance. This review will focus on the contribution of the polysaccharide capsule to the immunobiology of *C. neoformans*. In particular we will discuss the importance of this structure for interaction of *C. neoformans* with phagocytic cells and in the generation of cell-mediated immune responses essential for resistance in the immunocompetent host. Our own research interests focus on how the host attempts to overcome the anti-phagocytic properties of the capsule. We will describe recent experiments demonstrating how host cytokines can regulate ingestion of encapsulated yeasts in vitro and the importance of these cytokines in resistance to experimental infection in vivo. Only selected references have been cited in this discussion and more complete lists can be obtained from the reviews cited herein.

CHARACTERISTICS OF CAPSULE SYNTHESIS BY *C. NEOFORMANS*

C. neoformans var. *neoformans* can be isolated from the soil and is particularly enriched in areas contaminated with pigeon droppings, where concentrations of 10^6 viable yeasts/g have been reported (Ruiz & Bulmer 1981). Under these conditions, *C. neoformans* exists as a small, non-encapsulated or poorly encapsulated form with a mean diameter of $<5 \mu m$ (Ruiz & Bulmer 1981). This small particle and/or basidiospores of the sexual state of the organism are believed to be the infectious forms, allowing penetration into the broncho-alveolar spaces and avoiding the efficient clearing mechanisms of the upper respiratory tract (Ellis & Pfeiffer 1990). However, during infection in vivo, capsule synthesis by virulent *C. neoformans* is invariably seen and in some cases may extend to several times the diameter of the cell. The size of the capsule can be regulated according to the environmental conditions. Extended growth in soil is associated with a reduced capsule, and on synthetic media, capsule synthesis can be enhanced or suppressed according to factors such as osmolarity, pH and CO_2 concentration (e.g. Dykstra et al 1977). Furthermore, unencapsulated isolates of *C. neoformans* can synthesize capsular material within 5–10 h of incubation with human lung tissue (Farhi et al 1970). Although capsule size can be manipulated in vitro, such changes are not stable following injection into experimental animals (Dykstra et al 1977). However, stable, acapsular mutants of *C. neoformans* are available and together with their co-isogenic parent strains have been essential for studying the contribution of the capsule to virulence in vivo (Fig. 10.1; see below).

The polysaccharide capsule is predominantly composed of glucuro-no-xylomannan which consists of a linear $\alpha(1–3)$ mannose backbone substituted with D-xylose and D-glucuronic acid (Bhattacharjee et al 1984). The capsule polysaccharide is shed from viable yeasts during in vitro culture and is present in the serum and cerebrospinal fluid of infected individuals. Circulating levels of cryptococcal antigen can be exceedingly high, with titres up to $1:10^6$ being reported in cases of cryptococcal meningitis associated with AIDS. The detection of cryptococcal antigens at these sites allows a specific diagnosis of cryptococcal meningitis in over 90% of cases (Diamond 1991).

Antigenic differences in the capsule provide the basis for serotyping *C. neoformans*. Serotypes A and D are most prevalent and correspond to *C. neoformans* var. *neoformans*. These are the predominant isolates associated with opportunistic infections in Europe and North America and are readily cultured from environmental sources. Serotypes B and C correspond to *C. neoformans* var. *gatti* which is usually restricted to tropical and sub-tropical areas and has only been isolated

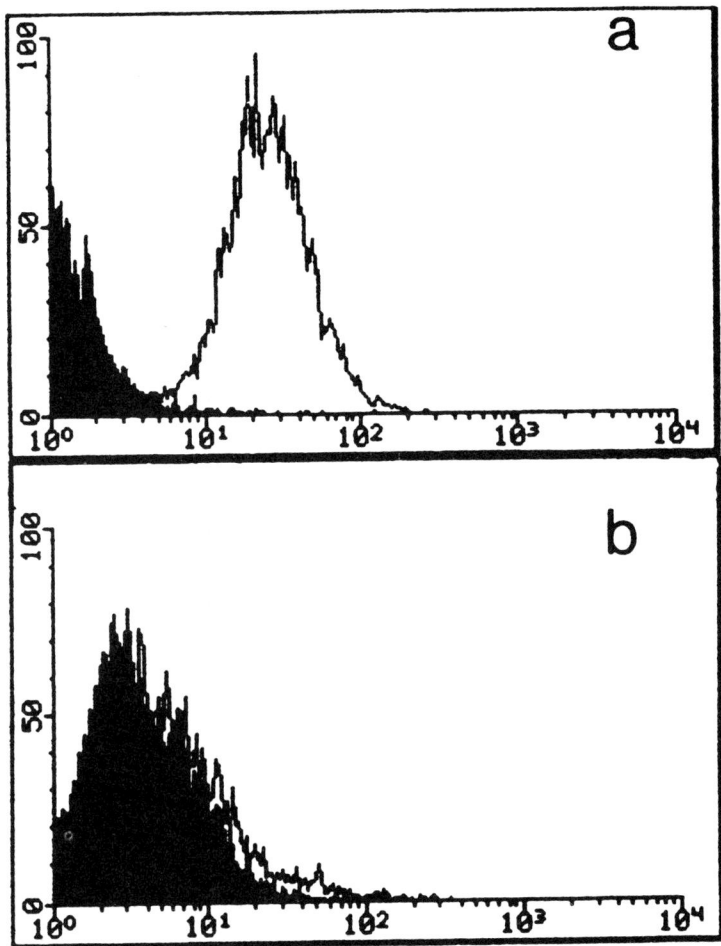

Fig. 10.1 Flow cytometric analysis of capsule expression by *C. neoformans*. 10^6 encapsulated (B3501; A) or acapsular (B4131; B) *C. neoformans* were stained with medium alone (solid histogram) versus rabbit anti-capsule antiserum (open histogram) followed by goat anti-rabbit-FITC. 5000 yeasts were analysed by FACScan flow cytometer and data expressed as the number of yeasts (*y* axis) versus fluorescent intensity (*x* axis).

from the environment in association with certain eucalyptus trees (Ellis & Pfeiffer 1990). Chemical analysis of polysaccharides from the four serotypes has revealed differences in the extent of xylose substitution of the common mannose backbone and in the extent of *o*-acetylation (Bhattacharjee et al 1984). Acetyl groups of microbial polysaccharides are usually immunogenic and for *C. neoformans*, de-*o*-acetylation reduces serological reactivity (Cherniak et al 1980).

The pathways of synthesis and extracellular organization of the cryptococcal polysaccharides are still being defined. Glucuronyltransferase and xylosyltransferase activities have recently been described in *C. neoformans* (White et al 1990) but the mechanism of secretion of the capsule components to the cell surface is still unknown. Important information has been obtained by studying the interaction of purified capsular polysaccharides with acapsular yeasts in vitro.

Binding of polysaccharide occurs in a rapid and specific manner, suggesting the presence of a receptor for the capsule polysaccharide on the fungal cell wall. It is possible that initial saturable binding of polysaccharides to the cell wall is followed by self association between polysaccharides resulting in an extensive capsule structure.

CAPSULE SYNTHESIS AS A DETERMINANT OF VIRULENCE

Synthesis of a polysaccharide capsule is a common determinant of virulence for many pathogenic microbes. Indeed, the major bacterial pathogens responsible for pulmonary and meningeal infection, including *Haemophilus influenzae, E. coli, N. meningitidis* and *Streptococcus pneumoniae,* all possess detectable capsules on their surface (Finlay & Falkow 1989). For *C. neoformans,* capsule production is the most established determinant of infectivity. Numerous studies have correlated the

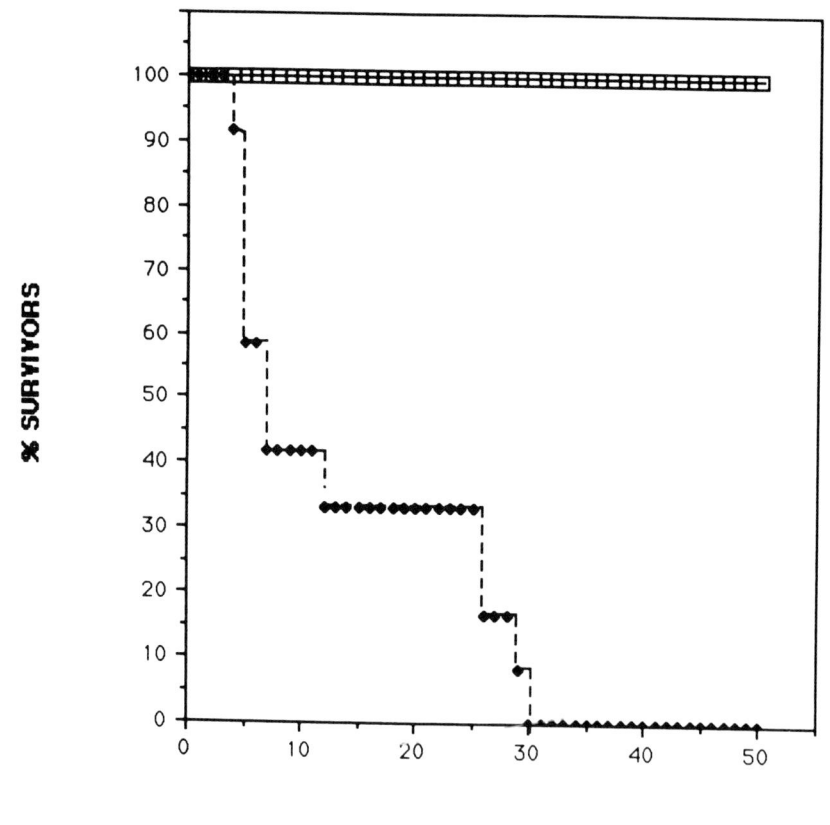

DAYS POST INFECTION

Fig. 10.2 Comparison of virulence in vivo of encapsulated *C. neoformans* and a stable acapsular mutant. CBA/Ca mice were injected i.p. with 3×10^7 encapsulated (B3501; ● ●) versus acapsular (B4131; ⊟) *C. neoformans.*

presence or absence of a capsule with virulence in experimental models of infection. Isolates obtained without detectable capsules are avirulent when injected into mice and reversion to the encapsulated state results in lethal infection (Mitchell & Friedman 1972). More direct comparisons of virulence can be made using stable acapsular mutants of *C. neoformans* generated by mutagenesis of an encapsulated parent strain. Again, the capacity to generate a detectable capsule structure is associated with lethal infection (Fig. 10.2; Fromtling et al 1982). Although controversial, it has been suggested that isolates of *C. neoformans* from AIDS patients have smaller capsules than those from patients infected with the organism in the absence of AIDS (Bottone & Wormser 1986). This may reflect the increased susceptibility of AIDS patients to potentially less virulent organisms which express smaller amounts of capsule.

It is important to note that while the capsule is the most extensively described, it is not the sole determinant of virulence for this organism. All members of the genus *Cryptococcus* possess capsules, yet only *C. neoformans* causes severe infection. The ability to synthesize melanin via a phenol oxidase enzyme system also influences infectivity of *C. neoformans* although this is not sufficient to confer virulence to non-encapsulated yeasts (Kwon-Chung & Rhodes 1986). The immunological consequences of melanin expression and its potential for protecting *C. neoformans* against oxygen-dependent killing by phagocytes (Jacobsen & Emery 1991) are important areas for further investigation.

Pathogenicity conferred by polysaccharide capsules is usually associated with (1) their anti-phagocytic action, (2) their poor immunogenicity and (3) their potential tolerogenic or immunosuppressive effects. All of these attributes have been described for the capsule of *C. neoformans* and may contribute to the pathogenicity of the organism. The anti-phagocytic action of the capsule has been extensively documented and inhibits ingestion of *C. neoformans* by neutrophils, monocytes and macrophages (Kozel et al 1988). An important exception to this is the alveolar macrophage, which can ingest unopsonized yeasts in vitro (Levitz & DiBenedetto 1989). In contrast, acapsular mutants are readily bound and ingested by phagocytic cells in the absence of exogenous opsonins. Thus it is believed that the capsule passively inhibits phagocytosis by masking phagocytosis-promoting structures on the cell wall (Kozel & Gotschlich 1982). This is confirmed in experiments where addition of purified polysaccharide to acapsular yeasts confers resistance to attachment and ingestion by phagocytes (Kozel & Mastronianni 1976). Purified polysaccharides from all four serotypes share this anti-phagocytic property and this can be removed by chemical modification of the capsule by periodate oxidation and reduction (Kozel & Hormerath 1984).

The anti-phagocytic action of the capsule can be partially overcome by opsonization of *C. neoformans* with either complement products or specific immunoglobulin (Kozel et al 1988). In the latter case, anti-capsule IgG binds to the capsule surface and promotes ingestion via interaction with Fc receptors expressed by phagocytic cells. IgG isolated from normal human serum is also opsonic for encapsulated yeasts, even though it is predominantly deposited below the capsule surface (Kozel et al 1988). Monoclonal antibodies directed against the capsule have also been shown to transfer protection against infection with *C. neoformans* in mice (Dromer et al 1987). Finally, anti-capsule antibodies are detected in patients with cryptococcosis, and their presence correlates with an improvement in response to treatment and a better long term prognosis (Diamond & Bennett 1974, Zuger et al 1986).

Other encapsulated pathogens employ a variety of strategies to avoid opsonization by components of the complement cascade and subsequent phagocytosis. The capsule can mask underlying structures which are efficient substrates for complement deposition, and may itself be a poor substrate for attachment of complement components. In contrast to these other models of evasion, the polysaccharide of *C. neoformans* is an efficient activator of the alternative complement pathway. Incubation in non-immune serum results in deposition of C3 components at or immediately below the capsule surface and therefore potentially available to complement receptors on phagocytic cells (Kozel et al 1988). Inactivation of C3b occurs rapidly at the capsule surface of *C. neoformans* and the predominant complement fragment generated is iC3b (Kozel & Pfrommer 1986). Most isolates of encapsulated *C. neoformans* show similar activation of the complement pathway, but considerable variation is found in the extent of phagocytosis that follows. This is not related to changes in the site of complement deposition, the number of C3 molecules per yeast or the type of C3 fragment which predominates (Kozel et al 1988). The basis of these differences in phagocytic potential are currently unresolved. Finally, the importance of complement for resistance is seen in vivo where depletion of C3 in guinea pigs by cobra venom factor increases susceptibility to infection with *C. neoformans* (Diamond et al 1973).

REGULATION OF PHAGOCYTOSIS OF *C. NEOFORMANS*

The deposition of complement at the surface of opsonized yeasts highlights the role of complement receptors in the interaction of virulent *C. neoformans* and phagocytic cells. Phagocytes express three distinct receptors capable of binding to fragments of C3, namely CR1, CR3 and CR4 (Ross 1989). CR1 (CD35) binds C3b, C4b and iC3b and is a member of the complement regulatory protein family. CR3 (CD11b/CD18) shows highest affinity for the inactivated form of C3b (iC3b), whilst CR4 (CD11c/CD18; p 150, 95) preferentially binds C3dg and under some conditions iC3b. In contrast to CR1, both CR3 and CR4 are members of the leucocyte integrin family, sharing the common features of a heterodimeric structure composed of membrane spanning α and β chains, and an obligate requirement for divalent cations for ligand binding (Springer 1990). The recognition site for CR3 binding to iC3b is determined by the tripeptide Arg-Gly-Asp (RGD) in humans, or Leu-Gly-Asp (LGD) in the mouse. CR3 is also reported to possess a binding site for β glucans and lipopolysaccharide, and is suggested to recognize additional non-complement ligands such as fibronectin, factor X and gp63 of *Leishmania* (Brown 1991).

Multiple complement receptors appear to be involved in binding of serum opsonized *C. neoformans* to phagocytes. Thus monoclonal antibodies to CR1, CR3 or CR4 can each inhibit binding to human monocyte-macrophages in vitro (Levitz & Tabuni 1991). Complement receptors cluster to the site of yeast binding and this interaction is blocked by disruption of the cytoskeleton with cytochalasin-D, or in the presence of azide. These results suggest that active migration of multiple receptors on the phagocyte surface is required for binding of the encapsulated yeast.

The factors which control whether these events then result in ingestion of the particle are not clear. Unlike Fc or mannose receptor dependent events, efficient ingestion of particles via complement receptors is not a constitutive feature of resting macrophages (Brown 1991). In the case of *C. neoformans*, only 23% of bound, complement opsonized yeasts were phagocytosed by human monocyte-macrophages compared to 64% following IgG opsonization (Levitz & Tabuni 1991). Efficient ingestion via complement receptors requires prior activation of the macrophage. This can be achieved in vivo by administration of thioglycollate or BCG and in vitro by stimulation with phorbol esters. Ingestion can also be enhanced by additional events at the phagocyte membrane such as binding to extracellular matrix proteins or purified C1q (Bobak et al 1988) and following co-operative interaction with mannose fucose receptors (reviewed in Brown 1991).

Griffin and colleagues have identified a low molecular weight cytokine which enhances ingestion of complement opsonized yeasts by murine peritoneal macrophages (Griffin 1981, Griffin & Mullinax 1984). This factor is secreted by T-cells but its precise biochemical characteristics have not been defined. We have developed a model system to study the effects of various macrophage activating cytokines on ingestion of encapsulated *C. neoformans*. Cytokines such as IFN-γ, GM-CSF, IL-4 and TNF can activate macrophages for tumoricidal and microbicidal functions, but until recently their effects on complement mediated phagocytosis had not been addressed. Here, incubation of macrophages with either murine rTNF-α, rGM-CSF and to a lesser extent rIL-1 increased ingestion of complement opsonized *C. neoformans* (Fig. 10.3). Maximal activation was observed after 3 days stimulation with the cytokines, although significant effects were observed by 24 h. This correlates with the known kinetics of these cytokines for activation of other macrophage functions and differentiates these events from those described by Griffin where activation occurred within minutes. In further experiments, suboptimal concentrations of TNF and GM-CSF which alone had no effect, showed clear synergy when added together at the initiation of culture. In contrast, addition of up to 1000 U/ml of IFN-γ had no effect on uptake despite enhancing Ia antigen expression and inducing morphological changes typical of macrophage activation. Activation of macrophages for phagocytosis also occurred with culture supernatants from *C. neoformans* primed T-cells responding to acapsular yeasts in vitro. This activity was neutralized by addition of the anti-TNF mAb TN319.12, and TNF per se was detected at low levels in the supernatants by ELISA assay. Thus, two known macrophage activating cytokines, TNF-α and GM-CSF but not IFN-γ, IL-4, or M-CSF increased the efficiency of ingestion of opsonized, virulent *C. neoformans*. Increased ingestion was only observed with serum opsonized yeasts and macrophage activation alone was unable to overcome the anti-phagocytic action of the capsule in the absence of opsonins. Ingestion was abrogated by addition of mAb M1/70 or 5C6, demonstrating the importance of CR3 in these events. In preliminary experiments, the increase in CR3-dependent ingestion could not be accounted for by changes in CR3 expression at the cell surface, consistent with the concept of receptor activation rather than quantitative changes in

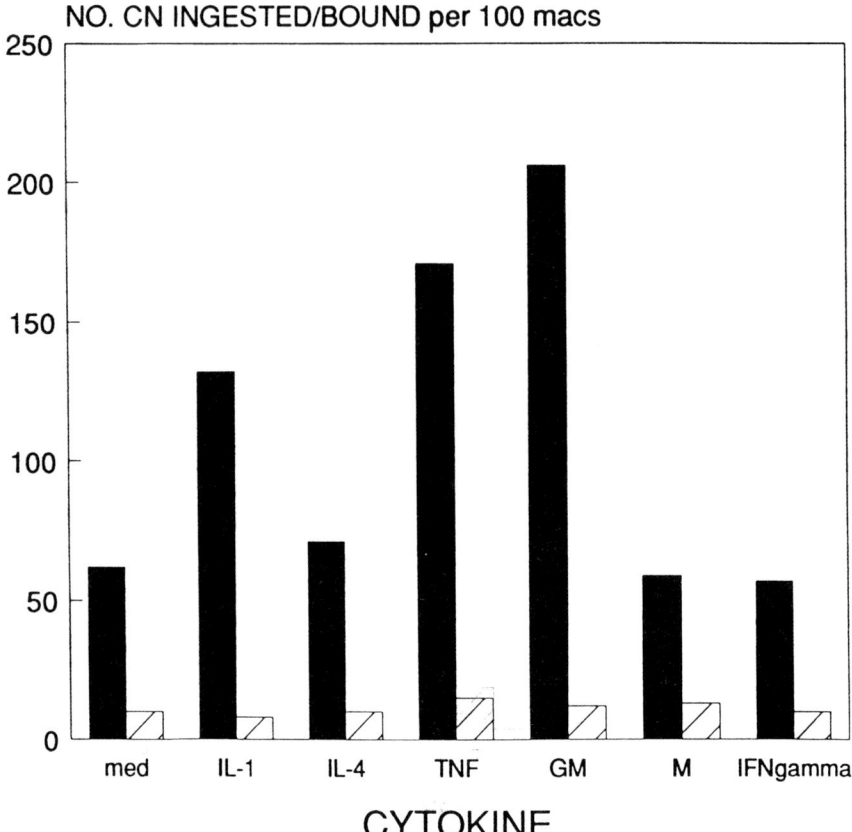

NO. CN INGESTED/BOUND per 100 macs

CYTOKINE

Fig. 10.3 Cytokine activation of macrophages enhances phagocytosis of encapsulated *C. neoformans*. Non-opsonized (▨) or normal mouse serum opsonized (■) *C. neoformans* were added to adherent peritoneal macrophage monolayers 3 days after activation with recombinant cytokines. Data are presented as the mean number of yeasts bound/ingested per 100 macrophages.

expression. The nature of this activation is a central issue in integrin biology and may involve upregulation of an independent receptor, increased mobility of CR3 in the cell membrane, alterations in cytoskeletal attachment or enhanced phosphorylation or other signalling events following CR3–ligand interactions.

An obvious advantage of using pathogens rather than inert phagocytic particles to study the regulation of phagocytosis is that mediators which enhance ingestion in vitro can be tested for their importance during infection in vivo. We have now investigated whether TNF is involved in resistance to virulent *C. neoformans* in vivo. Neutralizing mAb TN319.12 specific for murine TNF-α and β was administered to mice 1 day prior to injection with encapsulated *C. neoformans* and weekly during the course of infection (Sheehan et al 1989). As seen in Figure 10.4, neutralization of TNF in vivo increased the severity of infection and was associated with an increased number of yeasts in the brains of infected mice (data not shown). Although TNF may be involved in additional resistance mechanisms (such as the generation of reactive nitrogen intermediates) these results demonstrate the importance of this cytokine in resistance to experimental infection. Finally, injection of the anti-CR3

186

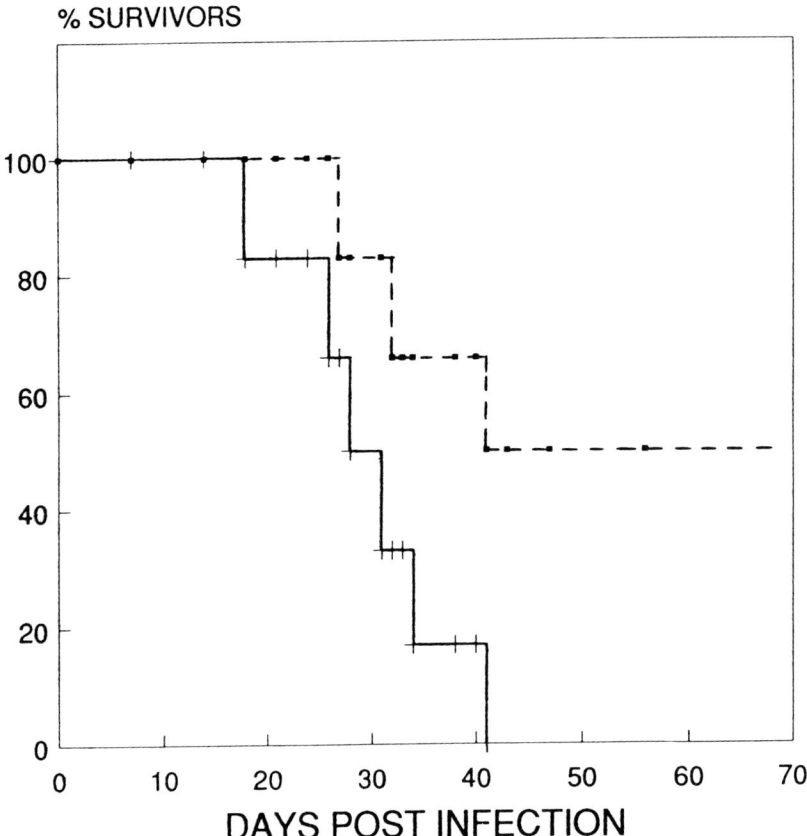

Fig. 10.4 Effect of anti-TNF mAb on *C. neoformans* infection in vivo. BALB/c mice were pretreated i.p. with 300 μg of either hamster anti-TNF mAb TN319.12 (++) or the control antibody L2 (●··●) one day prior to, and weekly following i.p. infection with 3×10^6 B3501 *C. neoformans*.

mAb 5C6, which blocks ingestion of opsonized *C. neoformans* in vitro and impairs the influx of inflammatory cells in vivo (Rosen et al 1989) also increased susceptibility to infection and reduced the average survival time of infected mice from 25.8 ± 4.8 to 7.7 ± 4.6 days (Collins & Bancroft, unpublished observations).

THE EFFECT OF CAPSULE SYNTHESIS ON CELL-MEDIATED IMMUNITY

Clinical and experimental evidence have demonstrated the importance of cell-mediated immunity in resistance to *C. neoformans* (e.g. Mody et al 1990). However, an important issue is the ability of the polysaccharide to interfere with development of T-cell immunity, thereby contributing to the virulence of the encapsulated yeast. Cryptococcal polysaccharide antigens can be found at high concentrations in the blood and CSF of infected individuals and this has led to the development of experimental models to test whether the capsular material is itself immunosuppressive. Non-antigen specific immunosuppression has been described during infection of experimental animals with *C. neoformans*, with reduction in delayed type hypersensitivity responses and primary humoral responses to heterologous antigens (e.g. Blackstock & Hall 1984, Masih et al 1986). These effects have been ascribed to the development of either adherent or non-adherent suppressor cells, although their precise characteristics and the mechanisms of action are unclear. In other studies, injection of capsular polysaccharides into inbred mice was found to generate a suppressor T-cell population which in vitro releases a soluble factor capable of inhibiting macrophage phagocytic activity (Blackstock et al 1987). Inhibition is rapid and specific for Fc and mannose-receptor-mediated events but not complement-dependent phagocytosis (Blackstock & Hernandez 1989). The inhibitory material has not been purified or sequenced and, in general, more information is needed about soluble mediators which inhibit macrophage phagocytosis.

The most extensively described model of immunosuppression concerns the cascade of suppressor T-cells induced following injection of mice with cryptococcal antigens or with sera from infected mice (reviewed in Murphy 1988). The series of suppressor cells induced regulate both the development and expression of delayed type hypersensitivity in vivo. Intravenous injection of polysaccharide containing *C. neoformans* antigens generates an $Lyt1,^+2^-$ T_s1-cell which inhibits the generation of T-cells mediating DTH in vivo (Murphy & Moorhead 1982, Murphy et al 1983). Additional suppressor cell subsets differing in their method of induction and the factors they produce are also observed in this system (Murphy 1988).

While the inhibitory effects of these cells are clear, their mechanism of action remains ill defined. The suppressor factors produced have not been purified to homogeneity or biochemically defined. Future experiments comparing their effects with known immunomodulatory cytokines should be informative. Recent advances in the definition of $CD4^+$ T-cells into Th1 and Th2 subsets may underlie some of these processes. Thus, Th1-cells which promote DTH reactions and secrete IFN-γ and IL-2 can be inhibited by products of Th2-cells including IL-4 and IL-10 (reviewed in Street & Mosmann 1991). The possible contribution of the Th1/Th2 network to the suppressive events described for *C. neoformans* is an important and exciting area for further investigation.

Finally, polysaccharides such as Ficoll and Dextran have been reported to inhibit the intracellular processing of protein antigens by macrophages (Leyva-Cobian & Unanue 1988). To assess whether cryptococcal polysaccharides may exert a similar immunosuppressive effect, we have investigated the effect of capsule synthesis on the processing and presentation of *C. neoformans* to specific T-cells. Lymph node cells from mice primed with acapsular *C. neoformans* in vivo proliferated in culture when stimulated with soluble antigens derived from either acapsular or encapsulated yeasts. In contrast, T-cell proliferation induced by intact encapsulated yeasts was greatly reduced in comparison to the acapsular mutant, suggesting that the capsule of intact *C. neoformans* inhibited T-cell activation. However, this effect was due to the anti-phagocytic action of the capsule preventing ingestion by antigen-presenting macrophages rather than an inhibitory effect on antigen processing per se. When T-cell proliferation was correlated with the rate of ingestion by purified macrophage antigen presenting cells, antigens of both forms of the organism were processed and presented with equal efficiency. Furthermore, addition of purified capsular polysaccharide had no effect on the processing of the heterologous antigen hen egg lysozyme by macrophages. Thus the capsule of *C. neoformans* interferes with T-cell stimulation via its anti-phagocytic action, without interfering with antigen processing and presentation (Collins & Bancroft 1991, in press).

SUMMARY

Cryptococcus neoformans is an encapsulated yeast which is emerging as an increasingly important opportunistic pathogen in association with the AIDS epidemic. Capsule production is an essential determinant of virulence and can interfere with ingestion by host phagocytic cells and the generation of cell-mediated immune responses. Future studies on the molecular biology of *C. neoformans* should provide important new insights into the genes which regulate capsule synthesis and their relationship to virulence. From an immunological perspective, further studies are needed to identify the mechanisms underlying suppression of macrophage and T-lymphocyte functions observed in vivo, and in vitro, *C. neoformans* also provides a fascinating opportunity to probe the events controlling ingestion of micro-organisms by phagocytic cells. Evidence that encapsulated and acapsular yeasts may differentially trigger certain macrophage functions also provides an important model to study the cell biology of receptor signalling at the macrophage cell surface (Levitz & DiBenedetto 1988). Finally, observations that cytokines such as IFN-γ (Levitz & DiBenedetto 1988, Salkowski & Balish 1991), GM-CSF and TNF are all essential for regulation of experimental immunity to *C. neoformans*, may provide the basis for future clinical trials on the effects of cytokine therapy in the immunocompromised host.

ACKNOWLEDGEMENTS

This work was supported by a Wellcome Trust University Award to GJB and an AIDS Directed Programme PhD Studentship to HLC. We gratefully acknowledge the support and advice of Prof. R. J. Hay.

REFERENCES

Bhattacharjee A K, Bennett J E, Glaudemans C P 1984 Capsular polysaccharides of *Cryptococcus neoformans*. Reviews of Infectious Diseases 6: 619–624
Blackstock R, Hall N K 1984 Non-specific immunosuppression by *Cryptococcus neoformans* infection. Mycopathologia 86: 35–43
Blackstock R, McCormack J M, Hall N K 1987 Induction of a macrophage-suppressive lymphokine by soluble cryptococcal antigens and its association with models of immunologic tolerance. Infection and Immunity 55: 233–239
Blackstock R, Hernandez N C 1989 Characterisation of the macrophage subset affected and its response to a T suppressor factor (TsFmp) found in cryptococcosis. Infection and Immunity 57: 2931–2937
Bobak D A, Washburn R G, Frank M 1988 C1q enhances the phagocytosis of *Cryptococcus neoformans* blastospores by human monocytes. Journal of Immunology 141: 592–597

Bottone E J, Wormser G P 1986 Poorly encapsulated *Cryptococcus neoformans* from patients with AIDS. II Correlation of capsule size observed directly in cerebrospinal fluid with that after animal passage. AIDS Research 2: 219–225

Brown E J 1991 Complement receptors and phagocytosis. Current Opinion in Immunology 3: 76–82

Cherniak R, Reiss E, Slodki M, Plattner R, Blumer S 1980 Structure and antigenic activity of capsular polysaccharide of *Cryptococcus neoformans* serotype A. Molecular Immunology 17: 1025–1032

Collins H L, Bancroft G J 1991 Encapsulation of *Cryptococcus neoformans* impairs antigen specific T cell responses. Infection and Immunity 52 (in press)

Deepe G S, Bullock W E 1990 Immunological aspects of fungal pathogenesis. European Journal of Clinical Microbiology and Infectious Disease 9: 377–380

Diamond R D, May J E, Kane M A, Frank M, Bennett J E 1973 The role of late complement components and the alternate complement pathway in experimental cryptococcosis. Proceedings of the Society for Experimental Biology and Medicine 144: 312–315

Diamond R D, Bennett J E 1974 Prognostic factors in cryptococcal meningitis. Annals of Internal Medicine 80: 176–181

Diamond R D 1991 The growing problem of mycoses in patients infected with the human immunodeficiency virus. Reviews of Infectious Disease 13: 480–486

Dromer F, Charriere J, Contrepois A, Carbon C, Veni P 1987 Protection of mice against experimental cryptococcosis by anti-*Cryptococcus* monoclonal antibody. Infection and Immunity 55:749–752

Dykstra M A, Friedman L, Murphy J W 1977 Capsule size of *Cryptococcus neoformans:* control and relationship to virulence. Infection and Immunity 16: 129–135

Ellis D H, Pfeiffer T J 1990 Ecology, life cycle, and infectious propagule of *Cryptococcus neoformans*. Lancet 336: 923–25

Farhi F, Bulmer G S, Tacker T R 1970 *Cryptococcus neoformans* iv. The not-so-encapsulated yeast. Infection and Immunity 1: 526–531

Finlay B, Falkow S 1989 Common themes in microbial pathogenicity. Microbiological Reviews 53: 210–230

Flesch I E A, Schwamberger G, Kaufman S H E 1989 Fungicidal activity of IFNγ activitated macrophages – extracellular killing of *Cryptococcus neoformans*. Journal of Immunology 142: 3219–3224

Fromtling R A, Shadomy H J, Jacobsen E J 1982 Decreased virulence in stable, acapsular mutants of *Cryptococcus neoformans*. Mycopathologia 79: 23–29

Griffin F M Jr 1981 Roles of macrophage Fc and C3b receptors in phagocytosis of immunologically coated *Cryptococcus neoformans*. Proceedings of the National Academy of Sciences, USA 78: 3853–3857

Griffin J R Jr, Mullinax P J 1984 Augmentation of macrophage complement receptor function in vitro. IV The lymphokine that activates macrophage C3 receptors for phagocytosis binds to a fucose bearing glycoprotein on the macrophage plasma membrane. Journal of Experimental Medicine 160: 1206-1218

Holmberg K, Meyer R D 1986 Fungal infections in patients with AIDS and AIDS-related complex. Scandinavian Journal of Infectious Diseases 18: 179–192

Jacobson E S, Emery H S 1991 Catecholamine uptake, melanization, and oxygen toxicity in *Cryptococcus neoformans*. Journal of Bacteriology 173: 401–403

Kozel T R, Mastronianni R P 1976 Inhibition of phagocytosis by cryptococcal polysaccharide: dissociation of the attachment and ingestion phases of phagocytosis. Infection and Immunity 14: 62–67

Kozel T R, Gotschlich E C 1982 The capsule of *Cryptococcus neoformans* passively inhibits phagocytosis of the yeast by macrophages. Journal of Immunology 129: 1660–1675

Kozel T R, Hermerath C A 1984 Binding of cryptococcal polysaccharide to *Cryptococcus neoformans*. Infection and Immunity 43: 879–886

Kozel T R, Pfrommer G 1986 Activation of complement system by *Cryptococcus neoformans* leads to binding of iC3b to the yeast. Infection and Immunity 52: 1–5

Kozel T R, Pfrommer G, Guerlain A, Highison B, Highison G 1988 The role of the capsule in phagocytosis of *Cryptococcus neoformans*. Reviews of Infectious Disease 10: S436–S439

Kwon-Chung K J, Rhodes J C 1986 Encapsulation and melanin formation as indicators of virulence in *Cryptococcus neoformans*. Infection and Immunity 51: 218–222

Levitz S M, DiBenedetto D J 1988 Differential stimulation of murine peritoneal cells by selectively opsonised encapsulated and acapsular *Cryptococcus neoformans*. Infection and Immunity 56: 2544–2551

Levitz S M, DiBenedetto D J 1989 Paradoxical role of capsule in murine bronchoalveolar macrophage mediated killing of *Cryptococcus neoformans*. Journal of Immunology 142: 659–665

Levitz S M, Tabuni A 1991 Binding requirements of *Cryptococcus neoformans* by cultured macrophages. Requirements for multiple complement receptors and actin. Journal of Clinical Investigation 87: 528–535

Leyva-Cobian F, Unanue E R 1988 Intracellular interference with antigen presentation. Journal of Immunology 141: 1445–1450

Masih D, Rubinstein H, Sotomayor C, Ferro M, Riera C 1986 Non-specific immunosuppression in experimental cryptococcosis in rats. Mycopathologia 94: 79–84

Mitchell T G, Friedman L 1972 In vitro phagocytosis and intracellular fate of variously encapsulated strains of *Cryptococcus neoformans*. Infection and Immunity 5: 491–498

Mody C H, Lipscomb M F, Street N E, Toews G B 1990 Depletion of CD4$^+$ (L3T4$^+$) lymphocytes in vivo impairs murine host defense to *Cryptococcus neoformans*. Journal of Immunology 144: 1472–1477

Murphy J W, Moorhead J 1982 Regulation of cell mediated immunity in cryptococcosis. 1. Induction of specific afferent T-suppressor cells by cryptococcal antigen. Journal of Immunology 128: 276–283

Murphy J W, Mosley R L, Moorhead J W 1983 Regulation of cell mediated immunity in cryptococcosis II Characterization of first order T suppressor cells (ts 1) and induction of second order suppressor cells. Journal of Immunology 130: 2876–2881

Murphy J W 1988 Influence of cryptococcal antigens on cell mediated immunity. Reviews of Infectious Disease 10: S432–S435

Rosen H, Milon G, Gordon S 1989 Antibody to the murine type 3 complement receptor inhibits T lymphocyte dependent recruitment of myelomonocytic cells in vivo. Journal of Experimental Medicine 169: 535–548

Ross G D 1989 Complement and complement receptors. Current Opinion in Immunology 2: 50–62

Ruiz A, Bulmer G S 1981 Particle size of airborne *Cryptococcus neoformans* in a tower. Applied and Environmental Microbiology 41: 1225–1229

Salkowski C A, Balish E 1991 A monoclonal antibody to gamma interferon blocks augmentation of natural killer cell activity induced during systemic cryptococcosis. Infection and Immunity 59:486–493

Sheehan K C F, Ruddle N F, Schreiber R D 1989 Generation and characterization of hamster monoclonal antibodies that neutralise murine tumour necrosis factors. Journal of Immunology 142: 3884–3893

Springer T A 1990 Adhesion receptors of the immune system. Nature 346: 425–433

Street N E, Mosmann T R 1991 Functional diversity of T lymphocytes due to secretion of different cytokine patterns. The FASEB Journal 5: 171–177

White C W, Cherniak R, Jacobsen E S 1990 Side group addition by xylosyltransferase and glucuronyltransferase in biosynthesis of capsular polysaccharide in *Cryptococcus neoformans*. Journal of Medical and Veterinary Mycology 28: 289–301

Zuger A, Louie E, Holzman R S, Simberkoff M S, Rahal J 1986 Cryptococcal disease in patients with the acquired immunodeficiency syndrome. Annals of Internal Medicine 104: 234–240

Discussion of paper presented by G. J. Bancroft

Discussed by T. R. Kozel
Reported by J. Verhoef

Dr Kozel, during his discussion, touched on three different subjects: capsule synthesis; complement activation by the capsule; and immunity related to the polysaccharide and some of its implications.

He said that one issue concerning capsule synthesis had troubled him for a number of years. The specific question was whether the polysaccharide studied in vitro was the same polysaccharide as that produced in vivo.

Dr Kozel said that there were many reports of serum antigen titres in the order of 1:500 000, 1:1 million, 1:2 million, sometimes as high as 1:8 million. In vitro, a preparation of cryptococcal polysaccharide, prepared from yeast culture filtrates, with an antigen titre of 1:500 000, which is a fraction of the maximum titres reported in the literature, is thick and viscous. This cannot be the case in vivo. Either the strains present in patients are producing polysaccharides that are different, or the polysaccharide is being processed in vivo.

Dr Peterson raised the point that some of the same arguments have been applied to the capsule of *S. aureus*.

The second question relates to the mechanism of complement activation, in electron micrographs of an encapsulated yeast incubated in normal human serum and stained for C3. There is a dense deposit of C3 at the periphery of the capsule. This reflects a possible concentration of 2×10^7 molecules per cell. This process is mediated by the alternative pathway. The C3 is almost entirely in the form of iC3b, and it is linked to the polysaccharide by a covalent ester bond. It takes about 8 min to completely cover the capsule of an encapsulated yeast with C3.

However, when the same experiment was completed with normal serum using non-encapsulated Cryptococci there was an early and simultaneous activation and binding of C3 around the cell wall of non-encapsulated Cryptococci. Coating with C3 is completed in 2 min. Complement in this case is activated by the classical pathway.

Normal serum contains an ubiquitous antibody to yeast cell walls. This serum with non-encapsulated *Cryptococci* can be converted back to complement activation via the alternative pathway. The same thing is repeated in serum that has been treated with EGTA to block the classical pathway. This work has all been done in vitro. The mechanism of complement binding has also been repeated in vivo in experimentally infected mice. In the lung there was activation and binding of C3 to the yeast. The same thing occurred in other tissues such as liver, spleen and prostate. The one organ in which there was no evidence of complement activation, i.e. binding of C3, was in the brain. Invariably no yeast cells with C3 bound to the capsule were found in brain tissue. The absence of complement in cerebrospinal fluid (CSF) clearly contributes to virulence.

Dr Kozel moved on to an entirely different point: the significance of the immune system, specifically the antibody response, to the polysaccharide. Normal subjects have antibody to the polysaccharide. Dr Kozel studied 30 normal subjects with an enzyme-linked assay specific for the soluble polysaccharide. All 30 subjects had IgM that was reactive with the polysaccharide. In contrast, only about 30% had IgG antibody reactive with the polysaccharide, and an even smaller proportion had appreciable amounts of IgA. All the top five IgG producers had IgG2 and only two of the five individuals had IgG1, which is very typical of what would be expected for human antibody responses to any polysaccharide.

What is the significance of this antibody? Is it simply due to an encounter with a cross reaction bacterial polysaccharide, or does it reflect a prior exposure to cryptococcal polysaccharide? As it has an unusual structure this possibility has to be considered.

Another factor related to the antibody to the polysaccharide was discussed: the prospects for passive immunization. It was shown several years ago that passive immunization was possible in a murine model of cryptococcosis. Dr Kozel has also studied the use of monoclonal antibodies for passive immunization and found that tissue levels of the yeast in lung and spleen may be decreased. But no effect on cryptococci in the brain was observed.

Dr Kozel concluded that in the future cytokines might be used in an immuno-suppressed patient to facilitate phagocytosis via complement receptors alone, or that it could be used in conjunction with passive immunization looking for possible synergy.

Dr Bennett raised the point that no cryptococcal polysaccharide has been described that could stimulate T-cells. Cryptococcal antigens that stimulate T-cells are presumably proteins. Dr Bancroft then added that everything known about the processing and presentation of antigens and binding to the T-cell receptor excludes the idea that T-cells could directly recognize polysaccharides because these events occur by peptides sitting in the groove of the MHC cleft and then being recognized by the T-cell receptor. It has not proved possible to block this phenomenon with polysaccharides.

The issue of serum levels of tumour necrosis factor (TNF) during experimental infections was raised. Dr Bancroft said that serum levels per se do not appear to signify much. (TNF can be easily absorbed by cells.) TNF should be measured at the mRNA level.

When the question of vaccines was raised, Dr Kozel answered that he did some work in this area 15 or 20 years ago and found those mice that were immunized were more susceptible to infection.

Dr Bennett then added that his group had made a conjugate of tetanus toxoid and cryptococcal polysaccharide and used passive and active immunization of mice to protect them against subsequent infection by high and low doses of *C. neoformans*. Both active and passive immunization schemes were able to protect against intravenous inoculation of 1000 but not against a million cryptococci. He concluded that even with high titres of antibody it is only possible to kill a small number of cryptococci, and this may be by the complement-mediated activity of the antibody enhancing phagocytosis and the intracellular killing process.

11. Recent advances in the molecular genetics of *Cryptococcus neoformans*

K. J. Kwon-Chung, J. C. Edman

INTRODUCTION

Cryptococcus neoformans is the aetiologic agent of cryptococcosis. The disease was first reported in 1894 by Busse, a pathologist who observed the round-to-oval 'corpuscle' in a sarcoma-like tumour of the tibia of a woman (Busse 1894). Busse isolated a culture from the lesion and Buschke, the physician who took care of the patient, thought it was a *Coccidia* (Buschke 1895). Soon after Busse's report, Sanfelice isolated *C. neoformans* from peach juice in Italy, and he realized that it was the same as Busse's fungus (Sanfelice 1894). Unlike the first cryptococcosis case, subsequent human isolates were obtained mainly from patients with meningoencephalitis, with cases reported from all parts of the world.

Cryptococcosis remained a rare disease until aggressive immunosuppressive therapy came into wide use (Diamond 1990). Since 1980, the occurrence of cryptococcosis has increased drastically, with AIDS becoming the leading predisposing factor for the disease. Currently, the frequency of cryptococcosis in AIDS patients is about 7–8% (Dismukes 1988).

After the heterothallic life cycle of *C. neoformans* was unveiled (Kwon-Chung 1975), factors such as the production of phenoloxidase and the polysaccharide capsule have been identified as virulence factors by classical genetic studies (Kwon-Chung & Rhodes 1986). With the high frequency of cryptococcosis in AIDS patients, research interest in *C. neoformans* has heightened, and considerable progress has been made with genetic studies of the organism.

In this paper, molecular biological studies with the emphasis on gene cloning, karyotyping, and the relationship between DNA-mediated transformation and virulence of *C. neoformans* will be discussed.

GENES CLONED FROM *C. NEOFORMANS*

To our knowledge, a total of 13 genes have been isolated from *C. neoformans* during the past 2 years (Table 11.1). Only five of these have been described in the literature. The first report of cloning a *C. neoformans* gene was made by Restrepo & Barbour (1989) for their isolation of rDNA encoding 5S, 18S, and 25S rRNA.

They used cloned *Saccharomyces cerevisiae* rDNA as a probe to isolate a single *Hind*III fragment containing the rDNA gene cluster. When we used this rDNA sequence as a probe to locate the gene on chromosomes of *C. neoformans* separated by pulsed-field electrophoresis, the probe hybridized to only one of the three largest chromosomes, depending on the isolate (Kwon-Chung et al 1991). Subsequently, 12 genes (or cDNA) have been cloned by four different methods: (1) complementing auxotrophs of *E. coli* or *S. cerevisiae*; (2) polymerase chain reaction (PCR); (3) difference cloning; and (4) using *S. cerevisiae* genes as heterologous probes. As listed in Table 11.1, *URA5, URA3, ADE1, ADE2, LEU2, HIS3, MDH1, TRP1,* and *DHFR* were cloned by the first method. In most of these cases, cDNA was used to complement *E. coli* or *S. cerevisiae*, with the cloned cDNA serving as a probe to isolate the genes from a genomic library. In the case of *TRP1* and *MDH1*, however, a *C. neoformans* genomic library constructed in a *S. cerevisiae* shuttle vector was used to transform yeast with appropriate markers. Among these nine genes, *URA5* (Edman & Kwon-Chung 1990), *ADE1*, and *ADE2* have been used for transformation of the corresponding *C. neoformans* auxotrophs. The size of the coding regions of these genes varied from 0.7 to 2.2 kbp. The *URA5* gene served as the first selective marker for transformation in *C. neoformans* var. *neoformans* and *C. neoformans* var. *gattii* (Edman & Kwon-Chung 1990). The gene

Table 11.1 *Cryptococcus neoformans* genes

Gene	Enzyme	Isolated by*	Size (kbp)	Reference
URA5	Orotidine monophosphate pyrophosphorylase	E. coli	0.7	Edman & Kwon-Chung 1990
URA3	Orotidine-5′-phosphate decarboxylase	S. cerevisiae	0.9	Edman, unpublished
TRP1	Phosphoribosylan-thranilate isomerase	S. cerevisiae	?	Perfect, Rude et al 1989b
MDH1	Mannitol dehydrogenase	S. cerevisiae	1.7	Perfect, Rude et al 1991
ADE1	Phosphoribosyl-amino imidazole succinocarboxamide synthetase	E. coli	2.2	Edman, unpublished
ADE2	Phosphoribosyl-amino imidazole carboxylase	E. coli	2.0	Edman, unpublished
LEU2	3-isopropylmalate dehydrogenase	S. cerevisiae	1.1	Edman, unpublished
HIS3	Imidazole glycerolphosphate dehydratase	S. cerevisiae	1.0	Moore & Edman, unpublished
DHFR	Dihydrofolate reductase	E. coli	0.6	Cao & Edman, unpublished
TS	Thymidylate synthase	PCR	0.9	Edman & Edman, unpublished
rDNA	—	Heterologous probe	8–9	Restrepo & Barbour 1989
Mating type	—	Difference cloning	15	Moore & Edman, unpublished
EF3	—	Heterologous probe	?	Myers et al 1991

* Gene or cDNA was isolated by complementation (*E. coli* or *S. cerevisiae*), the polymerase chain reaction (PCR), difference cloning, or heterologous probe (*S. cerevisiae* gene).

coding for thymidylate synthase (*TS*) was cloned by using PCR. The primers used were a mixture of synthetic oligonucleotides that contain all possible sequences of two highly-conserved regions of eukaryotic *TS*s. It was these same primers that enabled Edman et al to clone *TS* of *Pneumocystis carinii* (Edman et al 1989). The *EF3* gene was cloned by using the corresponding *S. cerevisiae* gene as a heterologous probe, since the DNA sequence of *EF3* is highly conserved among fungal species. Comparison of deduced amino acid sequences showed greater than 70% identity between the *C. neoformans* and *S. cerevisiae* genes (Myers et al 1991).

The mating type gene (*MATα*) was isolated by the difference cloning method. Since *C. neoformans* is heterothallic with a one-locus (*MAT*) two-allele (α and *a*) system, and the DNA sequences of *MATα* and *MATa* differ from each other to a considerable degree, the difference cloning method allowed the isolation of sequences that are present in DNA from *MATα* isolates and absent in *MATa*. Prior to the isolation of *MATα*, a congenic set of α and *a* reference strains that differ only in mating type was constructed using the widely-used tester strains B-3501 (α) and B-3502 (*a*) (Kwon-Chung 1976). Single-basidiospore cultures of *a* (B-4476) and α (B-4478) isolates were recovered from a cross of B-3501 × B-3502. B-4476 was mated with B-4478, and an α offspring from this union was back-crossed to B-4476 to yield second-generation progeny. The process of isolating α single-basidiospore and back-crossing the culture to B-4476 was repeated a total of 10 times to produce B-4500, an α strain that is congenic with B-4476.

To isolate *MATα*, DNA from B-4500 (α) cells was digested with the restriction endonuclease *Taq*I and hybridized to an excess of randomly-sheared and denatured DNA from B-4476 (*a*). Ligation of the hybridization mix to appropriately-digested plasmid vector selected fragments with two cohesive ends and allowed the formation of transformation-competent circles. Of 16 plasmid clones, one containing a 130 bp insert that hybridizes to *MATα* but not *MATa* genomic DNA, was isolated. The mating type-specific nature of this insert was confirmed by Southern blot analysis of B-4476 and B-4500, and 10 progeny were obtained from the cross B-4476 × B-4500. The probe hybridized to DNAs of B-4500 and all five *MATα* progeny, but not to DNAs of B-4476 and *MATa* progeny. This result indicated that the probe sequence is linked to the mating type locus and is unique for α strains. Using the 130 bp insert as a probe, overlapping genomic clones encompassing 15 kbp were isolated. Southern hybridization with fragments of these clones to DNA of *MATα* and *MATa* showed that this region contains sequences specific for *MATα*. The extent of the regions that are responsible for the determination of mating type will be confirmed by transformation experiments. The significance of the isolation and characterization of the *MATα* gene is three-fold: it will provide insight into the mating process, as well as the nature of genetic regulatory mechanisms. In addition, it will provide insight into the role of *MATα* in the pathogenicity of *C. neoformans*. Not only are the majority of clinical isolates of *C. neoformans* known to be α mating type (Kwon-Chung 1978), but our recent study indicated that α mating type strains produce fatal infections in mice more rapidly than *a* mating strains (unpublished data).

We have used 10 of the 13 genes listed in Table 11.1 as probes to hybridize with chromosomes of the two varieties of *C. neoformans*. The physical locations of these genes were very similar between the isolates of serotypes A and D of the *neoformans* variety, and differed from B and C serotypes of *C. neoformans* var. *gattii* (unpublished data).

ELECTROPHORETIC KARYOTYPE OF ENVIRONMENTAL AND CLINICAL ISOLATES

Karyotyping by pulsed-field electrophoresis has been used extensively for genetic, taxonomic, and epidemiological studies of eukaryotic organisms (Wickes et al 1991). The technique, first developed by Schwartz & Cantor (1982), had been continually modified so that chromosomes up to 12 Mb in size can be separated (Orbach et al 1988). Previous reports on karyotyping of *C. neoformans* either by the OFAGE system (Polacheck & Lebens 1989) or by the contour-clamped

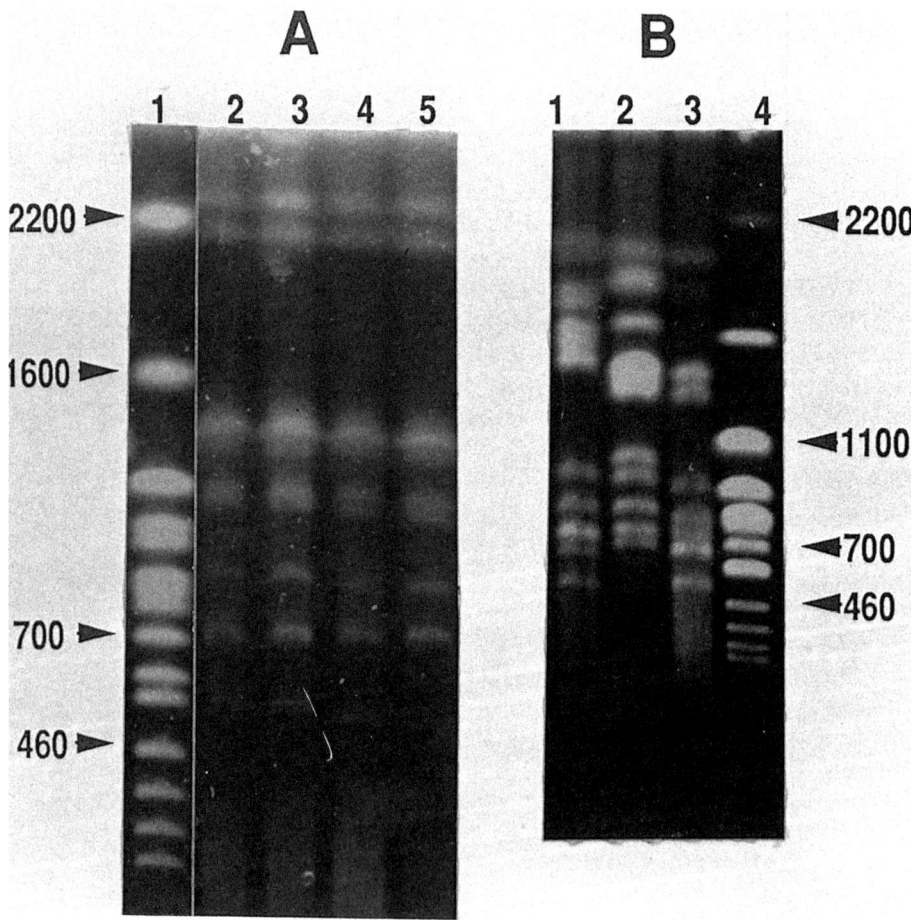

Fig. 11.1(A) Karyotype of *C. neoformans* var. *gattii*. Lane 1, a strain isolated from *E. camaldulensis* in San Francisco; lane. 2–4, strains isolated from *E. camaldulensis* in three different geographical locations in Northern Australia (B) Karyotype of *C. neoformans* var. *gattii* from patients in California (lanes 1, 3) and Africa (lane 2), type strain of *C. neoformans* var. *gattii*; *S. cerevisiae* (lane 4).

homogeneous field gel electrophoresis (CHEF) system (Perfect et al 1989a) indicated that each strain has a unique pattern of chromosome bands. Karyotyping, therefore, was suggested as a useful tool for distinguishing different strains (Perfect et al 1989a).

Unlike the previous studies with clinical isolates, the strains of *C. neoformans* var. *gattii* isolated from the red gum tree (*Eucalyptus camaldulensis*) found in California and three different geographic locations within Australia showed identical banding patterns by the CHEF system in our laboratory (Fig. 11.1A). Environmental isolates of *C. neoformans* var. *gattii* were not available until Ellis & Pfeiffer (1990) recently identified the ecological niche of this variety. The four isolates we have studied were of serotype B, and the number and size of their chromosomal bands were significantly different from the type strains of *C. neoformans* var. *gattii* (serotype B) (Fig. 11.1B) and *Filobasidiella neoformans* var. *bacillispora* (teleomorph of *C. neoformans* var. *gattii*), both isolated from human meningitis cases. Since the identification of *Eucalyptus*-originated *C. neoformans* var. *gattii* was made solely on the basis of biochemical characteristics (Kwon-Chung et al 1982, Kwon-Chung & Fell 1984) and the karyotype was significantly different from the type culture of *C. neoformans* var. *gattii*, further testing was necessary to confirm their identity. The commercially-available rDNA probe (AccuProbe by Gen-Probe, Inc., San Diego, CA) reported to be specific and sensitive for the identification of *C. neoformans* (Gordon et al 1991) was hybridized with the ribosomal RNA of various yeasts phylogenetically related to *C. neoformans* (Gueho et al 1989). The hybridization results of the various yeasts other than *C. neoformans* were far below the value considered to be positive, and that of the hybridization signals of *Eucalyptus*-originated isolates were of the same intensity as those produced by *C. neoformans* var. *gattii* strains isolated from cryptococcosis patients. Contrary to the environmental isolates, patient isolates of *C. neoformans* var. *gattii* revealed extensive polymorphism (size and number) in the chromosomal bands (Fig. 11.1B).

In isolates of *C. neoformans* var. *neoformans* studied in our laboratory, polymorphism exists among environmental as well as clinical isolates (Fig. 11.2). Variation is mostly seen in the size of chromosomes, and the extent of variation is much less than that seen among the clinical isolates of *C. neoformans* var. *gattii*. Overall, clinical and pigeon dropping isolates of *C. neoformans* var. *neoformans* yielded similar polymorphism patterns.

It appears that considerable DNA rearrangement, leading to an altered chromosome mobility, has occurred in these isolates. The gross genomic rearrangements, including high-level sequence amplification, extensive deletion, and random recombination between chromosomes carrying repeat sequences, have been known to generate karyotype polymorphism in a wide variety of organisms (Corcoran et al 1986, 1988, Shea et al 1986, Pologe & Ravetch 1988, Biggs et al 1989, Birch et al 1989, Janse et al 1989, Pagès et al 1989, Wagner & So 1990).

Observation of a uniform chromosome banding pattern in *Eucalyptus*-originated isolates, but not in patient isolates, is noteworthy. It is tempting to conclude that chromosome size and number polymorphism in clinical isolates of *C. neoformans* var. *gattii* occurred during asexual multiplication in human tissue. A similar phenomenon was reported in *Plasmodium berghei*. A high gametocyte-producing

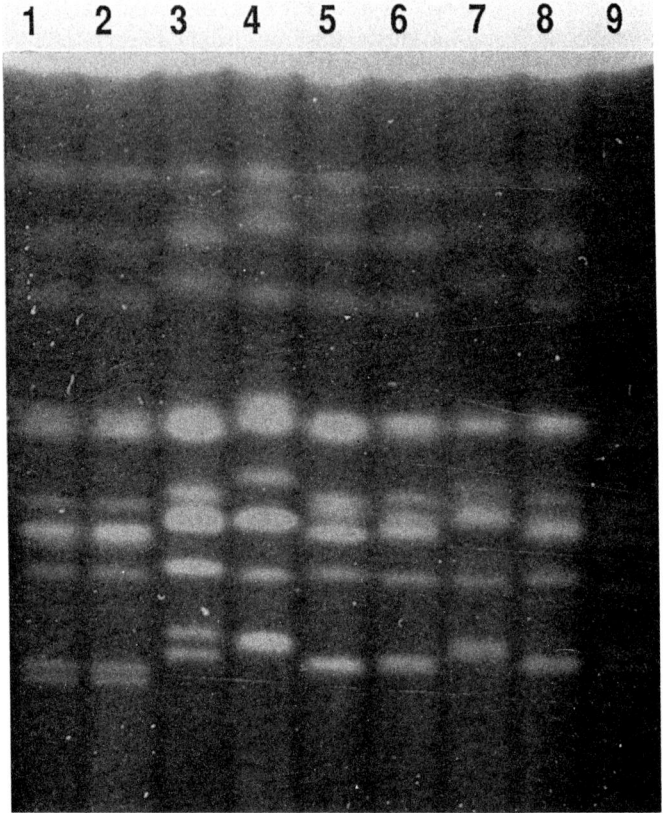

Fig. 11.2 Karyotype of *C. neoformans* var. *neoformans*. All environmental isolates except two patient isolates in lanes 3 and 9.

clone of *P. berghei* maintained in mice for prolonged periods showed karyotype changes, while those maintained in mosquitoes stayed stable (Janse et al 1989). Since chromosome size polymorphism was seen both in environmental and clinical isolates of *C. neoformans* var. *neoformans,* the situation may be similar to the low gametocyte-producing (LP) clone of *P. berghei.* Janse et al (1989) reported that the LP clones showed chromosomal instability during the passage in mosquitoes as well as in mice. Karyotypes of each isolate in both varieties of *C. neoformans,* however, were stable in vitro. The cultures maintained on agar for the past 15 years showed identical patterns to those kept in lyophilized form for 15 years.

DNA-MEDIATED TRANSFORMATION AND ITS EFFECT ON THE VIRULENCE OF *C. NEOFORMANS*

DNA-mediated transformation was achieved in *C. neoformans* by electroporating *ura5* cells in the presence of a plasmid vector containing the cloned *C. neoformans* *URA5* gene. Cloning of the *URA5* gene was accomplished by complementation of *pyrE E. coli* mutants with the *C. neoformans* cDNA library. The cDNA clone of

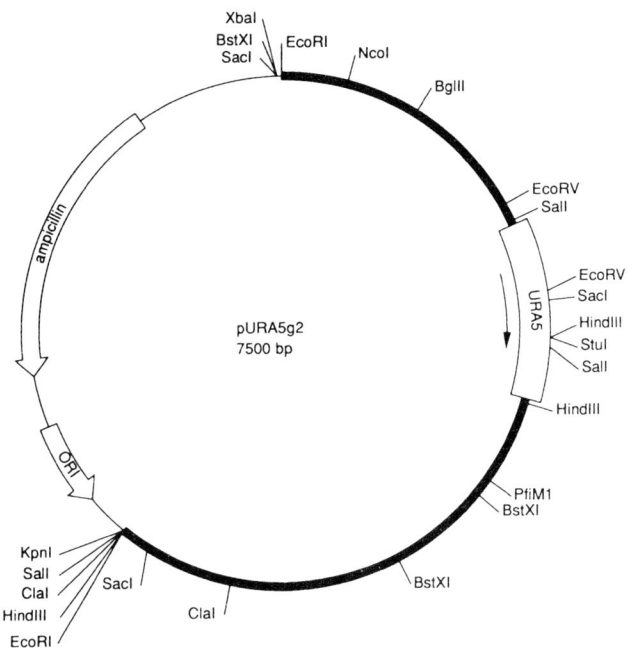

Fig. 11.3 Map of pURA5g2 (Edman & Kwon-Chung 1990).

orotidine monophosphate pyrophosphorylase (OMPpase) was then used as a probe to isolate the genomic clone of *URA5*. The plasmid pURA5g2 containing the entire *URA5* gene on a 4.5 kbp *Eco*RI insert (Fig. 11.3) was constructed and was introduced into the cells of the *ura5* mutant selected on 5-fluoro-orotic acid.

Transformation frequency with uncut pURA5g2 (supercoiled) was extremely low (1 or 2 transformants per μg DNA), and the transformants were all mitotically unstable (Edman & Kwon-Chung 1990). To increase transformation frequency, linearization of the plasmid was necessary and transformation frequency was increased by 2 to 3 logs when the plasmid was digested with *Eco*RI or *Nco*I. The *Eco*RI digest released the entire insert with no vector sequence, while the *Nco*I digest linearized the plasmid. Regardless of the enzyme used to prepare linear plasmids, transformants were always of three kinds: (1) highly unstable transformants with no evidence of integration but with extrachromosomal *URA5* sequences (Fig. 11.4); (2) stable transformants with ectopic integration; and (3) stable transformants with homologous integration into the resident *ura5* locus. Of the three types, the unstable transformants with extrachromosomal *URA5* sequences occurred most frequently, and stable transformants with homologous integration occurred with the least frequency. The extrachromosomal *URA5* sequences in the unstable transformants were autonomously replicating plasmids.

The autonomously replicating plasmids present in the transformants were of two kinds. Those in transformants with *Eco*RI-digested pURAg52 showed no apparent shift in molecular weight, because they all were 4.5 kb (the same size as the insert sequence); those in transformants with uncut or *Nco*I-digested pURA5g2 showed considerable alteration in molecular weight with new restriction sites.

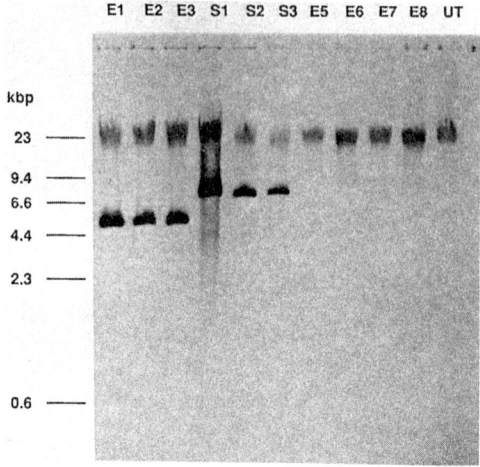

Fig. 11.4 Southern blot analysis of undigested DNA from URA⁺ transformants probed with pURA5g2. Lanes E1–E3, undigested DNA from three unstable transformants obtained with *Eco*RI-digested pURA5g2; S1 to S3, undigested DNA from three unstable transformants obtained with supercoiled pURA5g2; E5 to E8, undigested DNA from four stable transformants obtained with *Eco*RI-digested pURA5g2.Lane UT, undigested DNA from strain B-3501 (Edman & Kwon-Chung 1990).

Figure 11.5 shows the Southern blot analysis of *Eco*RI-digested (Fig. 11.5A) and *Stu*I-digested (Fig. 11.5B) transformants obtained with *Eco*RI-digested and uncut pURA5g2. All extrachromosomal plasmids within the transformed cells were in linear form as determined by exonuclease (*Bal*31 or T7 gene 6) digestion. Multiple attempts to rescue these plasmids in *E. coli* have failed. As expected, the stable transformants obtained using the *Eco*RI-digested vector showed that only the *C. neoformans* sequence (insert) had integrated. In the stable transformants obtained with *Nco*I-digested pURA5g2, the vector sequence was also integrated along with the insert sequence (Fig. 11.6).

To test the effect of transformation on virulence, several transformants (Table 11.2) from different categories were injected into mice, whose survival was recorded. The transformants used were phenotypically indistinguishable when grown on

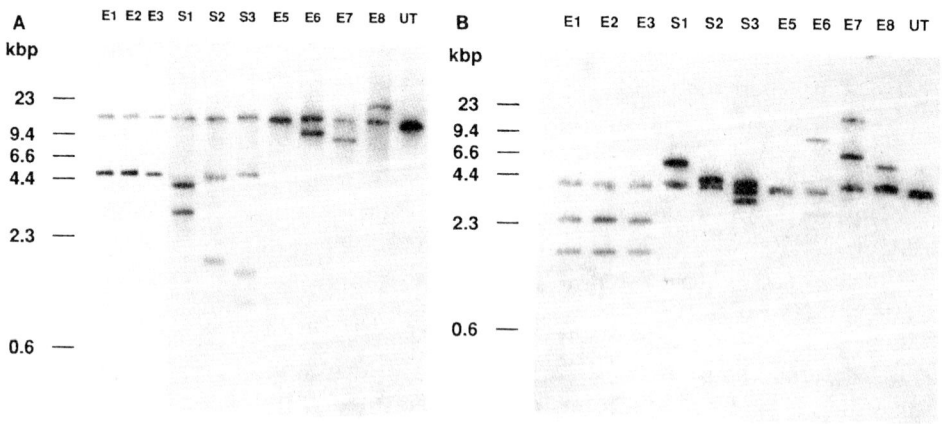

Fig. 11.5 Southern blot analysis of restricted (A, *Eco*RI; B, *Stu*I) DNA from Ura⁺ transformants. DNA samples and lanes are the same as Figure 11.4. The entire plasmid pURA5g2 was used as a probe (Edman & Kwon-Chung 1990).

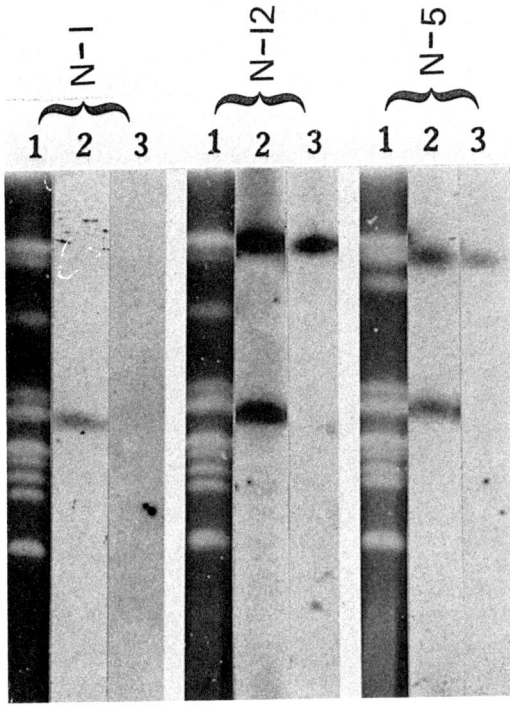

Fig. 11.6 Ethidium bromide stained gel of chromosomes separated by CHEF (lane 1) and Southern hybridization using pURA5g2 as a probe (lane 2) or vector sequence (lane 3) as a probe. N-1, unstable transformants obtained by *Nco*I-digested pURA5g2; N-12 and N-5, stable transformants with ectopic integration of *URA5* sequence as well as vector sequence.

complex media such as yeast extract peptone glucose agar. The *ura5* mutants and the transformants, however, produced drier colonies than the wild type when grown on minimal medium such as yeast nitrogen base agar with uracil. Figure 11.7 shows the survival of mice infected with the wild-type, *ura5* mutant, and *URA5* transformants obtained with *Nco*I-digested pURA5g2. The chromosomal positions of ectopically integrated *URA5* genes in these transformants are seen in Figure

Table 11.2 Wild-type, *ura5* mutants, and transformants used for animal study

Strain*	Chromosomal integration (position)*	Vector sequence	Extrachromosomal plasmid
B-3501 (wild type)	—	–	–
FOA-01-11-2 (*ura5*)	—	–	–
N-1		–	+
N-5	–Ectopic (2nd)	+	–
N-12	Ectopic (1st)	+	–
E-5	Homologous (5th)	–	–
E-6	Ectopic (4th)	–	–
E-7	Ectopic (9th)	–	–
E-8	Ectopic (1st)	–	–

* N and E strains are the transformants obtained with *Nco*-I-digested and *Eco*RI-digested pURA5g2, respectively.
† Chromosomes in which integration occurred.

203

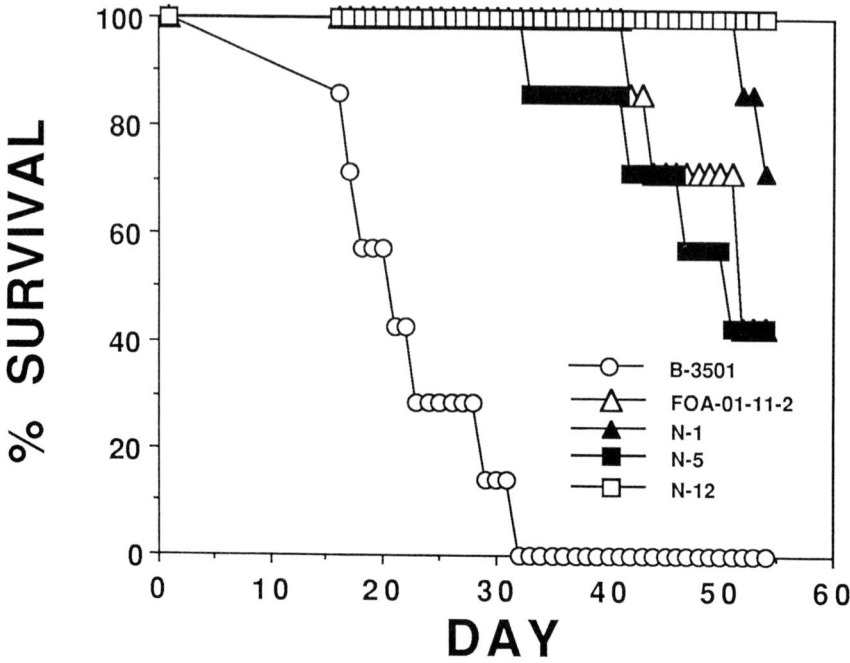

Fig. 11.7 Survival curve of mice infected with wild-type, *ura5* mutant, and transformants obtained with *Nco*I-digested pURA5g2.

11.6. The *ura5* mutant was significantly less virulent than the wild type ($P < 0.001$). The unstable *URA5* transformant with extrachromosomal plasmid (N-1) and the stable transformant with ectopic integration of the insert and vector sequence were equally less virulent compared to the *ura5* mutant (*ura5* vs. N-1, $P = 0.053$; *ura5*

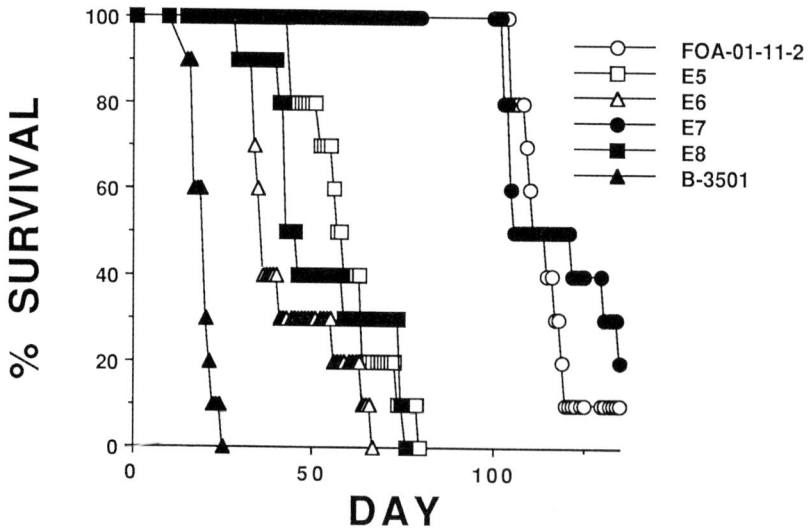

Fig. 11.8 Survival curve of mice infected with wild-type, *ura5* mutant, and transformants obtained with *Eco*RI-digested pURA5g2. Transformants carried no vector sequence.

vs. N-5, $P > 0.10$). The strain N-12 was even less virulent than the *ura5* mutant ($P < 0.001$). Figure 11.8 shows the survival of mice infected with the wild-type, *ura5* mutant, and *URA5* transformants obtained with *Eco*RI-digested pURAg2. All but one (E-7) transformant showed significantly higher virulence than the *ura5* mutant ($P < 0.001$), but they were still significantly less virulent than the wild type ($P < 0.001$). The transformant with homologous integration (E-5) did not show higher virulence than those with ectopic integration (E-6, E-8). The virulence of one transformant (E-7) remained the same as the *ura5* mutant ($P > 0.10$).

These results indicated that genetically manipulated *URA5* strains are less virulent than the wild-type *URA5* strains, regardless of the locus at which the *URA5* gene integrates, and that the integration of foreign DNA into the chromosomes lowers the virulence to a greater extent.

SUMMARY

The progress made in cloning *C. neoformans* genes for the past 2 years indicated that the majority of genes have been cloned by complementing *E. coli* or *S. cerevisiae* with the cDNA library of *C. neoformans,* and then using cDNA clones to isolate genomic sequences. In some cases, *S. cerevisiae* was used directly to clone the genomic sequence of *C. neoformans* by complementation. The genes highly conserved throughout the eukaryotic organism have been isolated by using cloned sequences of *S. cerevisiae* as a probe or using primers (for polymerase chain reaction) consisting of synthetic oligonucleotides based on conserved sequences.

Genomic rearrangement appears to take place in vivo in both varieties of *C. neoformans* in such a way that each patient isolate has a unique electrophoretic karyotype. This indicates that electrophoretic karyotyping cannot be used as an epidemiological tool to trace the environmental source of the infection.

DNA-mediated transformation systems showed that genetic manipulation is possible in *C. neoformans* and that molecular mechanisms for the factors associated with sexual differentiation or virulence can be identified. Studies show, however, that the insertion of foreign DNA (vector sequences) significantly lowers the virulence of *C. neoformans URA5*. Transformation by homologous integration did not show any advantage over the ectopic integration for the expression of virulence of *C. neoformans* in mice.

Since homologous integration is a rare event in *C. neoformans*, genetic manipulations including gene disruption or targeted insertion are difficult. Further progress in gene manipulation, therefore, awaits the techniques which enhance targeting of cloned fragments to their chromosomal locus.

ACKNOWLEDGEMENTS

We thank Brian L. Wickes for his technical assistance in the animal study and performance of karyotyping.

REFERENCES

Biggs B A, Kemp D J, Brown G V 1989 Subtelomeric chromosome deletions in field isolates of *Plasmodium falciparum* and their relationship to loss of cytoadherence in vitro. Proceedings of the National Academy of Sciences, USA 86: 2428–2432

Birch A, Häusler A, Vogtli M, Hütter R 1989 Extremely large chromosomal deletions are intimately involved in genetic instability and genomic rearrangements in *Streptomyces glaucescens*. Molecular and General Genetics 217: 447–458

Buschke A 1895 Über eine durch Coccidien hervorgerufene Krankhiet des Menschen. Deutsche Medizinische Wochenschrift 21: 14

Busse O 1894 Über parasitäre Zelleinschlüsse und ihre Züchtung. Zentralblatt für Bakteriologie 1 Abt Originale 16: 175–180

Corcoran L M, Forsyth K P, Bianco A A, Brown G V, Kemp D J 1986 Chromosome size polymorphisms in *Plasmodium falciparum* can involve deletions and are frequent in natural parasite populations. Cell 44: 87–95

Corcoran L M, Thompson J K, Walker D, Kemp D J 1988 Homologous recombination within subtelomeric repeat sequences generates chromosome size polymorphisms in *P. falciparum*. Cell 53: 807–813

Diamond R D 1990 *Cryptococcus neoformans*. In: Mandell G L, Douglas R G, Bennett J E (eds) Principles and practice of infectious diseases, 3rd edn. Churchill Livingstone, Edinburgh, pp 1980–1989

Dismukes W E 1988 Cryptococcal meningitis in patients with AIDS. Journal of Infectious Diseases 157: 624–628

Edman J C, Kwon-Chung K J 1990 Isolation of the *URA5* gene from *C. neoformans* var. *neoformans* and its use as a selective marker for transformation. Molecular and Cellular Biology 10: 4538–4544

Edman U, Edman J C, Lundgren B, Santi D V 1989 Isolation and expression of the *Pneumocystis carinii* thymidylate synthase gene. Proceedings of the National Academy of Sciences, USA 86: 6503–6507

Ellis D H, Pfeiffer T J 1990 Natural habitat of *Cryotococcus neoformans* var. *gattii*. Journal of Clinical Microbiology 28: 1642–1644

Gordon P C, Clark K A, Milliman C, Majlessi M, Talbot L A, Pusateri K D 1991 Development of rapid nonisotopic DNA probe assays for fungi: *Cryptococcus neoformans*. Abstract F81, American Society for Microbiology, p 421

Gueho E, Kurtzman C P, Peterson S W 1989 Evolutionary affinities of heterobasidiomycetous yeasts estimated from 18S and 25S ribosomal RNA sequence divergence. Systematic and Applied Microbiology 12: 230–236

Janse C J, Boorsma E G, van Vianen P H et al 1989 *Plasmodium berghei*: gametocyte production, DNA content, and chromosome-size polymorphism during asexual multiplication in vivo. Experimental Parasitology 68: 274–282

Kwon-Chung K J 1975 A new genus, *Filobasidiella*, the perfect state of *Cryptococcus neoformans*. Mycologia 67:1197–1200

Kwon-Chung K J 1976 Morphogenesis of *Filobasidiella neoformans*, the sexual state of *Cryptococcus neoformans*. Mycologia 688: 821–833

Kwon-Chung K J 1978 Distribution of α and *a* mating type of *Cryptococcus neoformans* among natural and clinical isolates. American Journal of Epidemiology 108: 337–340

Kwon-Chung K J, Polacheck I, Bennett J E 1982 Improved diagnostic medium for separation of *Cryptococcus neoformans* var. *neoformans* (serotype A and D) and *Cryptococcus neoformans* var. *gattii* (serotype B and C). Journal of Clinical Microbiology 15: 535–537

Kwon-Chung K J, Fell J W 1984 *Filobasidiella*. In: Kreger-van Rij N J K (ed) The yeasts: a taxonomic study. Elsevier Science Publishers, Amsterdam, pp 472–482

Kwon-Chung K J, Rhodes J C 1986 Encapsulation and melanin formation as indicators of virulence in *Cryptococcus neoformans*. Infection and Immunity 51: 218–233

Kwon-Chung K J, Varma A, Howard D H 1990 Ecology of *Cryptococcus neoformans* and prevalence of its two varieties in AIDS and non-AIDS associated cryptococcosis. In: Vande Bossche H, Mackenzie D, Cauwenbergh C, Van Cutsem J, Drouhet E, Dupont B (eds) Third symposium, Topics in mycology: mycoses in AIDS patients. Plenum Press, New York, pp 103–113

Kwon-Chung K J, Wickes B L, Edman J C 1991 Comparison of karyotype and linkage map of the two varieties of *Cryptococcus neoformans*. Abstract PS1.43, XI Congress of International Human and Animal Mycology, p 73

Merz W G, Connelly C, Hieter P 1988 Variation of electrophoretic karyotypes among clinical isolates of *Candida albicans*. Journal of Clinical Microbiology 26: 842–845

206

Myers K K, Ipma-Wong M F, Fonzi W A, Sypherd P S 1991 Isolation of translation elongation factor 3 gene from three opportunistic fungal pathogens: *Candida albicans, Pneumocystis carinii,* and *Cryptococcus neoformans.* Abstract F79, American Society for Microbiology, p 421

Orbach M J, Volrath D, Davis R W 1988 An electrophoretic karyotype for *Neurospora crassa.* Molecular and Cellular Biology 8: 1469–1473

Pagès M, Bastien P, Francisco V, et al 1989 Chromosome size and number polymorphisms in *Leishmania infantum* suggest amplification/deletion and possible genetic exchange. Molecular and Biochemical Parasitology 36: 161–168

Perfect J R, Magee B B, Magee P T 1989a Separation of chromosome of *Cryptococcus neoformans* by pulsed field gel electrophoresis. Infection and Immunity 57: 2624–2627

Perfect J R, Rude T H, Penning L M, Johnston S A 1989b Cloning of the *Cryptococcus neoformans* *Trp 1* gene by expression in *Saccharomyces cerevisiae.* Abstract P8, International Conference on *Cryptococcus* and cryptococcosis, Jerusalem, Israel

Perfect J R, Rude T H, Penning L M, Wong B 1991 Cloning of a *Cryptococcus neoformans* mannitol dehydrogenase gene. Abstract PS1.45, XI Congress of International Society for Human and Animal Mycology, p. 73

Polacheck I, Lebens G A 1989 Electrophoretic karyotype of the pathogenic yeast *Cryptococcus neoformans.* Journal of General Microbiology 135: 65–71

Pologe L G, Ravetch J V 1988 Large deletions result from breakage and healing of *P. falciparum* chromosomes. Cell 55: 869–874

Restrepo B I, Barbour A G 1989 Cloning of 18S and 25S rDNAs from the pathogenic fungus *Cryptococcus neoformans.* Journal of Bacteriology 171: 5596–5600

Sanfelice F 1894 Contributo alla morphologia e biologia dei blastomiceti che si sviluppano nei succhi di alcuni frutti. Annali dell'igiene sperimentale dell'Università di Roma 4: 463–495

Schwartz D C, Cantor C R 1982 Separation of yeast chromosome-sized DNAs by pulsed field gradient gel electrophoresis. Cell 37: 67–75

Shea C, Glass J D, Parengi S, Van der Paoeg L H T 1986 Variant surface glycoprotein gene expression site switches in *Trypanosoma brucei.* Journal of Biological Chemistry 261: 6056–6063

Wagner W, So M 1990 Genomic variation of *Trypanosoma cruzi:* involvement of multicopy genes. Infection and Immunity 58: 3217–3224

Wickes B L, Golin J E, Kwon-Chung K J 1991 Chromosome rearrangement in *Candida stellatoidea* results in a positive effect on phenotype. Infection and Immunity 59: 1762–1771

207

Discussion of paper presented by K. Kwon-Chung

Discussed by J. B. Hicks
Reported by J. Verhoef

Dr Hicks followed Dr Kwon-Chung's presentation with an appraisal of the advances that have been made towards a study of the pathogenesis of *Cryptococcus*. He pointed out the highlights in the data and compared these to the existing technologies used for work on *Saccharomyces cerevisiae* and other yeasts.

S. cerevisiae has a well understood and easily manipulated sexual cycle enabling the creation of stable haploid and diploid cell lines and the introduction of genetic markers in these strains. The elusiveness of such a system in *Candida* continues to frustrate workers and greatly increases the complexity of genetic manipulation. *Cryptococcus* has two haploid mating types, 'a' and 'α' cells, determined by DNA sequences encoded at the MAT locus. This allows manipulation of strains and an insight into the mating process. Interestingly, it may also provide an insight into the role of MAT 'α' in the pathogenicity of *C. neoformans*. Not only are the majority of clinical isolates of *C. neoformans* known to be 'α' mating type but recent studies indicated that the 'α' mating type strains produce fatal infections in mice more rapidly than 'a' mating strains. In response to a question from Dr Kozel, Dr Kwon-Chung said she could not distinguish between a MAT encoded or merely a MAT locus linked virulence factor. Dr Hicks reinforced the suggestion by Dr Kwon-Chung that mating sexual determinants which will be on the cell surface and will involve the cell wall could involve responses to the human environment and/or survival in other habitats. He summarized by saying that although genetic manipulations and karyotyping of *Cryptococcus* are still complicated, they are the foundations on which to improve these techniques.

DNA transformation systems were discussed, with *S. cerevisiae* being identified as the ideal. Shuttle plasmids are tractable, maintaining the same structures in *Escherichia coli* and yeast and are easily re-isolated from both organisms. Many of the most useful manipulations in *S. cerevisiae* are possible because of its ability to perform homologous recombination. This enables targeting of incoming DNA to homologous sequences in the genome and subsequent integration by recombination. Also possible is retrieval of genomic sequences by repair of plasmids, if they have homology with a gene, or by re-selection of integrated vectors through *E. coli* which contain sequences adjacent to the site of integration in yeast.

Dr Kwon-Chung's experiments have attempted to direct integration in a manner similar to that for *S. cerevisiae*. Later, prompted by a question from Dr Hobden,

Dr Kwon-Chung said these experiments were done in 'α' mating type strains but that preliminary experiments showed no difference in transformation frequency between the 'a' or 'α' strains. Two classes of events result from this. One is ectopic integration resulting in an unpredictable site of integration event of the incoming DNA without homologous recombination. This is coupled with an amplification event either before or after integration which results in catenates of the sequences forming large molecules (290 kb in the case of pURA5g2). These are linear and may be healed by telomere addition. These are not retrievable through *E. coli*, although Hicks foresees a means of constructing a shuttle vector which can be religated and retrieved in *E. coli*. The second type of event is that of homologous integration of the URA 5 sequence into the ura5 locus. This was directed in using a linearized plasmid with homologous DNA ends to the ura5 locus. Arguments that this has indeed occurred in this instance are difficult to uphold because the standard proof is to follow a co-integrated marker sequence. This has not yet been done. Dr Hicks pointed out that changes occur during transformation resulting in transformants with different karyotypes. This lack of a stable karyotype also complicated analysis of integration events. Dr Hicks concluded that *Cryptococcus* is more like other yeasts than like *S. cerevisiae*. It probably shows homologous integration, autonomous replication (albeit of linear sequences) and random integration. Methodologies to enable predictable genetic manipulation of this organism are improving.

Dr Shepherd raised the issue of the epidemiology of *C. gattii*. Dr Kwon-Chung believed that the organism was transferred from Australia to California. The Australian eucalyptus was extensively exported to the Pacific coast of southern California and central Africa as well as south-east Asia, where *C. gattii* is most prevalent. Her view supports Dr Ellis's hypothesis that *C. gattii* was transferred through seedlings or seeds of the eucalyptus.

Dr Edwards mentioned that there was a view that cryptococcal meningitis in California was more severe and difficult to manage clinically than the cases that are described from the east coast. He added that this was a clinical impression resulting from an analysis carried out several years ago. This could be explained by differences in serotype, i.e. BC versus AD. Dr Kwon-Chung added that it takes more amphotericin-B to eradicate the BC serotype and its recurrence rate is higher.

Plenary Lecture 2

Chairman: S. R. Norrby

12. Fungal evasion of host defences
R. J. Hay

INTRODUCTION

The ability to survive in order to achieve dispersal or reproduce is one of the principal characteristics of living organisms. Survival under adverse conditions is often achieved by a remarkable display of adaptive mechanisms which have become established by natural selection. Equally, the destruction of potentially harmful invaders is a property of all organisms, although the mechanisms involved have become more complex in the more evolutionarily advanced. While in the case of many pathogenic fungi adaptive mechanisms were presumably originally evolved to aid survival in the natural habitat, such as soil or vegetation, these same mechanisms may also prove useful in combating immunological defences where these organisms infect man as a secondary event. In addition, in those parasites which are confined to man the evolution of mechanisms for survival are no less important.

The range of adaptive mechanisms shown by fungi varies from changes in cell wall structure and width, the deposition of melanin, and capsule formation, to the production of toxins or biocides, and the elaboration of immunomodulatory substances; the existence of antigenic mimicry and antigenic variation seen with other micro-organisms has been reported in a few fungi and the convergence of complement and sterol receptor structures in mammalian and fungal cells may prove to be of protective advantage to fungi. These different mechanisms will be reviewed using examples of specific fungal infections although many have been shown to possess at least one, sometimes more, adaptive mechanisms.

CELL WALL CHANGES

As the outermost layer of most fungal cells, the cell wall plays a potentially important role in protection. A simple example is provided by a study of the differences in cell shape and wall thickness between the cells of vegetative hyphae and arthrospores in dermatophytes. The latter show an increase in width of at least five-fold compared to that seen in cells of hyphae grown in vitro. This can also be mimicked by growing dermatophyte cultures in a moist environment in the presence of 5% carbon dioxide (Zurita & Hay 1987).

The grossest changes in cell wall structure are those seen in fungal cells within mycetoma grains, particularly at the outer surface of the grain, where two main changes can be seen. The most obvious of these is gross cell-wall thickening. The main ultrastructural alterations are cell-wall thickening with alternating electron dense and electron lucent zones and fusion of adjacent cells (Hay & Collins 1983, Wethered et al 1987). At the periphery of grains, for instance, the cell walls may reach a size of up to 20 times their original thickness and the corrugated margin is formed by ruptured cells with fused walls. Fusion of adjacent cells obscures the definition of cell boundaries, particularly deeper within the grain.

It has been shown that these changes are accompanied by an apparent proliferation of the polysaccharide cytoskeleton of the cell wall (Wethered et al 1987). Within grains, PASTCH-positive staining fibrils can be seen extending beyond the outer cell-wall layer into the grain matrix and in some areas these overlap with those from adjacent fungal cells. These structures are similar to those produced by partial degradation of chitin in fungal cell walls. The onion skin appearance, suggesting cell wall reduplication, is probably based on a different mechanism. In experiments designed to reproduce the morphological arrangement of mycetoma grains, inert plastic implantation chambers sealed at one end with $4\,\mu m$ pore size filter discs were filled with *Madurella mycetomatis* or *Pseudallescheria boydii* mycelial fragments grown in vitro and surgically implanted subcutaneously in Balb/c mice hyperimmunized with the homologous organism. At the end of 6 weeks, chambers were removed and the fungal aggregates recovered from inside had undergone ultrastructural changes, including intrahyphal growth, which reproduce the early phase of 'onion skin thickening' seen in grains (D Wethered, R J Hay 1987, unpublished data). Intrahyphal growth is produced by other fungi under conditions of nutritional and oxygen deprivation. This appears to be a different mechanism to that seen with the formation of dermatophyte arthrospores in 5% carbon dioxide described previously.

Cell-wall thickening is likely to hinder host resistance by a number of mechanisms. Cell aggregates are less penetrable by drugs and oxidative, as well as nonoxidative, killing products produced by host polymorphonuclear leukocytes (PMNs). The cell wall changes may also alter the expression of polysaccharide adhesin molecules on the fungal surface hindering the fungus/leucocyte interaction. Thickening of the cell wall is not the only change seen within mycetoma grains, and with experimental mycetoma infections with the actinomycete, *Nocardia caviae*, loss of cell wall constituents and formation of L-forms appears to favour resistance to destruction by macrophages (Beaman & Scates 1981).

The rim of many mycetoma grains has an eosinophilic refractile fringe similar to that referred to as Splendore-Hoeppli material, seen around a number of other large parasites from schistosome ova to *Sporothrix schenckii* yeasts forming asteroid bodies. Using immunogold labelling it has been found that human immunoglobulin, mainly IgM, is deposited around the outside of grains in the area of the eosinophilic fringe, suggesting that antibody deposition plays a part in the formation of the grain periphery. However, no immunoglobulin can be identified

214

within the centre of the grain, showing that human immunoglobulin is not required for the formation of the matrix of mycetoma grains (Wethered et al 1987).

THE FORMATION OF AN EXTRACELLULAR MATRIX

In some organisms a further adaptive measure appears to be the formation of a cocoon of an impermeable substance which surrounds the organisms in vivo. This is best illustrated once again by the example of certain mycetoma agents which elaborate an extracellular matrix whose structural integrity imparts strength to the grain. Grains from these mycetoma agents are difficult to cut with a microtome and often sections show ragged transverse fracture lines which crisscross each grain. Filaments or hyphae can be seen with electron microscopy to be surrounded by amorphous or fibrillar electron-dense material. The fungi, *M. mycetomatis* and *Neotestudina rosatii* as well as an actinomycete, *Streptomyces somaliensis*, are examples of this pattern of structural adaptation. The matrix, often called cement, produced by *M. mycetomatis* is a complex phenol or fungal melanin. It has been shown (Findlay & Vismer 1974) to give strength and resilience to material such as rat collagen permeated by diffusing melanin in vitro. In infections caused by this organism the cement can be seen to surround live or effete fungal hyphae and contains numerous cytoplasmic remnants (Hay & Collins 1983). The material is non-antigenic and with immunogold labelling appears free from antigenic components derived from the fungus, confirming that it is a combination of inert fungal melanin, possibly with host derived material (Wethered et al 1987). Polyclonal rabbit antisera to *M. mycetomatis* do not react with diffusible melanin extracts in two-dimensional crossed immunoelectrophoresis (Wethered et al 1988). There have been no studies of the 'cement' surrounding *N. rosattii* grains.

Cement formation is not a property of many pathogenic organisms, but is a subtle adaptation for invading organisms as it shields them from host immunity within, in the case of *M. mycetomatis*, an 'antigen free' zone. The latter may explain the low titre antibody responses seen even in well established infections (Zaini et al in press).

CAPSULE FORMATION

Encapsulation is a property which conveys protection on many micro-organisms, particularly bacteria, but is seldom seen with pathogenic fungi apart from *Cryptococcus neoformans*. This organism and its capsule is the subject of a presentation in this symposium (Ch. 10) and it will not be discussed further here.

MELANIN BIOSYNTHESIS

The formation of pigment either within the cell wall, or its extracellular excretion is a property of many pathogenic fungi. The principle fungal melanins are either derived from tyrosine and related precursors following a similar pathway to human melanin biosynthesis (DOPA melanins) or from pentaketides (DHN melanins) (Wheeler & Bell 1988). DHN melanin biosynthesis is blocked by a number of agents, including tricyclazole. Other forms of melanin biosynthesis include the catechol melanins (GDHB melanins). In addition, some phenol melanins are secreted by the organism and polymerize outside the cell (extracellular melanins). The cement of *M. mycetomatis* is formed in this way. The human and plant pathogen *Natrassia mangifera* (*Hendersonula toruloidea*) also produces extra-cellular melanins.

Fungal melanins protect the organism by permeating the cell wall or the environ-ment. They may also bind drugs and some contain superoxide dismutase activity. Melanin-defective mutants of the organism *Wangiella dermatitidis*, a cause of chromomycosis are less pathogenic than pigmented strains in mice and are more easily eliminated from experimentally infected animals than the pigmented forms (Dixon et al 1987).

A number of other fungi which cause cutaneous or subcutaneous infections produce melanins. Some are DHN melanin producers, e.g. *Cladosporium carrioni*, which causes chromomycosis whereas others, including *M. mycetomatis* elaborate extracellular melanin from different precursors. Hyphal fragments of *C. carrioni* grown on media containing tricyclazole, which inhibits DNA melanin formation, are more susceptible in vitro to the myeloperoxidase (lactoperoxidase) halide system, which forms one of the killing mechanisms found in polymorphonuclear leucocytes, suggesting that in this organism the presence of cell wall melanin may be a defence against PMN attack. The phenomenon is seen at various con-centrations of hydrogen peroxide, with the greatest difference in viability between untreated and tricyclazole treated cells being seen at a concentration of 10^{-4} M (Hay 1989). A similar phenomenon can be seen with *Sporothrix schenckii* strains where the more heavily pigmented conidia from mycelial phase organisms are less easily killed by the myeloperoxidase/halide killing system. The way in which the pigment acts as a protective factor is not clearly understood but melanin, in addition to any other function, appears to convey structural strength to the cell wall.

TOXIN PRODUCTION

With most other micro-organisms the production of toxins has always been regarded as an important means of protective adaptation. An example is the production of mycotoxins, such as aflatoxin, by *Aspergillus* species. It has been shown that aflatoxins from organisms on stored foodstuffs, such as aflatoxin B, will cause acute hepatic necrosis in experimentally treated animals.

The longstanding controversy over the existence of *Candida* toxins is also of relevance. In a study of extracts of *C. albicans* which were assessed for toxic reactions in animals, a cell wall glycoprotein fraction was found to have two main effects (Cutler et al 1972). It would induce pyrexia in rabbits and when injected in greater concentrations was lethal in mice. It must be emphasized that the concentrations used were higher than those likely to be found in human infections. Further evidence on toxins from *Candida* has been demonstrated by another group of investigators although activity is associated with a single isolate of the organism (Iwata 1977). It has been characterized as a heat-labile protein with a molecular weight of 75 kDa which can cause anaphylactic shock in mice. Other workers have not been able to demonstrate a similar active compound in other *C. albicans* isolates.

Generally, although it is possible to demonstrate that some pathogenic fungal species produce potentially toxic substances, these are present in low concentrations which do not approach in potency, for instance, the mycotoxins of fungi associated with stored grain. Conversely, although a number of pathogenic fungi produce mycotoxins in vitro or as saprophytes – *A. flavus* (aflatoxins), *T. rubrum* (rubratoxin) – there is no evidence that they do so in vivo. There is no experimental data, for instance, to support a role for aflatoxins in the pathogenesis of the sclerosing tumour – paranasal *Aspergillus* granuloma.

IMMUNOMODULATION BY FUNGI

The process of the development of an immune response to all invasive organisms is modulated by regulatory mechanisms inherent in the host's immune system. In addition it has become clear that many micro-organisms directly affect the functioning of immunological pathways. The study of immunomodulation directly associated with pathogenic fungi can be illustrated by studies of experimental and human dermatophytosis. These comprise a group of common infections, some of which are acute and self-resolving, whereas others fail to respond to therapy and patients remain infected for months, if not years, with non-inflammatory indolent skin lesions. The clinical expression of the different patterns of skin disease seen in this group includes: tinea pedis, corporis, and tinea imbricata. The chief organisms particularly associated with chronic disease of this type in man are *Trichophyton rubrum* and *T. concentricum*. Previous work has indicated that patients with chronic dermatophytosis usually have either immediate or absent delayed type hypersensitivity reactions to intradermal antigens prepared from dermatophytes (Jones et al 1973). In addition some, but not all studies, have suggested that defective in vitro responses to dermatophyte antigens using lymphocyte transformation responses or leucocyte migration inhibition can be seen (Hanifin et al 1974). This work suggests that there are defective immune responses in man in some infections, particularly those caused by *T. rubrum*. By contrast, studies in mice have shown that animals with experimentally induced dermatophytosis with *T. quinckeanum* have a short-lived infection (10–16 days) associated with the appearance of specifically activated T lymphocytes and that resistance can be transferred to naive recipient animals with Thy-1 positive lymphocytes (Calderon & Hay 1984a). However, a small proportion of the infected population of animals develop a more prolonged infection lasting for over 35 days; their lymphocyte transformation responses to mitogens or dermatophyte antigens in heterologous serum are not altered, while they are depressed in homologous serum. Prolonged infection can be induced by pretreatment of animals with the specific dermatophyte antigen in Freund's incomplete adjuvant or alum. It is possible, therefore, that the dermatophyte antigen itself, may act as an immunomodulator (Calderon & Hay

1984b). Circulating dermatophyte antigen detected using a radiometric assay employing TQ-1, a monoclonal antibody, has shown that both infected mice and humans with chronic dermatophytosis due to *T. rubrum* and *T. concentricum* have circulating levels of an antigen derived from dermatophytes and in severe cases this may disappear with therapy (Calderon et al 1987, Mayou et al 1987).

In a study of cell-mediated immune responses carried out recently, a number of new observations have been made (McGregor et al 1990). Patients with chronic dermatophytosis due to *T. rubrum* have normal cell-mediated immunity to common antigens as measured by lymphocyte transformation in vitro. This is at variance with other studies which purport to demonstrate a widespread alteration in cellular immunity as a susceptibility factor to dermatophyte infection (Hanifin et al 1974). However, these may be reconciled, as at even comparatively low concentrations of antigen there is inhibition of lymphocyte transformation. No significant difference in lymphocyte responses to any antigen was demonstrable when heterologous as compared to autologous serum was used in the assay system.

A consistent observation was that lymphocyte transformation to both cytoplasmic and soluble exoantigen derived from *T. rubrum* decreased at protein concentrations above $5\,\mu g/ml$ of antigen until, at protein concentrations above $25\,\mu g/ml$, there was complete inhibition of lymphocyte proliferation. This decrease in lymphocyte transformation did not occur at high concentrations of other mitrogens or antigens although a plateau in blastogenesis was observed with these.

Addition of inhibitory concentrations of *T. rubrum* antigen to lymphocytes stimulated with candida and PPD antigens and the mitogen PHA as well as the lower, stimulatory, concentrations of *T. rubrum* antigen completely abolished lymphocyte proliferation. This suggests that the antiproliferative effect of the *T. rubrum* antigen in vitro is not specific for T lymphocytes responsive to the dermatophyte antigen but generally affects lymphocyte blastogenesis. When lymphocytes were incubated with PHA, and the inhibitory effect of adding *T. rubrum* antigen $> 25\,\mu g/ml$ was assessed at different time points of incubation, the inhibitory effect of *T. rubrum* antigen was strongest when it is added at time 0 in the incubation. Reduction in lymphocyte proliferation also occurs if *T. rubrum* antigen is added in the first 24 h of incubation with PHA but thereafter has no effect on the assay.

FACS analysis of lymphocytes incubated with PHA and inhibitory concentrations of *T. rubrum* showed evidence of activation such as the expression of HLA-DR on lymphocytes in culture as well as increases in cell size even though they were not able to proliferate. This suggests that the mechanism does not interfere with this stage of activation.

Reversal of lymphocyte inhibition occurs if cells are washed after incubation with inhibitory concentrations of *T. rubrum* antigen for up to 48 h. Lymphocyte inhibition by *T. rubrum* can be overcome by stimulation of cultures by increasing the concentrations of PHA and PPD. This may explain why different dermatophyte species show different inflammatory responses and why those producing highly inflammatory lesions show the greatest lymphocyte transformation responses in vitro. The inhibitory activity appears to reside in a fraction of cytoplasmic antigen produced from *T. rubrum* with a molecular weight of over 30 kDa. It is also apparent that both *T. mentagrophytes* and *Epidermophyton floccosum* produce similar factors although as yet it is not known whether these are identical to that seen with *T. rubrum*. In experimental infections there is evidence that factor(s) affecting the development of resistance to infection may be specific to a single organism. In experimental murine infections, preconditioning of animals with *T. quinckeanum*, but not *Pseudallescheria boydii*, led to prolongation and increased severity of subsequent infections with *T. quinckeanum* in naive mice. This suggests that a shared determinant such as a mannose-containing sugar, implicated in immunomodulation with other fungi (see below), may not be the only factor responsible for altering the immune responses to infection. In addition, humans with *T. rubrum* or *T. concentricum* infections have a circulating antigen detectable with a monoclonal antibody with affinity to phosphorylcholine (Calderon et al 1987). Phosphorylcholine-containing antigenic fractions of nematodes are well recognized as having immunomodulatory properties (Perry et al 1974). It is likely, therefore, that a number of different factors affecting lymphocyte blastogenesis may exist. It is also not clear whether immunological effects of dermatophyte products are simply confined to lymphocytes. An important effector cell for resistance to dermatophytes is the PMN (Calderon & Hay 1987) and there is some evidence that defective PMN killing seen in some patients with severe infections may be restored to normal after elimination of the fungus (Mayou et al 1987).

Immunomodulation by fungi is not confined to the dermatophytes. It is also seen in *Candida* infections. In chronic dermatophytosis, failure to induce lymphocyte transformation by patients' lymphocytes has been correlated with a circulating antigen which can be removed from autologous serum with an anti-*Candida* polyclonal antibody or concanavalin A (Fischer et al 1978). Recent work here suggests that mannose-containing sugars are the most likely candidates for immunomodulatory factors, with oligosaccharides bearing 2–6 residues being the most potent inhibitors of lymphocyte blastogenesis (Podzorski et al 1990). Once again, immunomodulation in candidiasis is a complex pattern. Other antigens and mechanisms are involved, including mannan and unidentified serum factors as well as the induction of suppressor lymphocytes (Garner et al 1990). The targets of suppression are also varied. While many investigators have concentrated on T-cell mechanisms, there is evidence that *Candida* products may also affect other immune pathways. For instance, one group (Wright et al 1984) demonstrated that mannan would suppress PMN-killing by interfering with myeloperoxidase via a physico-chemical interaction between the two molecules, thus blocking yeast binding to the enzyme. With *Aspergillus fumigatus* another factor, gliotoxin, produced in vitro affects the phagocytosis of peritoneal macrophages (Mullbacher et al 1985).

CONCLUSIONS

The adaptive mechanisms associated with fungi causing disease in humans are varied. Some affect the structures of the fungal cell producing key alterations in its specifications as a potential target for host immune cells and drugs. Others involve the direct inhibition of host effector mechanisms. The implications of these findings are equally wide, as they influence the validity of drug testing and the study of immunology as well as the efficacy of host resistance and therapy. However, they may also provide new targets for the development of drugs or immunological therapy. Certainly the study of these adaptive mechanisms is important in furthering our understanding of the factors affecting the pathogenesis of fungal infection.

ACKNOWLEDGEMENTS

I would like to acknowledge the invaluable assistance of the following investigators in studies described in this section: Raquel Calderon, Diana Wethered, Michelle Bartholomew, Mary Moore, Andy Hamilton, Jane MacGregor, Jeanette Zurita.

REFERENCES

Beaman B L, Scates S M 1981 Role of L forms of *Nocardia caviae* in the development of chronic mycetomas in normal and immunodeficient murine models. Infection and Immunity 33: 893–907

Calderon R A, Hay R J 1984a Cell-mediated immunity in experimental murine dermatophytosis. I: T-suppressor activity elicited in dermatophyte infections caused by *T. quinckeanum*. Immunology 53: 457–464

Calderon R A, Hay R J 1984b Cell-mediated immunity in experimental murine dermatophytosis. II: Adoptive transfer of immunity to dermatophyte infections by lymphoid cells from donors with acute or chronic infections. Immunology 53: 465–472

Calderon R A, Hay R J 1987 Fungicidal activity of human neutrophils and monocytes on dermatophyte fungi, *Trichophyton quinckeanum* and *Trichophyton rubrum*. Immunology 61: 289–296

Calderon R A, Hay R J, Shennan G I 1987 Circulating antigens and antibodies in human and mouse dermatophytosis. Use of monoclonal antibody reactive to phosphoryl-choline-like epitopes. Journal of General Microbiology 133: 2699–2705

Cutler J E, Friedman L, Milner K C 1972 Biological and chemical characterization of toxic substances from *Candida albicans*. Infection and Immunity 6: 616–627

Dixon D M, Polak A M, Szaniszlo P J 1987 Pathogenicity and virulence of wild type and melanin deficient *Wangiella dermatitidis*. Journal of Medical and Veterinary Mycology 25: 97–106

Findlay G H, Vismer H F 1974 Black grain mycetoma. A study of the chemistry, formation and significance of the tissue grain in *Madurella mycetomi* infection. British Journal of Dermatology 91: 297–303

Fischer A, Ballet J J, Griscelli C 1978 Specific inhibition of the in vitro *Candida*-induced lymphocyte proliferation by polysaccharide antigens present in serum of patients with chronic mucocutaneous candidiasis. Journal of Clinical Investigation 62: 1005–1013

Garner R E, Childress A M, Human L G, Domer J E 1990 Characterization of *Candida albicans* mannan induced mannan specific delayed hypersensitivity suppressor cells. Infection and Immunity 58: 2613–2620

Hanifin J M, Ray L F, Lobitz W C 1974 Immunological reactivity in dermatophytosis. British Journal of Dermatology 90: 1–8

Hay R J, Collins M J 1983 An ultrastructural study of pale eumycetoma grains. Sabouraudia 21: 261–269

Hay R J 1989 A thorn in the flesh – a study of the pathogenesis of subcutaneous infections. Clinical and Experimental Dermatology 14: 407–415

Iwata K 1977 Toxins produced by *Candida albicans*. Contributions to Microbiology and Immunology 4: 77–85

Jones H E, Reinhardt J H, Rinaldi M G 1973 A clinical, mycological and immunological survey for dermatophytosis. Archives of Dermatology 1078: 61–70

Mayou S, Calderon R A, Hay R J, Goodfellow A 1987 Deep dermatophyte infection. Clinical and Experimental Dermatology 12: 385–388

MacGregor J M, Hamilton A J, Hay R J 1990 Inhibition of lymphocyte blastogenesis by a factor derived from *Trichophyton rubrum*. British Journal of Dermatology 123(6): 86

Mullbacher A, Waring P, Eichner R D 1985 Identification of an agent in cultures of *Aspergillus fumigatus* displaying antiphagocytic and immunomodulating activity in vitro. Journal of General Microbiology 131: 944–951

Perry P, Petit A, Poulain J, Luffau G 1974 Phosphorylcholine bearing components in homogenates of nematodes. European Journal of Immunology 4: 637–639

Podzorski R P, Gray G R, Nelson R D 1990 Different effects of native *Candida albicans* mannan and mannan derived oligosaccharides on antigen-stimulated lymphocyte proliferation in vitro. Journal of Immunology 144: 707–716

Wethered D B, Markey M A, Hay R J, Mahgoub E S, Gumaa S A 1987 Ultrastructural and immunogenic changes in the formation of mycetoma grains. Journal of Medical and Veterinary Mycology 25: 39–46

Wethered D B, Markey M A, Hay R J, Mahgoub E S, Gumaa S A 1988 Humoral immune responses to mycetoma organisms: characterisation of specific antibodies by the use of enzyme-linked immunosorbent assay and immunoblotting. Transactions of the Royal Society of Tropical Medicine and Hygiene 82: 918–923

Wheeler M K, Bell A A 1988 Melanins and their importance in pathogenic fungi. Current Topics in Medical Mycology 2: 338–389

Wright C D, Bowie J U, Nelson R D 1984 Influence of yeast mannan on release of myeloperoxidase by human neutrophils: determination of structural features of mannan required for formation of myeloperoxidase-mannan neutrophil complexes. Infection and Immunity 43: 467–474

Zaini F, Moore M K, Hay R J, Campbell C K, Noble W C 1991 The antigenic structure of mycetoma agents and a study of their immunogenicity. Mycoses 34: 19–28

Zurita J, Hay R J 1987 The adherence of dermatophyte microconidia and arthroconidia to human keratinocytes in vitro. Journal of Investigative Dermatology 82: 529–534

Discussion of paper presented by R. J. Hay

Reported by S. R. Norrby

The issue of atopy and IgE as an aggravating factor in patients infected with *T. rubrum* was brought up by Dr Bennett. Dr Hay agreed that such infections are more common in atopic patients and that there seems to be a clear relationship between chronicity and IgE reactivity. However, the mode by which IgE or other factors involved in atopy influence the course of a *T. rubrum* infection is still unknown. An untested hypothesis is that increased IgE levels turn on production of interleukin-4, which, in turn, could depress the normal immune reaction to the organism.

Dr Walsh asked if anyone had seen an increased incidence of mycetoma or chromoblastomycosis in patients with symptomatic HIV infections in Africa. Such reports also seem to be absent from those countries in Africa which have high frequencies of the mycoses and in which HIV infections are common.

Dr Schaffner inquired about the effector mechanisms for the T-cell mediated immunity demonstrated in Dr Hay's model for dermatomycoses. Dr Hay suggested some possible explanations for this phenomenon. The first is that activated T-cells trigger a variety of events including activation of kerotinocytes which are immunologically highly active cells. This would result in a release of cytokines which, in turn, would attract macrophages and neutrophils. A second possibility is that the epidermal proliferation is increased, thus shedding the dermatophytes into the environment.

In this context it was also discussed whether the same immune mechanisms which have been observed in dermatomycoses also apply to mucosal candidiasis. Dr Hay pointed out that a recently observed problem in patients with chronic mucocutaneous candidiasis is that some of them develop very serious dermatophyte infections with deep crusted lesions. These patients seem to have switched organisms from a controllable *Candida* infection to a dermatophyte infection which is much more difficult to control.

The nature of the id reactions seen in patients with dermatomycoses was discussed by Dr McAdam and Dr Hay. The id reaction is a secondary rash which occurs in patients with inflammatory athlete's foot or inflammatory ringworm. In conjunction with the reaction, the dermatophyte infection becomes more inflamed. The secondary rash, which can be triggered by treatment, never contains the causative organisms. Histologically, two forms of id reaction are seen: an eczema-

222

tous one which seems to be a manifestation of T-cell activation and a cutaneous vasculitis which could be precipitated by massive release of antigen, for example during treatment. Dermatophyte antigen has been demonstrated in id lesions.

Session V:
Serodiagnosis

Chairman: D. W. R. Mackenzie

ERRATA

The correct keys should be noted for the captions on the following pages:

Page 233, Figure 13.1
($\blacksquare$) = sensitivity; ($\boxtimes$) = positive predictive value; ($\square$) = negative predictive value.

Page 234, Figure 13.2
($\blacksquare$) = sensitivity; ($\boxtimes$) = positive predictive value; ($\square$) = negative predictive value.

Page 235, Figure 13.3
($\boxtimes$) = analysis by cases; ($\blacksquare$) = analysis by sample.

Page 236, Figure 13.4
($\blacksquare$) = blood cultures alone; ($\boxtimes$) = antigenaemia alone; ($\square$) = blood culture and antigenaemia.

13. Immunodiagnosis of invasive candidiasis in patients with neoplastic diseases

T. J. Walsh, J. W. Lee, P. A. Pizzo

INTRODUCTION

Invasive candidiasis is difficult to diagnose and is the cause of substantial morbidity and mortality in hospitalized patients, especially those with neoplastic diseases (Meunier-Carpentier et al 1981, de Repentigny & Reiss 1984, Solomon 1984, Burnie et al 1985, Horn et al 1985, Walsh & Pizzo 1988, Armstrong 1989). The current approach to its diagnosis consists of a high index of clinical suspicion, use of blood cultures, diagnostic imaging techniques [e.g. computerized ultrasonography (US), tomography (CT) scans and magnetic resonance imaging (MRI)] and biopsy of infected tissues. Depending upon the diagnostic modality, these approaches, however, may lack sensitivity, may be positive only in more advanced stages of infection, and may be unduly invasive in compromised patients.

Detection of cell wall, cytoplasmic or metabolic components may facilitate diagnosis of invasive candidiasis. Such potential markers for invasive candidiasis include *Candida* cell wall antigens, such as mannans (Bousgnoux et al 1990, Lemieux et al 1990), *Candida* metabolites, such as D-arabinitol (Gold et al 1983, Wong & Brauer 1988), and *Candida* cytoplasmic antigens (Taschdjian et al 1973, Jones 1980, Araj et al 1982, Strockbine et al 1984a, b, Matthews et al 1987, Matthews & Burnie 1988). One of these cytoplasmic antigens is a *Candida* enolase (Strockbine et al 1984a, b) and another is a breakdown produce of a *Candida* heat shock protein (HSP 90) (Matthews et al 1987, Matthews & Burnie 1988). While several reviews have discussed many of these potential diagnostic markers (de Repentigny & Reiss 1984, Bennett 1987, Jones 1990), the purpose of this review will be to discuss these markers as they pertain to invasive candidiasis in patients with neoplastic diseases, paying particular attention to immunodiagnostic techniques and newer understanding of *Candida* enolase.

DEFINITIONS AND CLASSIFICATION

A classification of candidiasis is important in understanding the patterns of expression of diagnostic markers in different conditions of the disease. Comparative interpretation of different studies of diagnostic modalities is critically dependent

227

upon the uniformity of definitions and classification. In order to provide a uniform understanding of terms used in this chapter, the following classification and definitions are provided. *Invasive candidiasis* may be defined as infection due to *Candida* spp. in blood or deep non-mucosal tissue sites. It may be classified further as either *deep candidiasis* (tissue-proven invasive candidiasis) or *fungaemia* (invasive candidiasis proven by blood culture only). *Deep candidiasis* may be *localized* to a single organ or be *disseminated* to involve two or more non-contiguous foci. Tissue-proven deep candidiasis by this classification excludes mucosal candidiasis. *Mucosal candidiasis* is defined as infection by *Candida* limited to invasion of mucosal surfaces, including those of the alimentary, genitourinary or tracheobronchial mucosa. *Colonization* may be defined as the presence of *Candida* isolated from mucosal surfaces (oropharynx, rectum, and vagina) with no evidence of active infection. Specifically excluded from this study were five neutropenic patients with urine cultures positive for *Candida*, as these patients may have had upper urinary tract infection that could not be reliably proven or excluded as a diagnosis.

The increasing usage of cytotoxic chemotherapy, immunosuppressive regimens, and broad spectrum antibacterial therapy has contributed substantially to the expanding frequency of invasive candidiasis, particularly in patients with cancer. Several conditions that are particularly associated with patients with neoplastic diseases include acute haematogenous disseminated candidiasis with cutaneous and skeletal muscle infection (Jarowski et al 1978, Arena et al 1981), hepatosplenic candidiasis (chronic disseminated candidiasis) (Thaler et al 1988), and fungaemia related to chronic in-dwelling silastic venous catheters. Mucosal diseases, including oropharyngeal and oesophageal candidiasis, are also commonly observed in these patients. Mucosal candidiasis commonly serves as the portal of entry of invasive candidiasis involving deep non-mucosal tissues and disseminated infection. Most cases of invasive candidiasis are nosocomial infections that appear to arise from endogenous flora, i.e. they are hospital-associated and less commonly hospital-acquired (Walsh & Pizzo 1988). Nevertheless, well-characterized outbreaks of nosocomial candidiasis have been reported in immunosuppressed patients.

CLINICAL EVALUATION

Bedside clinical evaluation is the cornerstone of assessment of a patient with possible invasive candidiasis. Table 13.1 summarizes the conventional and investigative diagnostic modalities for approaching patients with possible invasive candidiasis. Recognition of the sub-population of patients with neoplastic diseases at high risk for invasive candidiasis heightens the clinical index of suspicion of deep mycosis. Several findings on physical examination should suggest or strongly indicate the presence of invasive candidiasis. These findings include persistent or recurrent fever, despite antibacterial therapy (Pizzo et al 1982, Walsh et al 1991), erythematous cutaneous lesions, especially when associated with myalgias (Jarowski et al 1978, Areua et al 1981), tenderness in the right or left upper quadrants, suggestive of hepatic or splenic infection (Thaler et al 1988). Detection of *Candida* endophthalmitis, while particularly valuable in non-neutropenic patients (Edwards

Table 13.1. Conventional and investigative modalities for diagnosis of invasive candidiasis

Conventional
Clinical evaluation
Detection of fungaemia
Diagnostic imaging of invasive candidiasis
Histopathological identification of invasive candidiasis
Investigational
Detection of anti-*Candida* antibodies
Detection of *Candida* antigens
Cell wall mannan
Cytoplasmic antigens
Detection of *Candida* metabolites
Detection of cell wall components of *Candida* by *Tachypleus* assay
Amplification of *Candida* DNA by polymerase chain reaction

1985), is seldom possible in granulocytopenic hosts because of the lack of granulocytes contributing to vitreal opacifications.

DETECTION OF FUNGAEMIA

The lysis centrifugation (Isolator, Dupont, DE) system is one of the most important technical developments in detection of fungaemia during the past decade. Several studies have demonstrated that the time to recovery of *Candida* is earlier and the frequency of recovery of *Candida* is greater in comparison to conventional broth and diphasic systems (Henry et al 1983, Bille et al 1984, Brannon & Kiehn 1986, Guerra-Romero et al 1987). More recent preliminary data suggest that a large volume (30 ml) broth system, which contains lytic agents, may be comparable to the lysis centrifugation system in detection of candidaemia (Mirrett 1991).

DIAGNOSTIC IMAGING OF INVASIVE CANDIDIASIS

The recent advances in diagnostic imaging by MRI, and US have substantially contributed to the diagnosis of deep tissue invasive candidiasis in patients with neoplastic diseases. Perhaps the most dramatic example of the utility of diagnostic imaging is evident in evaluation of hepatosplenic candidiasis, wherein US, CT imaging, and MRI serve as complementary tools in detection of lesions measuring $\geqslant 5\text{--}10$ mm in liver, spleen and, occasionally, lung and kidney. As most patients with hepatosplenic candidiasis have negative blood cultures at the time of diagnosis, the demonstration of such lesions may be the only conventional laboratory evidence consistent with invasive candidiasis.

HISTOPATHOLOGICAL IDENTIFICATION OF INVASIVE CANDIDIASIS

The findings of lesions comparable with invasive candidiasis should lead to confirmation by biopsy of the infected tissue. Tissue diagnosis is important for several reasons. It eliminates other processes in the differential diagnosis, especially other fungal infections and neoplastic disease. Tissue diagnosis unequivocally confirms the presence of *Candida*, thereby permitting aggressive therapy without reservations in the event of treatment-related toxicity. Tissue diagnosis also fulfils the requirements stipulated for the acquisition of investigational agents (e.g. liposomal formulations of amphotericin B) in cases which eventually prove refractory to therapy. Cultures of biopsied tissue in hepatosplenic candidiasis usually are negative. Thus recognition of fungal elements within such tissue becomes paramount. Methenamine silver and periodic acid–Schiff (PAS) stains may be the only means of detecting fungal elements within tissue. Biopsies of suspicious skin lesions may reveal fungal elements deep within or invading the dermal blood vessels. Cultures of these biopsies, especially in patients not receiving antifungal therapy, may yield the aetiological agent.

DETECTION OF ANTI-*CANDIDA* ANTIBODIES

Anti-*Candida* antibodies were studied extensively in the two decades spanning the 1960s and 1970s (Taschdjian et al 1971, Stickle et al 1972, Harding et al 1976, Kozinn et al 1978, Gulnan et al 1979). These assays consisted of precipitin tests or passive haemagglutination methods. Because of technical limitations at the time, the antigenic extracts were crude and not well-standardized. These antigen preparations consisted of cell wall or cytoplasmic constituents. However, subsequent work demonstrated that some cytoplasmic antigen preparations contained cell wall mannan (Jones 1980).

Ensuing work during the next decade investigated the antibody response to defined antigens. Anti-cell-wall mannan antibodies were the most extensively studied (Jones 1980, Greenfield et al 1983, Meckstroth et al 1981). These antibodies were found in most human sera. Patients with invasive candidiasis were found to have a trend toward more elevated levels of anti-cell-wall mannan antibodies; however, a clearly delineated bimodal distribution of antibody levels was not found.

Various investigators have examined the human antibody response to cytoplasmic extracts (treated to remove cell wall mannans) (Jones 1980, Greenfield & Jones 1981, Strockbine et al 1984a, Matthews et al 1984). When these cytoplasmic extracts of *C. albicans* were resolved with polyacrylamide gel electrophoresis and Western blots (immunoblots) were performed with sera from both patients with invasive candidiasis and non-infected controls, antibodies to several immunodominant cytoplasmic antigens ranging from 40 to 60 kDa were found.

DETECTION OF *CANDIDA* ANTIGENS

The advent of the *Cryptococcus* latex agglutination (LA) assay for detection of circulating cryptococcal polysaccharide antigen led to the expectation that a similar system could be developed for detection of invasive candidiasis. Unfortunately, detection of circulating *Candida* antigens has proved to be substantially more complex and formidable. An assay with the same facility, sensitivity, and specificity as the *Cryptococcus* LA assay has yet to be developed for detection of invasive candidiasis and does not appear to be forthcoming in the near future. Thus far, most immunodiagnostic studies for antigen detection have been directed towards identifying *Candida* cell wall mannans or cytoplasmic antigens.

Cell wall mannan

Numerous studies (de Repentigny & Reiss 1984, Bennett 1987, Jones 1990) have attempted to employ radioimmunoassay (RIA), enzyme-linked immunosorbent assay (ELISA), and LA to identify circulating cell wall mannan. Anti-cell-wall mannan antibodies and other binding proteins have prevented the detection of this antigen unless the immune and other circulating complexes are disrupted by hydrolysis followed by heating (Jones 1980, Ferreira et al 1990, Weiner & Coats-Stephen 1979). As cell wall mannan antigen is cleared rapidly from serum and the serum levels are small (usually ≤ 100 ng/ml), repeated serum sampling is necessary in order to improve sensitivity (Jones 1980). More profoundly immunocompromised patients, such as patients with acute leukaemia, would be less likely to produce neutralizing antibody and, indeed, this patient population has detectable cell wall mannan antigenaemia during invasive candidiasis (Meckstroth et al 1981).

A commercially available LA assay (CAND-TEC, Ramco Laboratories, Inc., Houston, TX) that detects an antigen of unknown identity has been studied in a variety of trials with widely varying results. While the utility of the assay has been controversial, some of the disparity of results observed in different centres also may reflect differences in study design, patient populations, definitions, classification, and sampling frequency (Gentry et al 1983, Burnie & Williams 1985, Bailey et al 1985, Fung et al 1986, Kahn & Jones 1986, Ness et al 1989).

Cytoplasmic antigens

Defined cytoplasmic antigens may offer other markers for detection of invasive candidiasis. Two such potential cytoplasmic markers, described as immunodominant antigens, were a *Candida* enolase and a breakdown product of a 90 kDa heat shock protein (HSP-90).

Strockbine et al (1984a) identified an immunodominant cytoplasmic 48 kDa antigen of *Candida*, to which antibody production was strongly associated with deep candidiasis in patients without neoplastic diseases. This 48 kDa antigen was subsequently found to be *Candida* enolase (Mason et al 1988, Franklyn et al 1990). Studies of experimental disseminated candidiasis in mice and rabbits demonstrated that antigenaemia due to the 48 kDa antigen detected by ELISA was expressed in the absence of fungaemia, correlated with deep tissue infection, distinguished superficial involvement from deep involvement, and declined in response to antifungal therapy (Walsh et al 1988).

Initial studies of immunocompromised cancer patients receiving cytotoxic chemotherapy revealed circulating antigen in serum of those patients with invasive candidiasis. Thus, in order to investigate the expression of this *Candida* cytoplasmic antigen in the serum of a carefully defined population of high-risk cancer patients with deeply invasive candidiasis and its potential for diagnosis of these infections, a prospective clinical trial among patients from four medical oncology centres over a 2-year period was conducted (Walsh et al 1991). Antigen was detected by using a double sandwich liposomal immunoassay for *Candida* enolase in serially collected sera. Expression of antigenaemia was studied in known cases of invasive candidiasis proven by presence of *Candida* spp. in deep non-mucosal tissue and/or blood cultures. Careful attention was directed towards classification and definitions of study populations as well as patterns of infection. Table 13.2 summarizes these definitions and the classification.

Table 13.2 Classification of patients and control populations for investigation of diagnostic markers of invasive candidiasis

I. Candidiasis
  A. Invasive candidiasis
    1. Deep candidiasis: tissue-proven invasive candidiasis
    2. Fungaemia: invasive candidiasis proven by blood culture only
  B. Colonization
    The presence of *Candida* spp. isolated from mucosal surfaces (oropharynx, rectum, and vagina) with no evidence of deep visceral infection in neutropenic cancer patients

II. Control populations
  A. Bacteraemia
    Bacteria isolated from blood cultures from febrile patients with no evidence of candidiasis
  B. Non-*Candida* fungal infections
    Fever and microbiologically or histopathologically proven deep fungal infection due to fungi other than *Candida* spp.
  C. No evidence of infection
    No microbiologically or clinically proven infection
  D. Normal blood bank donors

170 cancer patients were entered into the study and 684 serum samples assayed. 24 patients were found to have invasive candidiasis; 13 of these patients had deep candidiasis (tissue-proven invasive candidiasis) and 11 had fungaemia (blood culture-proven invasive candidiasis). 50 patients diagnosed with *Candida* colonization and 96 patients with no evidence of candidiasis were included as negative control groups.

Among the 24 cases of invasive candidiasis in patients with neoplastic diseases, the overall sensitivity of detecting *Candida* enolase antigenaemia per serum sample was 54% (Fig. 13.1). Multiple serum sampling improved detection of antigenaemia, which was found in 11 (85%) of 13 known cases of deep tissue-proven infection and in 7 (64%) of 11 known cases of fungaemia. The overall sensitivity of *Candida* enolase antigenaemia in these patients was 75% (18/24) (Fig. 13.2). Specificity was 96% in comparison to control groups, which included patients with mucosal colonization, bacteraemia, and other deep mycoses (Fig. 13.3). Antigenaemia was detected in the absence of fungaemia in five cases of tissue-proven invasive candidiasis, but was not detected in six cases of fungaemia alone. Antigenaemia complemented but did not replace blood cultures in the diagnosis of invasive candidiasis (Fig. 13.4).

The findings of enolase antigenaemia in the absence of fungaemia in this study are consistent with the results of earlier in vivo studies which showed that mice infected intraperitoneally or intravenously with *C. albicans* had deep visceral infection and enolase antigenaemia but minimal-to-absent fungaemia (Walsh et al 1988). These animal studies showed a correlation between the level of circulating antigen and the extent of deep tissue infection (as measured by CFU/g of tissue infection) suggesting that enolase antigenaemia may be a reflection of deep visceral candi-

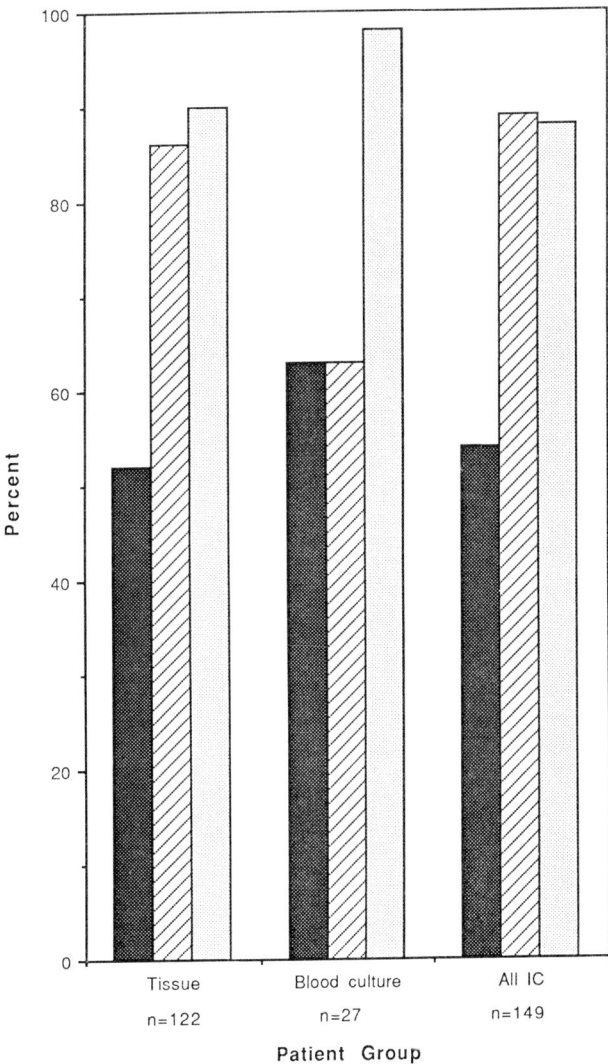

Fig. 13.1 *Candida* enolase antigenaemia in cancer patients with invasive candidiasis (IC): analysis by number of samples and according to the method of diagnosis [tissue confirmation (histopathology) and blood culture]. (■) = sensitivity; (□) = positive predictive value; (□) = negative predictive value.

diasis. The mechanisms of release, regulation, and plasma kinetics of *Candida* enolase are not known. If the release of *Candida* enolase is active in vivo during deep tissue infection, then enolase antigenaemia may be an important marker of deep visceral infection in the absence of fungaemia. A febrile cancer patient, for example with antigenaemia but without fungaemia, and with hepatic and splenic lesions consistent on CT scan with hepatosplenic candidiasis, might be spared a biopsy procedure to establish the diagnosis. With improvement of the assay's single-sample sensitivity, it may prove to be a useful indicator of deep infection in neutropenic cancer patients and may complement the diagnostic utility of blood cultures.

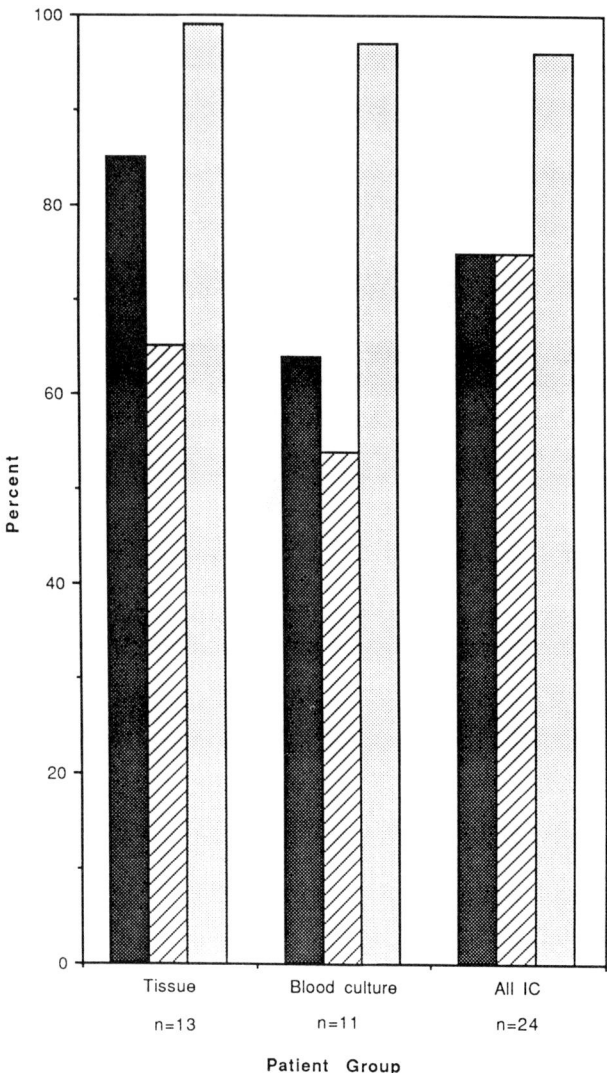

Fig. 13.2 *Candida* enolase L antigenaemia in cancer patients with invasive candidiasis (IC): analysis by number of patients and according to the method of diagnosis [tissue confirmation (histopathology) and blood culture]. (■) = sensitivity; (□) = positive predictive value; (□) = negative predictive value.

Several factors may contribute to enolase antigen-negative cases of invasive candidiasis: (1) antibody-mediated clearance of antigen, (2) low tissue concentrations of *Candida*, whether by antifungal therapy or recovery from granulocytopenia, and (3) infrequent sampling. Antibody-mediated clearance of *Candida* enolase through immune complex formation may be an important factor in causing false-negative results of the assay. Strockbine et al (1984a) found that *Candida* enolase antigen was the immunodominant cytoplasmic antigen of *Candida* in relatively non-immunocompromised patients with invasive candidiasis, in whom high titres of antibody were detected by Western blot. Indeed, if a study for

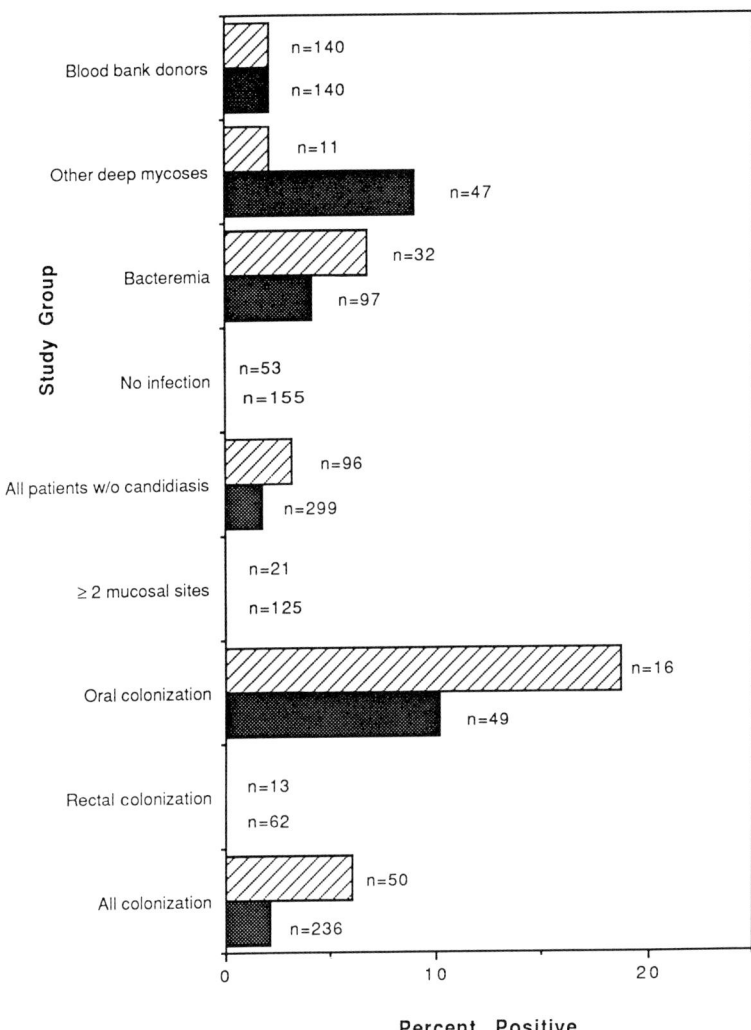

Fig. 13.3 *Candida* enolase antigenaemia in cancer patients and control populations without invasive candidiasis. (□) = analysis by cases; (■) = analysis by sample.

detection of *Candida* enolase antigenaemia was conducted in patients with *Candida* endocarditis and strongly reactive Western blots, it could be predicted virtually no circulating antigen would be detected. Patients who are profoundly immuno-compromised or who are neutropenic but who do not have significant impair-ment of immunoglobulin responsiveness may be able to mount a sufficient level of neutralizing antibody. Recent data from our laboratory indicate that elevated titration values (absorbance × dilution) of > 1:20 of anti-enolase antibody in serum of less severely immunocompromised patients are elevated in those with invasive candidiasis. A combination of antigen and antibody detection systems will be necessary to optimally utilize *Candida* enolase as a marker of invasive candidiasis. Antigenaemia may be most useful in profoundly immunocompromised patients

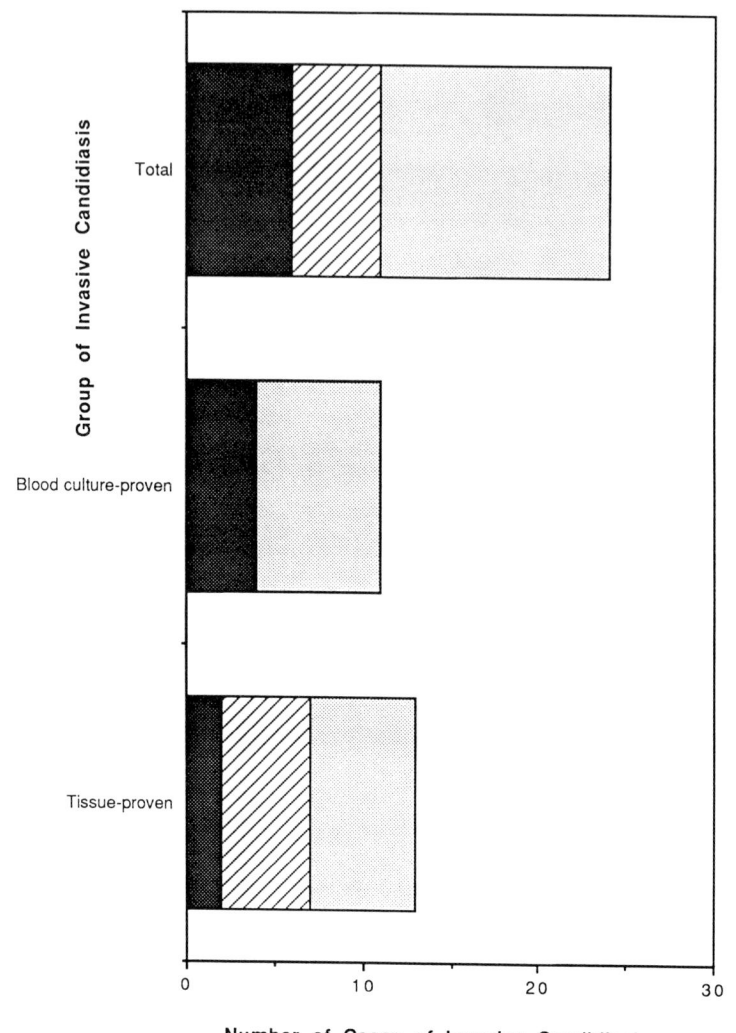

Fig. 13.4 Complementarity of blood cultures and enolase antigenaemia in detection of invasive candidiasis in cancer patients; (■) = blood cultures alone; (□) = antigenaemia alone; (□) = blood culture and antigenaemia.

with impaired B- and T-cell immunity. Antibody detection may be most appropriate in less compromised patient populations such as surgical patients undergoing organ transplantation or gastrointestinal surgery. *Candida* enolase may serve as a model for other immunodominant antigenic markers of invasive opportunistic mycoses, such as aspergillosis and candidiasis. Table 13.3 summarizes this concept of immunodominant antigen and antibody detection. Thus, a combination of antigen *and* antibody detection systems will be necessary to utilize *Candida* enolase optimally as a marker of invasive candidiasis (Abstract).

Detection of *Candida* enolase in the urine of high-risk patients may serve as another approach towards diagnosing invasive candidiasis. For example, gran-

Table 13.3 Potential populations for use of *Candida* enolase antigen and antibody detection

Patient population	Antigen detection	Antibody detection
Leukaemia/lymphoma	+	+/−
Allogeneic bone marrow transplantation	+	+/−
Recovery from granulocytopenia	+	+
Organ transplantation	+/−	+
General surgery	−	+

+ likely to be detected; +/− possibly detectable; − unlikely to be detected

ulocytopenic rabbits with disseminated candidiasis were found to have antigenuria due to *Candida* enolase (Walsh et al 1988). Patients with fungaemia recently were found to have a 47 kDa cytoplasmic antigen detected in urine by immunoblot (Ferreira et al 1990). The exact identity of this urinary antigen is unknown. Detection of antigenuria is non-invasive, may be advantageous in the presence of neutralizing antibody, and may complement the detection of enolase antigenaemia. Urinary *Candida* enolase would probably not be useful in distinguishing between patients with upper and lower urinary tract candidiasis.

The multicentre *Candida* enolase study was not specifically designed to determine whether detectable enolase antigenaemia preceded positive blood cultures (or vice versa) as the first indicator of invasive candidiasis. Among the 24 patients with invasive candidiasis, only 6 patients had simultaneous blood cultures and antigen determinations, allowing comparison of time of detection. Among these evaluable patients with comparable samples for antigenaemia and fungaemia, all had antigenemia (1–8 days) before fungaemia. Among the remaining 18 patients, 6 others had no detectable antigenaemia, 5 had no detectable fungaemia, and 7 had blood drawn for culture and antigen on different days, which prevented adequate comparison. Given that experimental and clinical data indicate that *Candida* enolase is not usually detectable in mucosal candidiasis, one would expect limitations of this marker in early diagnosis because of the inability to identify high-risk patients with invasive mucosal candidiasis. The utility of enolase antigenaemia in early detection is currently undergoing further study.

There are many basic and clinical aspects of *Candida* enolase antigenaemia that require investigation. The role of elevated anti-enolase antibody not only in clearing antigen but also in serving as a concomitant marker for invasive candidiasis must be studied. The principles learned from the use of combined antigen and antibody detection systems may guide later studies on the development of other immunodominant markers for fungal pathogens. Among the basic aspects that require investigation are the molecular and cellular regulation of expression of *Candida* enolase in the cell and in the host, antigen processing, and antigen clearance. Other clinical questions to be addressed are its expression in different conditions of systemic candidiasis in various high-risk patient populations, its prognostic significance, its role for monitoring antifungal therapy, and its potential for complementing other investigational diagnostic markers.

Another immunodominant cytoplasmic antigen (ICA) has been extensively studied by Matthews et al (1987). The 47 kDa antigen has been identified as an immunodominant breakdown product of a 90 kDa heat shock protein (HSP-90) of *C. albicans*. As Western blot patterns may not sufficiently resolve the bands of antigens within the range of 47 to 52 kDa, the 48 kDa *Candida* enolase antigen and the 47 kDa antigen may be distinguished by their pattern on Western blots with monoclonal antibodies. Monoclonal antibodies that recognize the enolase antigen cross-react on immunoblot with antigenic bands at 120–135 kDa and 35–38 kDa (Strockbine et al 1984b). By comparison, antibodies reactive to the 47 kDa antigen or a synthetic peptide epitope derived from the antigen react with a band at 92 kDa (Matthews et al 1987, Matthews & Burnie 1989). An enzyme-linked dot immunobinding assay has been employed for detection of this 47 kDa antigen in patients with invasive candidiasis (Matthews & Burnie 1988).

Both the *Candida* enolase antigen and the 47 kDa antigen are ICAs. As ICAs of *C. albicans*, both antigens also share the property of eliciting a detectable antibody response, especially upon recovery from immunosuppression and during resolution of infection. There is no convincing evidence, however, that antibodies to these antigens are protective. Instead, such antibodies may be markers of improved immune response in immunocompromised patients or may reflect the ability of an infected host who survives long enough to elaborate antibodies to these ICAs.

DETECTION OF *CANDIDA* METABOLITES

The cyclopentol D-arabinitol is the most extensively studied metabolite of *C. albicans* (Wong et al 1982). Serum concentrations of D-arabinitol detected by gas–liquid chromatography may be determined by comparison of serum concentrations to known internal standards. Care must be taken in utilizing proper extraction and derivitization techniques (de Repentigny et al 1985, Wong et al 1985). As arabinitol is cleared by glomerular filtration, arabinitol concentrations must be corrected against serum creatinine (Gold et al 1983). Circulating levels of D-arabinitol clearly are detectable in cases of invasive candidiasis. However, the demands imposed by the time, cost, and complexity of the GLC assay prohibit routine clinical application of these methods for detection of D-arabinitol. Other techniques under development may greatly facilitate detection of D-arabinitol.

DETECTION OF CELL WALL COMPONENTS OF *CANDIDA* BY *TACHYPLEUS* ASSAY

The Japanese horseshoe crab, *Tachypleus tridentatus*, has provided a source for an amoebocyte lysate assay for diagnosis of fungal infecion. The *Tachypleus* clotting cascade has two pathways which are differentially activated by fungal cell wall products and by endotoxin (Obayashi et al 1985, 1986). The gelation reaction of the amoebocyte lysate assay, which is well known to be initiated by bacterial endotoxin, is now also known to be triggered by the synthetic carbohydrate, carboxymethyl-1,3-β-D-glucan in concentrations of $\geqslant 1$ ng/ml (Morita et al 1981). Given the potential application of the amoebocyte lysate assay, different activating factors were selectively removed from the lysate in order to generate more specific preparations. Removal of factor G from the lysate permitted activation only by endotoxin; in contrast, retaining factor G and removing factors B and C results in a 1,3-β-D-glucan-activated system, which may be useful in the detection of fungus. As more consistent data have been generated by use of the *Tachypleus* (Japanese horseshoe crab) in comparison to *Limulus polyphemus* (American horseshoe crab), an assay using this system has been applied to a limited group of patients (Ikegami et al 1988). Additional clinical trials are currently being conducted in the United States.

AMPLIFICATION OF *CANDIDA* DNA BY POLYMERASE CHAIN REACTION (PCR)

The use of *Candida* DNA amplication by PCR in clinical specimens is yet another strategy for improving diagnosis of invasive candidiasis. Amplification of the genome of C14-demethylase as a fungus-specific gene was recently utilized by Buchman and colleagues (1990). Further investigation of this modality is currently in progress.

SUMMARY

Early treatment of invasive candidiasis is an important factor in the successful outcome of patients with neoplastic diseases. Clinical evaluation, blood cultures, and biopsies are the diagnostic standard tools in management of invasive candidiasis. Unfortunately, these methods may lack sensitivity in early recognition of this infection. Recognition in serum or urine of molecular markers of invasive candidiasis may greatly facilitate patient management. Immunodiagnosis of circulating mannans, enolase, or breakdown products of heat shock protein 90 may identify invasive *Candida* infection. Detection of D-arabinitol by gas–liquid chromatography or enzyme-linked reaction may also recognize invasive candidiasis. The recent use of *Candida* DNA amplification by polymerase chain reaction in clinical specimens is yet another strategy for improving diagnosis. These systems, however, are investigational and require further research; no single system will supplant the standard diagnostic tools, but data derived from a combination of systems might prove most useful in managing invasive candidiasis in patients with neoplastic diseases.

Invasive candidiasis is a complex disease in which these markers of invasive candidiasis may be expressed at different stages of infection. There is no single marker which can identify all cases of invasive candidiasis in all patient populations. Instead, development of a panel of diagnostic markers would perhaps enhance the clinician's assessment in patients who might benefit from the early treatment of invasive fungal infections.

REFERENCES

Araj G F, Hopfer R L, Chesnut S, Fainstein V, Bodey G P 1982 Diagnostic value of the enzyme-linked immunosorbent assay for detection of *Candida albicans* cytoplasmic antigen in sera of cancer patients. Journal of Clinical Microbiology 16: 46–52

Arena F P, Perlin M, Brahman H, Weiser B, Armstrong D 1981 Fever, rash and myalgias of disseminated candidiasis during antifungal therapy. Archives of Internal Medicine 141: 1233

Armstrong D 1989 Problems in management of opportunistic fungal diseases. Reviews of Infectious Diseases 2 (Suppl. 7): S1591–S1599

Bailey J W, Sada E, Brass C, Bennett J E 1985 Diagnosis of systemic candidiasis by latex agglutination for serum antigen. Journal of Clinical Microbiology 21: 749–752

Bennett J E 1987 Rapid diagnosis of candidiasis and aspergillosis. Review of Infectious Diseases 9: 398–401

Bille J, Edson R, Roberts G 1984 Clinical evaluation of the lysis centrifugation blood culture system for the detection of fungemia and comparison with a conventional biphasic broth blood culture system. Journal of Clinical Microbiology 19: 126–128

Bousgnoux M E, Hill C, Moissenet D, De Chauvin M F et al 1990 Comparison of antibody, antigen, and metabolite assays for hospitalized patients with disseminated or peripheral candidiasis. Journal of Clinical Microbiology 28: 905–909

Brannon P, Kiehn T E 1986 Large scale clinical comparison of lysis centrifugation and radiometric systems for blood culture. Journal of Clinical Microbiology 24: 886–887

Buchman T G, Rossier M, Merz W G, Charache P 1990 Detection of surgical pathogens by in vitro DNA amplification. Part I. Rapid identification of *Candida albicans* by in vitro amplification of a fungus specific gene. Surgery 108: 338–346

Burnie J P, Williams J D 1985 Evaluation of the Ramco latex agglutination test in the early diagnosis of systemic candidiasis. European Journal of Clinical Microbiology 4: 98–101

Burnie J P, Odds F C, Lee W, Webster C, Williams J D 1985 Outbreak of systemic *Candida albicans* in intensive care unit caused by cross infection. British Medical Journal 290: 746–748

de Repentigny L, Reiss E 1984 Current trends in immunodiagnosis of candidiasis and aspergillosis. Reviews of Infectious Diseases 6: 301–312

de Repentigny L, Marr L D, Keller J W, Carter A W, Kuykendall R J, Kaufman L, Reiss E 1985 Comparison of enzyme immunoassay and gas–liquid chromatography for the rapid diagnosis of invasive candidiasis in cancer patients. Journal of Clinical Microbiology 21: 972–979

Edwards J E 1985 *Candida* endophthalmitis. In: Bodey G P, Fainstein V (eds) Candidiasis. Raven Press, New York, pp. 211–225

Ferreira R P, Yu B, Niki Y, Armstrong D 1990 Detection of *Candida* antigenuria in disseminate candidiasis by immunoblotting. Journal of Clinical Microbiology 28: 1075–1078

Franklyn K M, Warmington J R, Ott A K, Ashman R B 1990 An immunodominant antigen of *Candida albicans* shows homology to the enzyme enolase. Immunology and Cell Biology 68: 173–178

Fung J C, Donta S T, Tilton, R C 1986 *Candida* detection system (CAD-TEC) to differentiate between *Candidia albicans* colonization and disease. Journal of Clinical Microbiology 24: 542–547

Gentry L O, Wilkinson I D, Lea A S, Price M F 1983 Latex agglutination test for detection of *Candida* antigen in patients with disseminated disease. European Journal of Clinical Microbiology 2: 122–128

Gold J W M, Wong B, Bernard E M, Klehn T E, Armstrong D 1983 Serum arabinitol concentrations and arabinitol/creatinine ratios in invasive candidiasis. Journal of Infectious Diseases 147: 504–513

Greenfield R A, Jones J M 1981 Purification and characterization of a major cytoplasmic antigen of *Candida albicans*. Infection and Immunity 34: 469–477

Greenfield R A, Bussey M J, Stephens J L, Jones J M 1983 Serial enzyme-linked immunosorbent assays for antibody to *Candida* antigens during induction chemotherapy for acute leukemia. Journal of Infectious Diseases 148: 275–283

Guerra-Romero L, Edson R S, Cockerill III F R, Horstmeier C D, Roberts G D 1987 Comparison of Du Pont Isolator and Roche Septi-chek for detection of fungemia. Journal of Clinical Microbiology 25: 1623–1625

Guinan M E, Portas M R, Hill H R 1979 The candida precipitin test in an immunosuppressed population. Cancer 43: 299–302

Harding S A, Sanford G R, Merz W G 1976 Three serologic tests for candidiasis: diagnostic value in distinguishing deep or disseminated infecion from superficial infection or colonization. American Journal of Clinical Pathology 65: 1001–1009

240

Henry N K, McLimans C A, Wright A J, Thompson R L, Wilson W R, Washington II J A 1983 Microbiological and clinical evaluation of the isolator lysis centrifugation blood culture tube. Journal of Clinical Microbiology 17: 864–869

Horn R, Wong B, Kiehn T E, Armstrong D 1985 Fungemia in a cancer hospital: changing frequency, earlier onset, and results of therapy. Reviews of Infectious Diseases 7: 646–655

Ikegami K, Ikemura K, Shimazu T, Shibuya M, Sugimoto H, Yoshioka T, Sugimoto T 1988 Early diagnosis of invasive candidiasis and rapid evaluation of antifungal therapy by combined use of conventional chromogenic *Limulus* test and a newly developed endotoxin specific assay. Journal of Trauma 28: 1118–1126

Jarowski C I, Flalk M A, Murray H W, Gottlieb G J, Coleman M, Steinberg C R, Silver R T 1978 Fever, rash and muscle tenderness. Archives of Internal Medicine 138: 544–546

Jones J M 1980 Kinetics of antibody responses to cell wall mannan and a major cytoplasmic antigen of *Candida albicans* in rabbits and humans. Journal of Laboratory and Clinical Medicine 96: 845–860

Jones J M 1990 Laboratory diagnosis of invasive candidiasis. Clinical and Microbiological Review 3: 32–45

Kahn F W, Jones J M, 1986 Latex agglutination tests for detection of *Candida* antigens in sera of patients with invasive candidiasis. Journal of Infectious Diseases 153: 579–585

Kozinn P J, Taschdjian C L, Goldberg P K et al 1978 Efficiency of serologic tests in the diagnosis of systemic candidiasis. American Journal of Clinical Pathology 70: 893–898

Lemieux C, St Germain G, Vincelette J, Kaufman L, deRepentigny L 1990 Collaborative evaluation of antigen detection by a commercial latex agglutination test and enzyme immunoassay in the diagnosis of invasive candidiasis. Journal of Clinical Microbiology 28: 249–253

Mason A B, Brandt M E, Buckley H R, 1988 Enolase activity associated with *Candida albicans* cytoplasmic antigen. Yeast 5: S231–S240

Matthews R, Burnie J 1988 Diagnosis of systemic candidiasis by an enzyme-linked dot immunobinding assay for a circulating immunodominant 47-kilodalton antigen. Journal of Clinical Microbiology 26: 459–463

Matthews R C, Burnie J P 1989 Cloning of a DNA sequence encoding a major fragment of the 47 kilodalton stress protein homologue of *Candida albicans*. FEMS Microbiology Letters 60: 25–30

Matthews R C, Burnie J P, Tabaqchall S, 1984 Immunoblot analysis of the serological response in systemic candidosis. Lancet ii: 1415–1418

Matthews R C, Burnie J P, Tabaqchall S 1987 Isolation of immunodominant antigens from sera of patients with systemic candidiasis and characterization of serological response to *Candida albicans*. Journal of Clinical Microbiology 25: 230–237

Meckstroth K L, Reiss E, Keller J W, Kaufman L 1981 Detection of antibodies and antigenemia in leukemic patients with candidiasis by enzyme-linked immunosorbent assay. Journal of Infectious Diseases 144: 24–32

Meunier-Carpentier F, Kiehn T E, Armstrong D 1981 Fungemia in the immunocompromised host. American Journal of Medicine 71: 363–370

Mirrett S, Davis T, Wilson M, Reynolds J, Fuller D, Koontz F, Allen S, Reller B 1991 Controlled evaluation of BACTEC selective fungal medium for detection of fungemia Abstract C-351 Abstracts of the American Society of Microbiology p. 400

Moritz T, Tanaka S, Nakamura T, Iwanaga S 1981 A new 1,3-β-D-glucan-mediated coagulation pathway found in *Limulus* amebocyte FEBS Letters 129: 318–321

Ness J J, Vaughn W P, Woods G L 1989 *Candida* antigen latex test for detection of invasive candidiasis in immunocompromised patients. Journal of Infectious Diseases 159: 495–501

Obayashi T, Tamura H, Tanaka S et al 1985 A new chromogenic endotoxin-specific assay using recombined *Limulus* coagulation enzyme and its clinical applications. Clinica Chemica Acta 149: 55–65

Obayashi T, Tamura H, Tanaka S, Ohki M, Takahashi S, Kawal T 1986 Endotoxin-inactivating activity in normal and pathological human blood samples. Infection and Immunity 53: 294–297

Pizzo P A, Robichad K J, Gill F A, Witebsky F G 1982 Empirical antibiotic and antifungal therapy for cancer patients with prolonged fever and granulocytopenia. American Journal of Medicine 72: 101–111

Solomon S L, Khabbaz R F, Parker R H, Anderson R L, Geraghty M A, Furman R M, Martone W J 1984 An outbreak of *Cryptococcus parapsilosis* bloodstream infections in patients receiving parenteral nutrition. Journal of Infectious Diseases 149: 98–102

Stickle D, Kaufman L, Blumer S O, McLaughlin D W 1972 Comparison of a newly developed latex agglutination test and an immunodiffusion test in the diagnosis of systemic candidiasis. Applied Microbiology 23: 490–499

Strockbine N A, Largen M T, Zweibel S M, Buckley H R 1984a Identification and molecular weight characterization of antigens from *Candida albicans* that are recognized by human sera. Infection and Immunity 43: 715–721

Strockbine N A, Largen M T, Buckley H R 1984b Production and characterization of three monoclonal antibodies to *Candida albicans* proteins. Infection and Immunity 43: 1012–1018

Taschdjian C L, Kozinn P J, Cuesta M V, Tobi E F 1971 Serodiagnosis of candidal infections. American Journal of American Pathology 57: 195–203

Taschdjian C L, Seelig M S, Koznin P J 1973 Serological diagnosis of candidal infections. Critical Reviews in Laboratory Sciences 4: 19–59

Thaler M, Pastakia B, Shawker T H, O'Leary, Pizzo P A 1988 Hepatic candidiasis in cancer patients: the evolving picture of the syndrome. Annals of Internal Medicine 108: 88–100

Walsh T J, Pizzo P A 1988 Nosocomial fungal infections: a classification for hospital acquired fungal infections and mycoses arising from endogenous flora or reactivation. Annual Review of Microbiology 42: 517–546

Walsh T J, Buckley H, Hom-Eng M, Johnson D E, Maret M, Gary P 1988 Analysis of a 48-kilodalton cytoplasmic antigen of *Candida albicans* in experimental candidiasis (abstract 0–111). In: Abstracts of the 10th Congress of the International Society for Human and Animal Mycology, Barcelona

Walsh T J, Hathorn J W, Sobel J D et al 1991 Detection of circulating *Candida* enolase by immunoassay in patients with cancer and invasive candidiasis. New England Journal of Medicine 324: 1026–1031

Walsh T J, Lee J, Lecciones J et al 1991 Empirical amphotericin B in febrile granulocytopenic patients. Reviews of Infectious Diseases 13: 496–503

Weiner M H, Coats-Stephen M 1979 Immunodiagnosis of systemic candidiasis: mannan antigenemia detected by radioimmunoassay in experimental and human infections. Journal of Infectious Diseases 140: 989–993

Wong B, Bernard E M, Gold J W M, Fong D, Silber A, Armstrong D 1982 Increased arabinitol levels in experimental candidiasis in rats: arabinitol appearance rate, arabinitol/creatinine ratios, and severity of infection. Journal of Infectious Diseases 146: 346–352

Wong B, Bernard E M, Armstrong D, Roboz J, Suzuki R, Holland J F 1985 Letter. Journal of Clinical Microbiology 21: 478–479

Wong B, Brauer K L 1988 Enantioselective measurement of fungal D-arabinitol in the sera of normal adults and patients with candidiasis. Journal of Clinical Microbiology 26: 1670–1674

Discussion of paper presented by T. J. Walsh

Discussed by R. C. Matthews
Reported by D. W. R. Mackenzie

Dr Matthews began her discussion by noting that the 47kDa (identified as HSP90) and 48kDa antigens of *Candida albicans* banded very close together on immunoblots, and could only be distinguished biochemically or by monoclonal antibodies. Homologues to this heat shock protein have been found in other microorganisms by using antibodies raised against specific epitopes on the candidal HSP90. An immunodot assay based on 47kDa purified by affinity chromatography was positive in 87% of non-neutropenic patients. In contrast to results reported by Dr Walsh with enolase, antigen sensitivity was reduced in neutropenic patients (77%).

Levels of antigenaemia may be related to presence of specific antibody. In patients producing IgG, good levels of antigen may be present, but in those producing mainly IgM, tests are likely to be negative.

By mapping epitopes along the major carboxy fragment of HSP90 and measuring their reactivity against sera from patients containing antibody to 47kDa antigen, a major epitope (C) has been identified and synthesized. Dr Matthews presented further data suggesting not only that specific anti-*Candida* antibody is protective in experimentally infected rabbits, but that resistance might be associated with a specific epitope. Conceivably, humanized monoclonal antibody might prove useful in the treatment of systemic candidiasis in conjunction with antifungal therapy.

Candida HSP90 is primarily intracellular, immunogold studies showing an association with the cell membrane. It has a homology with human HSP in excess of 50%. Although apparently not expressed on the cell surface, it may be released from the cell, where it binds with a number of extra-cellular proteins. Dr Matthews suggested that the *Candida* HSP90 might be considered a virulence factor. If released in large amounts into serum, it may mediate some of the effects seen in systemic candidiasis. Specific antibody might therefore neutralize the effects of fungal HSP90 on serum proteins.

A common problem in tests for detection of *Aspergillus* and *Candida* antigenaemia is their transient nature. In one reference laboratory an antigen test for aspergillosis was made unavailable because clinicians were excluding the diagnosis of invasive aspergillosis on the basis of a single negative test.

Dr Walsh pointed out that different antigens and antibodies, as well as metabolites, are likely to be expressed at different points in the course of invasive candidiasis, and emphasized that comparisons of test systems based on enolase versus HSP90 may be less productive than viewing them as potentially complementary. By analogy with tests for hepatitis B or Epstein–Barr viruses, laboratory testing for *Candida* infections might benefit by incorporating different systems in a panel of tests, possibly including PCR and metabolite detection as well as antigen and antibody assays.

PCR procedures for candidiasis are under development and Dr Shepherd reported an encouraging approach involving a probe which hybridizes with a DNA segment with a minimum of 500 copies per cell, and the polymerase-ligase reaction. A different approach has been taken by Dr Walsh and his colleagues, using a probe for C14 demethylase. Progress in this area would appear to depend on selection of the most suitable copy. One possibility suggested was the 5.2kb intermediate segment present as a repeated copy in a ribosomal gene.

The question of sensitivity, in terms of detectable reactants, is relevant not only to PCR and antigen detection but also to blood cultures. Dr Walsh emphasized the lack of correlation between the level of fungaemia and antigenaemia, reporting that some 70–80% of patients with proven disseminated candidiasis had fewer than five colonies on culture plates.

Detection of *Candida* antigenuria was reviewed briefly by Dr Walsh, who found about 60% of urines of experimentally infected rabbits positive for enolase. Presence of the 47kDa antigen in urine has also been reported in the literature. One possible reason for the failure to focus on antigen detection in urine for *Candida* infections, as opposed to aspergillosis, is the common occurrence of *Candida* as a cause of localized urinary tract infection, or simply as a colonizer.

The presence on the market of a test (Hybritech *Directigen*) for enolase raises the question of its target population. This test has at present a limited geographical availability, and is also specifically recommended only for highly immuno-compromised neutropenic patients. A broader application would clearly be desirable. At present, the test is considered to be complementary to blood cultures. With sensitivity in the range of 75% with repeated sampling, and 54% on single samples, improvement to 90–95% might be achieved by introducing a complementary test for homologous antibody. Increased costs might be reduced by changing the detecting system to an ELISA-based immunodot on urine. The need to accept that a single test is unlikely to achieve complete success was emphasized repeatedly, as was the accompanying need to ensure that limitations of procedures are appreciated by clinicians, and that repeated testing is required.

14. Serodiagnosis of aspergillosis

V. T. Andriole

INTRODUCTION

During the recent past, the incidence of certain opportunistic systemic fungal infections has increased, particularly in immunocompromised patients (Marier et al 1979, Rinaldi 1983, Sabetta et al 1985, Burnie & Matthews 1989, Saral 1991). Of these, infections caused by *Candida* species, particularly *C. albicans*, and by *Aspergillus* species, particularly *A. fumigatus*, are the most troublesome because of current difficulties in establishing their diagnosis (de Repentigny & Reiss 1984, Sabetta et al 1985, Hopwood & Warnock 1986, Bennett 1987, de Repentigny 1989). Thus, recent investigations in many laboratories have concentrated on the serological diagnosis of invasive candidiasis and aspergillosis in an attempt to provide clinicians with a non-invasive technique that might serve as a reliable diagnostic test (Sabetta et al 1985, Bennett 1987, Burnie & Matthews 1989, de Repentigny 1989). This paper will concentrate on the serodiagnosis of invasive aspergillosis.

The first reported cases of human aspergillosis appeared almost 150 years ago (Bennett 1844, Sluyter 1847, Virchow 1856, Rinaldi 1983). However, the importance and variety of distinct clinical entities caused by aspergillosis was not appreciated until 1952 (Rippon 1982, Rinaldi 1983). Since that time we have learned that both allergic aspergillosis and colonization with aspergillus organisms are common diseases. Furthermore, during the past quarter century invasive aspergillosis has also been recognized, primarily in immunocompromised patients, and particularly in patients receiving cytotoxic therapy for acute leukaemia, or undergoing organ or bone marrow transplantation (Tan et al 1966, Bodey 1966, Young et al 1970, Meyer et al 1973, DeGregorio et al 1982, Sherertz et al 1987, Robertson & Larson 1988, Denning & Stevens 1990).

Invasive aspergillosis is associated with significant morbidity, and mortality rates may be as high as 90% despite therapy with amphotericin B (Aisner et al 1977, DeGregorio et al 1982, Burnie & Matthews 1989, Denning & Stevens 1990). However, the death rate may be reduced by early diagnosis and treatment (Aisner et al 1977). For this reason many believe that a reliable diagnostic test, capable of detecting invasive aspergillosis in its very early stages, may improve survival if patients receive prompt, aggressive therapy. Thus, methods were developed to evaluate the presence, in body fluids, of either antibody or antigen as a diagnostic test for invasive aspergillosis.

ANTIBODY DETECTION IN ASPERGILLOSIS

A number of serological tests for detecting antibodies in patients with aspergillosis have been developed. These tests have been reviewed thoroughly in an excellent and recent publication by de Repentigny (1989), and will not be reviewed in detail again here. In general, anti-aspergillus antibodies are not commonly found in sera from healthy persons unless highly sensitive immunoassays are used (Rinaldi 1983). Immunodiffusion and counterimmunoelectrophoresis are probably the most widely used assays for the measurement of antibody (Meyer et al 1973, Schaefer et al 1976, Marier et al 1979, Fisher et al 1981, Rinaldi 1983, Burnie & Matthews 1989, de Repentigny 1989, Fratamico & Buckley 1991). Radioimmunoassay (Marier et al 1979), passive haemagglutination (Gold et al 1980), enzyme-linked immunosorbent assay (Holmberg et al 1980), and immunoblotting (Matthews et al 1985, de Repentigny et al 1991) have been used. Current experience with these tests indicate that they are of value for the diagnosis of allergic bronchopulmonary aspergillosis, and aspergilloma, whereas they are not uniformly reliable in the *early* diagnosis of invasive aspergillosis even when the more sensitive radioimmunoassay (Marier et al 1979) or enzyme-linked immunosorbent assays are used (de Repentigny 1989, Fratamico & Buckley 1991). In this context, immunocompromised patients with invasive aspergillosis are likely to have little capacity to react to infection with high concentrations of specific antibody (Marier et al 1979, Rinaldi 1983, de Repentigny 1989, Fratamico & Buckley 1991). In earlier studies from our laboratory, a solid-phase radioimmunoassay was developed to measure antibody responses to *A. fumigatus* and *A. flavus* antigens in 19 patients with invasive aspergillosis. This method was compared with immunodiffusion and counterimmunoelectrophoresis (Marier et al 1979). We found significant elevations in aspergillus antibody levels in 15 (79%) of 19 patients with invasive aspergillosis when measured by radio-immunoassay, as compared with 5 of 19 and 4 of 19 when measured by immuno-diffusion or counterimmunoelectrophoresis, respectively. Only 7 of 58 patients with other fungal or bacterial infections were positive by radioimmunoassay, as was 1 of 20 by immunodiffusion and counterimmunoelectrophoresis. However, none of the patients had significant elevations of antibody level on the day of onset of their invasive aspergillosis, but by day 14 or later all had significant rises in antibody level. Furthermore, a four-fold rise in antibody level was specific for aspergillosis and was not seen in patients with candidiasis or bacterial infection. These data indicated that our radioimmunoassay was more sensitive than immunodiffusion or counterimmunoelectrophoresis in detecting an antibody response in patients with invasive aspergillosis, and that a rise in antibody level, rather than an elevated level, was more important and specific for invasive aspergillosis. However, since serial antibody determinations were required for the specific diagnosis of invasive aspergillosis, it was not possible to establish a diagnosis at an early stage in the course of this infection.

Recent investigations have identified and characterized immunodominant components of *A. fumigatus* which appear to be recognized in the sera of some patients with invasive aspergillosis (Matthews et al 1985, Fratamico & Buckley 1991, Fratamico et al 1991, de Repentigny et al 1991). Matthews et al (1985) used the immunoblot technique to analyse the serological responses in 14 patients with invasive pulmonary aspergillosis, diagnosed by histology and culture of pulmonary tissues. Antibody was detected against nine components of the fungus, ranging in molecular weight from 33 to 88 kDa. Antibody to one band of 40 kDa was present in the sera from 11 of 14 patients with invasive pulmonary aspergillosis and was absent in 10 healthy control sera. Unfortunately, the time course of the appearance of the antibody response in relation to the onset of invasive pulmonary aspergillosis was not evaluated. Thus, the potential for this procedure to serve as a more sensitive and specific serodiagnostic test early in the course of invasive aspergillosis remains to be determined.

More recently, Fratamico & Buckley (1991) described the identification, by Western immunoblotting, and the characterization of an immunodominant antigen with a molecular weight of 58 kDa present in mycelial extracts of a strain of *A. fumigatus*, which was recognized by antibodies in the sera of patients with invasive aspergillosis. They studied 172 serum samples from 38 patients with invasive aspergillosis and observed that all serum samples had antibodies to this 58 kDa antigen, including some from patients with invasive aspergillosis due to *A. flavus*. Thus, this 58 kDa antigen of *A. fumigatus* is shared apparently by both of these species of *Aspergillus*. Pooled normal human serum obtained from healthy adults did not react. However, the criteria used to establish a diagnosis of invasive aspergillosis in the patients studied was not defined, nor was the time course of the appearance of the antibody to the onset of invasive aspergillosis evaluated.

Immunoblot analysis of the antibody response to protein antigens of an *A. fumigatus* mycelial homogenate has also been studied recently by de Repentigny et al (1991) in an experimental rabbit model of invasive aspergillosis. Sero-conversion was observed against antigens of 41, 54, and 71 kDa in some infected animals that survived for 10 or more days. The 41 kDa antigen was not often recognized by sera from rabbits before infection, but seroconversion was observed in half of the infected rabbits that survived for 10 or more days. The very valuable time course for the development of antibody was carefully studied in these experiments, in contrast to antibody responses studied by others. However, this serodiagnostic test, as with other methods for measuring antibody, would also require serial antibody determinations and may be of less value if detecting the early onset of invasive aspergillosis.

ANTIGEN DETECTION IN INVASIVE ASPERGILLOSIS

A number of methods have been developed and tested in an attempt to detect circulating aspergillus antigen, either free or in the form of immune complexes. Dissociation of antigen–antibody complexes by treatment with heat, boiling in trichloroacetic acid, or heat, acid and enzymatic digestion are important in order to increase the sensitivity of antigen detection. Counterimmunoelectrophoresis was used by Lehmann & Reiss (1978) to detect aspergillus polysaccharide antigen in the serum (obtained postmortem) of a leukaemic child, and in the serum and urine of immunosuppressed rabbits with invasive aspergillosis. Shaffer et al (1979a, b) described a radioimmunoassay that detected an undefined polysaccharide antigen in the serum of three patients with invasive aspergillosis and in a rabbit model 3 days after infection with *A. fumigatus*. The sensitivity of the radioimmunoassay was 500 ng/ml.

Weiner & Coats-Stephen (1979) also evaluated a radioimmunoassay to detect circulating aspergillus carbohydrate antigen in experimentally infected rabbits and identified antigen in 78% of animals with invasive aspergillosis. In early clinical studies, Weiner (1980) reported antigenaemia detected by radioimmunoassay in 4 of 7 patients, and in 4 of 6 patients in a later study (Weiner et al 1983). In their most recent report (Talbot et al 1987), antigen was detected by radioimmunoassay in 74% of 22 high-risk patients with invasive aspergillosis. Importantly, they showed that antigenaemia was detected prior to clinical suspicion of disease in 30% of patients, and prior to histopathological or microbiological evidence of disease in 46% of patients. They found the sensitivity of the method was 74% with a specificity of 90%, and a positive and negative predictive value of 82 and 85% respectively.

Dupont et al (1987) detected purified *A. fumigatus* galactomannan antigen by radioimmunoassay and enzyme-linked immunoassay in the serum and urine of patients and rabbits with invasive aspergillosis. However, this antigen was detected in the serum from only 2 of 12 patients (in concentrations of 150 and 500 ng/ml), and in the urine from only 7 of 13 patients with invasive aspergillosis (in concentrations of 1–83 ng/ml). Furthermore, galactomannan was detected in the serum from only 4 of 12 lethally infected rabbits, whereas urinary galactomannan was detectable throughout the course of lethal aspergillosis in all 16 rabbits in concentrations of 24–1900 ng/ml. Both the radioimmunoassay and enzyme-linked immunoassay gave comparable results. The difficulty in detecting galactomannan in the serum of lethally infected rabbits, experienced by these investigators, was explained by the rapid clearance of *A. fumigatus* galactomannan from the bloodstream via renal excretion and by macrophage mannose receptor-mediated endocytosis by Kupffer cells in the liver (Bennett et al 1987).

Detection of circulating aspergillus antigen in other experimental animal models of invasive aspergillosis has also been reported by other groups of investigators (Sabetta et al 1985, de Repentigny et al 1987, Patterson et al 1988, 1989b, 1990, Phillips & Radigan 1989, Ste-Marie et al 1990). In one brief report (Phillips & Radigan 1989), immunoaffinity chromatography was used to identify an 80 kDa immunoreactive component of *A. fumigatus* in the serum of 6 of 15 experimentally infected rabbits. However, this 80 kDa antigen could not be demonstrated in the serum of three human cases of invasive aspergillosis documented by histopathology.

A sensitive enzyme-linked immunoassay was used by de Repentigny et al (1987) to detect *A. fumigatus* galactomannan antigenaemia in 4 of 4 experimentally infected, immunosuppressed rabbits. The circulating antigen bound to concanavalin A and had a molecular weight of 50–100 kDa. More recent studies by this group of investigators described the detection of circulating aspergillus antigen in the serum of an immunosuppressed, experimentally infected rabbit by inhibition enzyme-linked immunoassay with a murine monoclonal antibody (mAb 1) of the immunoglobulin (IgM) class (Ste-Marie et al 1990). Furthermore, characterization of mAb 1 indicated it did not cross-react with candida mannan, and it did bind to the inner cell wall and intracellular membranes of hyphae and conidia of *A. fumigatus* as determined by immunelectron microscopy. The results of these experiments also suggested that mAb 1 recognized the immunodominant oligo-galactoside side chains of *A. fumigatus* galactomannan. However, the utility of this and other monoclonal antibodies as useful techniques for the serodiagnosis of invasive aspergillosis in patients remains to be determined.

Detection of circulating aspergillus antigen in experimental invasive aspergillosis has been studied extensively in our laboratory (Sabetta et al 1985, Patterson et al 1988, 1989b, 1990, Andriole et al in press). In our studies, the time course of the appearance of circulating aspergillus antigen following lethal or sub-lethal challenge with *A. fumigatus*, and the impact of treatment with various antifungal agents on the kinetics of aspergillus antigenaemia, as well as the relationship of antigenaemia to the extent of invasive aspergillosis in each animal, have been characterized in detail. Circulating aspergillus antigen is measured by an inhibition enzyme-linked immunosorbent assay, which detects the carbohydrate component of the aspergillus antigen in concentrations as low as 10 ng/ml (Sabetta et al 1985). The antibody used in our method is polyclonal, was prepared in rabbits immunized with aspergillus conidia, and does not cross-react with candida mannan. We have repeatedly and invariably demonstrated the ability of this test to detect aspergillus carbohydrate antigen at minimum serum levels of 50 ng/ml. Thus, the inhibition enzyme-linked immunosorbent assay has been consistently reproducible, with a sensitivity of 63% at 10 ng/ml and 100% at 50 ng/ml. Of note, in the rabbit 500 ng or more of aspergillus carbohydrate antigen per ml of serum completely binds all of the available aspergillus antibody (Sabetta et al 1985).

In our immunosuppressed rabbit model of lethal invasive aspergillosis, circulating aspergillus antigen first appeared in low concentrations by 48 h after onset of infection, and then in rapidly increasing amounts up to the time of death. Also, the level of aspergillus antigen in serum correlated directly with the number of *Aspergillus* organisms per gram of tissue in liver, lung, kidney and brain. Furthermore, treatment with the antifungal agents amphotericin B, liposomal amphotericin B, fluconazole, saperconazole, and a combination of amphotericin B plus fluconazole, was observed to either reduce significantly or eliminate completely the circulating antigen in treated animals as compared with untreated control rabbits. Again, circulating aspergillus antigen levels in the treated animals correlated directly with the number of *Aspergillus* organisms in tissue and with a reduction in mortality from invasive aspergillosis. Of importance, we noted that the persistence of low levels of aspergillus antigen in the serum of treated animals indicated residual presence of viable *Aspergillus* organisms in tissue. This observation suggested that persistent antigenaemia, even at low levels, might be a reliable indicator of inadequately treated invasive aspergillosis in patients.

In contrast to the studies described above which have detected circulating aspergillus antigen in animals with invasive aspergillosis, Wong et al (1989) used gas chromatography and gas chromatography/mass spectrometry to measure levels of D-mannitol in the serum and tissues of rats given a rapidly lethal dose of *A. fumi-*

gatus conidia intravenously. They observed increased amounts of D-mannitol in the livers and sera of infected rats, and significantly higher serum D-mannitol/creatinine ratios than were observed in uninfected controls, and suggested that D-mannitol might be a potential marker for aspergillosis. Although these preliminary studies may lead to more definitive data to support this concept, the unpredictability of the kinetics of in vivo metabolites of infecting organisms, with the possible exception of overwhelming rapidly fatal disease, makes this approach much less attractive as a potential diagnostic test for early invasive aspergillosis.

Other groups of investigators (Le Pape & Deunff 1986, Wilson et al 1987, Johnson et al 1989, Burnie & Matthews 1989, Rogers et al 1990) have also detected circulating aspergillus antigen in patients with proven or highly probable invasive aspergillosis. Some of these patients have had localized infection, i.e. invasive pulmonary aspergillosis, whereas others have had disseminated infection. This distinction is important with regard to the level of detectable circulating aspergillus antigen (Andriole 1988, unpublished observations).

Le Pape & Deinff (1986) found 9 out of 10 patients positive for aspergillus antigen from 28 serum samples using an enzyme-linked immunosorbent assay inhibition system. Wilson et al (1987) also used an inhibition enzyme-linked immunosorbent assay to detect aspergillus antigen in 3 of 5 bone-marrow transplant patients studied retrospectively, and 1 liver transplant patient studied prospectively, who died of disseminated aspergillosis proven at autopsy. Circulating antigen was also detected retrospectively in the serum of 3 other bone-marrow transplant patients who died with suspected disseminated aspergillosis. They also observed that tests on single serum samples were often negative whereas multiple specimens from the same patient increased the frequency of detection. Similarly, Johnson et al (1989) detected aspergillus antigenaemia, in a retrospective survey, using a competitive inhibition biotin-streptavidin-linked immunosorbent assay in 3 of 4 bone marrow transplant patients with histopathologically proven invasive aspergillosis, and in 1 patient with suspected infection. No antigen was detected in 17 bone-marrow transplant patients without proven or suspected invasive aspergillosis or in 16 healthy control subjects. They also observed that detection of antigen rose with an increasing number of samples tested.

Rogers et al (1990) evaluated two different inhibition enzyme-linked immunosorbent assays to detect serum and urinary aspergillus antigen in 121 neutropenic patients after leukaemia therapy or bone-marrow transplantation. The anti-aspergillus antibody used was either high-titre human anti-aspergillus serum (polyclonal), or rat IgM monoclonal antibody to *A. fumigatus* galactomannan. Antigen was detected in the serum or urine of 16 of 19 patients early in the course of invasive pulmonary aspergillosis and in 11 of 13 episodes of clinically suspected fungal infection. Significantly more urine samples than sera from patients with invasive pulmonary aspergillosis were positive for antigen. Specifically, with the human anti-aspergillus antibody only 13% of 482 serum samples and 20% of 173 urine samples were positive for antigen; with the rat monoclonal antibody only 18% of 345 serum samples and 44% of 170 urine samples were positive for antigen. Antigen was also detected in 1 of 90 patients with no evidence of invasive pulmonary aspergillosis. The authors state that antigen detection did not correlate with antifungal therapy or the isolation of *Aspergillus* sp. from sputum or other specimens.

However, antigen was detected early in serum or urine in 84% of 19 patients with proven invasive pulmonary aspergillosis, but in only a small percentage of urine and serum samples obtained from these patients throughout the course of their disease. These discordant observations are not easily explained. Burnie & Matthews (1989) used a reverse passive latex agglutination method, in a prospective study in febrile neutropenic patients who had failed to respond to broad spectrum antibiotics, to detect circulating aspergillus antigen. They studied 20 patients in whom a definitive diagnosis was made histopathologically, and 13 patients with a suspected diagnosis of invasive aspergillosis. Circulating antigen was detected in the initial serum sample in only 5 of 20 proven cases of invasive aspergillosis, and in 7 of the 13 with suspected infection, whereas antigen was detected in terminal serum specimens in 12 of the 20 proven cases and in 11 of the suspected cases. Thus an early false negative result was obtained in 21 of 33 of the proven or suspected cases of invasive aspergillosis. In only 12 cases was there a reasonable level of detectable antigen in the initial serum sample.

Clinical studies from our laboratory were first reported by Sabetta et al (1985) in which our competitive inhibition enzyme-linked immunosorbent assay was used. This assay was developed to detect circulating aspergillus carbohydrate antigen in serum using high titred polyclonal rabbit anti-aspergillus antibody, which was capable of detecting 10 ng of carbohydrate antigen per ml of serum. Circulating antigen was detected in 11 of 19 patients with invasive aspergillosis proven histopathologically at autopsy or by biopsy when the method was applied retrospectively to single serum samples from each patient. No circulating antigen was detected in serum from 34 patients with *C. albicans* sepsis, 28 patients with other non-aspergillus infections, and 18 healthy control hospital personnel. In a follow-up study from our group, Patterson et al (1989a) determined the positive predictive value of aspergillus antigen testing with our modified inhibition enzyme-linked immunosorbent assay by reviewing our laboratory records for a 2-year period and identifying all patients with 50 ng or more of antigen detected per ml of serum. We identified 30 patients, all of whom were immunosuppressed, with at least one serum sample positive for over 50 ng of aspergillus antigen per ml. Histopathologically proven invasive aspergillosis was present in 16 of the 30 patients (57%), with maximum antigen values of 70–3500 ng/ml; 7 of the 30 had probable invasive aspergillosis defined by a positive culture for *Aspergillus* sp. and a clinical illness compatible with the disease; 20% had an indeterminate diagnosis, defined by no microbiologically proven cause of infection in the presence of persistent fever despite antibiotic therapy, and there was no evidence of invasive aspergillosis in only 1 of the 30 patients. However, there were no false positive results in 23 of the 30 patients who had serum samples tested serially and who had 50 ng of antigen or more per ml of serum. In addition, when we analyzed the maximum antigen values detected in patients with proven invasive aspergillosis, those with proven *disseminated* aspergillosis had a median antigen values of 600 ng/ml, which was significantly higher than the median antigen value of 93 ng/ml seen in patients with proven invasive *pulmonary* aspergillosis. Also, the course of antigenaemia in these patients correlated with outcome. Specifically, 18 of 23 patients with proven or probable invasive aspergillosis had serial serum samples tested for aspergillus antigen. Clearance of antigenaemia was seen in 5 patients and all 5 survived their infection. In contrast, persistent or rising aspergillus antigen levels were seen in 13 patients who died of invasive aspergillosis. In this study, the positive predictive value of our method for proven or probable invasive aspergillosis was 77%, and may be as high as 97% if all patients with a proven, probable or an indeterminate diagnosis were true positives (Patterson et al 1989a). Our observations suggest that, with our method, detection of 50 or more ng/ml of aspergillus antigen in the serum of patients is highly predictive of invasive aspergillosis and that a rise or fall in antigenaemia correlates with the clinical course of this infection. Furthermore, high antigen values are seen in disseminated disease.

FUTURE DIRECTIONS

Significant progress has been made in the serodiagnosis of invasive aspergillosis, but much more work must be done. Recently, more than 30 antigenically-active components of *A. fumigatus* have been demonstrated (Hearn 1988). The identification of the most important of these, if any, in the serum of patients with invasive aspergillosis must be determined. Such identification may lead to standardization of a method for early diagnosis of invasive aspergillosis. The present data do not support serial antibody determinations in patients with invasive aspergillosis as an optimal diagnostic test for the early detection of this infection. In contrast, antigen detection, by the testing of serial samples in serum or urine in high-risk patients by inhibition enzyme-linked immunosorbent assay, offers great promise as a moderately sensitive but highly specific method of detecting early infection in many high-risk patients. We have learned that the detection rate for aspergillus antigen in serum and urine is increased by testing frequently obtained samples, dissociating immune complexes in the method employed, and by developing a sensitive assay technique. The latter, in my view, is directly dependent upon the affinity of the antibody used for the antigen detected in the patients body fluids, whether it be serum or urine or bronchial lavage fluid.

The use of monoclonal antibodies provides an opportunity for standardization of an assay and may improve the diagnostic utility of aspergillus antigen detection. However, monoclonal antibodies directed against specific antigens, which may not always be present in invasive aspergillosis, may reduce the sensitivity of the test. Also, a major use of antigen detection, at least in our experience, may be in guiding treatment. Although correlation of antigen levels in predicting remission or relapse of infection has not been established, our preliminary observations suggest that falling aspergillus antigen levels in the serum of patients with invasive aspergillosis on proper antifungal therapy correlate with survival from this devastating infection.

SUMMARY

The recent advances and future directions which may be important in the development of a highly sensitive and specific serodiagnostic test for the early diagnosis of invasive aspergillosis have been reviewed. Also, the difficulties that have emerged during the development of newer diagnostic methods for the detection of either

Aspergillus antibody or antigen in the body fluids of patients at high risk of acquiring invasive aspergillosis have been emphasized. Much progress has been made despite these difficulties.

We have learned that anti-aspergillus antibody detection is not likely to lead to early diagnosis of invasive aspergillosis, whereas sensitive methods which reliably detect small but significant amounts of aspergillus carbohydrate antigen in body fluids of immunosuppressed high-risk patients may provide us with a non-invasive early diagnostic technique which is both sensitive and specific.

REFERENCES

Aisner J, Schimpff S C, Wiernik P H 1977 Treatment of invasive aspergillosis: relation of early diagnosis and treatment to response. Annals of Internal Medicine 86: 539–543

Andriole V T 1988 Unpublished observations

Andriole V T, Miniter P, George D et al (in press) Animal models: their usefulness of studies of fungal pathogenesis and drug efficacy in aspergillosis. Reviews of Infectious Diseases

Bennett J E 1987 Rapid diagnosis of candidiasis and aspergillosis. Reviews of Infectious Disease 9: 398–402

Bennett J E Friedman M M, Dupont B 1987 Receptor-mediated clearance of aspergillus galactomannan. Journal of Infectious Diseases 155: 1005–1010

Bennett J H 1844 On the parasitic vegetable structures found growing in living animals. Transactions of the Royal Society of Edinburgh 15: 277–294

Bodey G P 1966 Fungal infections complicating acute leukemia. Journal of Chronic Diseases 19: 667–687

Burnie J P, Matthews R C 1989 Recent laboratory observations in the diagnosis of systemic fungal infection: *Candida* and *Aspergillus*. In: Holmberg K, Meyer R (eds) Diagnosis and therapy of systemic fungal infections. Raven Press, New York, p 101

DeGregorio M W, Lee W M F, Linker C A et al 1982 Fungal infections in patients with acute leukemia. American Journal of Medicine 73: 543–548

Denning D W, Stevens D A 1990 Antifungal and surgical treatment of invasive aspergillosis: review of 2121 published cases. Reviews of Infectious Diseases 12: 1147–1201

de Repentigny L, Reiss E 1984 Current trends in immunodiagnosis of candidiasis and aspergillosis. Reviews of Infectious Diseases 6: 301–312

de Repentigny L, Boushira M, Ste-Marie L et al 1987 Detection of galactomannan antigenemia by enzyme immunoassay in experimental invasive aspergillosis. Journal of Clinical Microbiology 25: 863–867

de Repentigny L 1989 Serologic techniques for diagnosis of fungal infection. European Journal of Clinical Microbiology and Infectious Diseases 8: 362–375

de Repentigny L, Kilanowski E, Pedneault L et al 1991 Immunoblot analyses of the serologic response to *Aspergillus fumigatus* antigens in experimental invasive aspergillosis. Journal of Infectious Diseases 163: 1305–1311

Dupont B, Huber M, Kim S J et al 1987 Galactomannan antigenemia and antigenuria in aspergillosis: studies in patients and experimentally infected rabbits. Journal of Infectious Diseases 155: 1–11

Fisher B D, Armstrong D, Yu B et al 1981 Invasive aspergillosis: progress in early diagnosis and treatment. American Journal of Medicine 71: 571–577

Fratamico P M, Buckley H R 1991 Identification and characterization of an immunodominant 58-kilodalton antigen of *Aspergillus fumigatus* recognized by sera of patients with invasive aspergillosis. Infection and Immunity 59: 309–315

Fratamico P M, Long W K, Buckley H R 1991 Production and characterization of monoclonal antibodies to a 58-kilodalton antigen of *Aspergillus fumigatus*. Infection and Immunity 59: 316–322

Gold J W M, Fisher B, Yu B et al 1980 Diagnosis of invasive aspergillosis by passive hemagglutination assay of antibody. Journal of Infectious Diseases 142: 87–94

Hearn V 1988 Serodiagnosis of aspergillosis. In: Vanden Bossche H, Mackenzie D W R, Cauwenbergh G (eds) Aspergillus and aspergillosis, Plenum Press, New York, p. 43

Holmberg K, Berdischewsky M, Young I S 1980 Serologic immunodiagnosis of invasive aspergillosis. Journal of Infectious Diseases 141: 656–664

Hopwood V, Warnock D W 1986 New developments in the diagnosis of opportunistic fungal infection. European Journal of Clinical Microbiology 5: 379–388

Johnson T M, Kurup V P, Resnick A et al 1989 Detection of circulating *Aspergillus fumigatus* antigen in bone marrow transplant patients. Journal of Laboratory and Clinical Medicine 114: 700–707

Lehmann P F, Reiss E 1978 Invasive aspergillosis: anti-serum for circulating antigen produced after immunization with serum from infected rabbits. Infection and Immunity 20: 570–572

Le Pape P, Deunff J 1988 Detection of aspergillus glycoprotein antigen in sera of patients with invasive aspergillosis: an enzyme-linked immunosorbent assay inhibition technique. In: Drouhet E, Cole G T, de Repentigny L et al (eds) Fungal antigens, 1st international symposium. Plenum Press, New York, p. 382

Marier R, Smith W, Jansen M et al 1979 A Solid-phase radioimmunoassay for the measurement of antibody to aspergillus in invasive aspergillosis. Journal of Infectious Diseases 140: 771–779

Matthews R, Burnie J P, Fox et al 1985 Immunoblot analysis of serologic responses in invasive aspergillosis. Journal of Clinical Pathology 38: 1300–1303

Meyer R D, Young L S, Armstrong D et al 1973 Aspergillosis complicating neoplastic disease. American Journal of Medicine 54: 6–15

Patterson T F, Miniter P, Ryan J L et al 1988 Effect of immunosuppression and amphotericin B on aspergillus antigenemia in an experimental model. Journal of Infectious Diseases 158: 415–422

Patterson T F, Miniter P, Andriole V T 1989a Predictive value of serum aspergillus antigen detection in the diagnosis of invasive aspergillosis. 89th Annual Meeting of the American Society for Microbiology, New Orleans, LA, May 14–18, 1989, p 458

Patterson T F, Miniter P, Dijkestra J et al 1989b Treatment of experimental invasive aspergillosis with novel amphotericin B/cholesterol-sulfate complexes. Journal of Infectious Diseases 159: 717–724

Patterson T F, Miniter P, Andriole V T 1990 Efficacy of fluconazole in experimental invasive aspergillosis. Reviews of infectious Diseases 12: S281–S285

Phillips P, Radigan G 1989 Antigenemia in a rabbit model of invasive aspergillosis. Journal of Infectious Diseases 159: 1147–1150

Rinaldi M G 1983 Invasive aspergillosis. Reviews of Infectious Disease 5: 1061–1077

Rinaldi M G 1991 Problems in the diagnosis of invasive fungal diseases. Reviews of Infectious Diseases 13: 493–495

Rippon J W 1982 Medical mycology. The pathogenic fungi and the pathogenic actinomycetes, 2nd edn. W B Saunders, Philadelphia, pp. 565–594

Robertson M J, Larson R A 1988 Recurrent fungal pneumonias in patients with acute nonlymphocytic leukemia undergoing multiple courses of intensive chemotherapy. American Journal of Medicine 84: 233–239

Rogers T R, Haynes K A, Barnes R A 1990 Value of antigen detection in predicting invasive pulmonary aspergillosis. Lancet 336: 1210–1213

Sabetta J R, Miniter P, Andriole V T 1985 The diagnosis of invasive aspergillosis by an enzyme-linked immunosorbent assay for circulating antigen. Journal of Infectious Diseases 152: 946–953

Saral R 1991 *Candida* and *Aspergillus* infections in immunocompromised patients: an overview. Reviews of Infectious Diseases 13: 487–492

Schaefer J C, Yu B, Armstrong D 1976 An aspergillosis immunodiffusion test in the early diagnosis of aspergillosis in adult leukemia patients. American Review of Respiratory Diseases 113: 325–329

Shaffer P J, Kobayashi G S, Medoff G 1979a Demonstration of antigenemia in patients with invasive aspergillosis by solid phase (protein A-rich *Staphylococcus aureus*) radioimmunoassay. American Journal of Medicine 67: 627–630

Shaffer P J, Medoff G, Koboyashi G S 1979b Demonstration of antigenemia by radioimmunoassay in rabbits experimentally infected with *Aspergillus*, Journal of Infectious Diseases 139: 313–319

Sherertz R J, Belani A, Kramer D S et al 1987 Impact of air filtration on nosocomial *Aspergillus* infections. American Journal of Medicine 83: 709–718

Sluyter 1847 De vegetabilibus organismi animalis parasitis ac de novo epiphyto in pityriasi versicolore obvio. Inaug. Diss. Berolini. In: Barthelat G-J (ed) 1903 Les mucorinees pathogenes et les mucormycoses chez les animaux et chex l'homme. Archives de Parasitologie 7: 1–6

Ste-Marie L, Senechal S, Boushira M et al 1990 Production and characterization of monoclonal antibodies to cell wall antigens of *Aspergillus fumigatus*. Infection and Immunity 58: 2105–2114

Talbot G H, Weiner M H, Gerson S L et al 1987 Serodiagnosis of invasive aspergillosis in patients with hematologic malignancy: validation of the *Aspergillus fumigatus* antigen radioimmunoassay. Journal of Infectious Diseases 155: 12–27

Tan K K, Sugai K, Tan K L 1966 Disseminated aspergillosis. Case report and review of the world literature. American Journal of Clinical Pathology 45: 697–703

Virchow R 1856 Beitrage zur Lehre von den beim Menschen vorkommenden pflanzlicken parasiten. Archiv für Pathologische Anatomie und Physiologie und für Klinische Medicin 9: 557–593

Weiner M H, Coats-Stephen M 1979 Immunodiagnosis of systemic aspergillosis. I. Antigenemia detected by radioimmunoassay in experimental infection. Journal of Laboratory and Clinical Medicine 93: 111–119

Weiner M H 1980 Antigenemia detected by radioimmunoassay in systemic aspergillosis. Annals of Internal Medicine 92: 793–796

Weiner M H, Talbot G H, Gerson S L et al 1983 Antigen detection in the diagnosis of invasive aspergillosis: utility in controlled, blinded trials. Annals of Internal Medicine 99: 777–782

Wilson E V, Hearn V M, Mackenzie D W R 1987 Evaluation of a test to detect circulating *Aspergillus fumigatus* antigen in a survey of immunocompromised patients with proven or suspected invasive disease. Journal of Medical and Veterinary Mycology 25: 365–374

Wong B G, Brauer K L, Tsai R R 1989 Increased amounts of the *Aspergillus* metabolite D-mannitol in tissue and serum of rats with experimental aspergillosis. Journal of Infectious Diseases 160: 95–103

Young R C, Bennett J E, Vogel C L et al 1970 Aspergillosis: the spectrum of the disease in 98 patients. Medicine 49: 147–173

Discussion of paper presented by V. T. Andriole

Discussed by L. de Repentigny
Reported by D. W. R. Mackenzie

Dr de Repentigny began by pointing out that although antigens of *Aspergillus fumigatus* have been characterized in numerous publications, very few have come into widespread use. Attempts to identify immunodominant antigens have not yet led to the introduction of highly sensitive and specific tests. *Aspergillus* galactomannan has attracted much attention, and has been detected in sera and urine of patients with invasive aspergillosis. However, problems are created by its ephemeral nature in sera, and by the lack of sufficient clinical data to substantiate improved predictive values. As a consequence, only marginal improvement can be anticipated by introducing tests of increased sensitivity.

More recently, other antigens with lower molecular weights than galactomannan, e.g. 41, 54, and 71kDa, have been detected in urine of both experimentally infected animals and humans with invasive aspergillosis. The relationship between these antigens and those previously described by Matthews, Brouwer or Calvanico remains to be determined. Other studies by Haynes et al (1990) on patients with invasive aspergillosis have reported the detection in urine of protein antigens with molecular weights of 11, 18 and 29kDa.

Because of the rapidity with which invasive aspergillosis develops in profoundly immunocompromised hosts, tests for invasive aspergillosis in patients with acute leukaemia who are neutropenic are likely to be of limited value. They may be more helpful where progression of the disease is slower, for example in patients with chronic granulomatous disease. Since antibody is not universally absent prior to infection, serial determinations of antibodies to *A. fumigatus* would appear to be mandatory.

Sensitivity of existing tests for *Aspergillus* antigen is proving more difficult to improve than specificity. Focus of future attention on the presence of antigens in urine would be justified, since the relatively prolonged excretion of galactomannan compared with serum provides it with improved sensitivity. In the past few years, immunoassays have been improved for invasive aspergillosis in terms of greater simplicity and sensitivity.

Monoclonal antibodies are now being introduced, and a commercial latex agglutination kit has been marketed in Europe. This new test is of interest but, at the present state of development, problems with its reproducibility have been encountered in some centres. Dr Dupont reported that it was effective in experimentally infected rabbits, but false positives, possibly caused by contamination with bacterial enzymes, were relatively common in human urines, even after removal of protein followed by dialysis against glycine buffer. Dr Bennett, however, suggested that analysing urine is not an attractive procedure if it has to be concentrated and dialysed. Infected patients are acutely ill, and results from laboratory tests are needed without the delay imposed by concentration and overnight dialysis. ELISA tests may not be easily reproducible in a diagnostic laboratory, particularly when not used for some time, and the simpler latex agglutination test has obvious advantages.

Limitations of existing tests for invasive aspergillosis include suboptimal sensitivity, dependency on serial examinations, cost, restricted availability, problems related to technology transfer, and a comparatively low perceived market priority by commercial organizations.

Dr Andriole commented on preliminary serological findings in a large prospective, double-blind study in the USA, involving 20 leukaemia centres where sera were obtained twice-weekly from patients undergoing induction chemotherapy, and 16 bone marrow centres. Sera were examined for antigen conversion. This occurred in 9% of leukaemic patients and 10.6% of bone marrow recipients. A considerable amount of testing is therefore required to detect a relatively small number of patients with antigenaemia.

Dr Bennett pointed out that antigen is present in patients with large numbers of organisms, and that this is not necessarily reflected in the chest X-ray. When patients with chronic granulomatous disease have pulmonary aspergillosis, there are usually very dense inflammatory reactions and very few organisms. In such patients, tests for antigen are negative. This also occurs in patients with aspergillosis of the paranasal sinuses, who can have very serious disease, eroding into the brain. In these cases, the number of organisms is small, and antigen tests are often negative. The patients whose sera react are those who are markedly neutropenic, with rapidly advancing pulmonary disease and a readily discernible infiltrate. When the infiltrate is very small, the antigen test is typically negative, but as the infiltrate becomes bigger, the test becomes positive. In evaluating a test, the type of disease is therefore important, not just the percentage of positive results obtained.

Metabolite detection has been investigated for aspergillosis and Dr Walsh suggested that the D-mannitol reported earlier by Dr Wong and his associates appeared promising. He reported that this has recently been found in serum and broncho alveolar lavage of experimentally infected rabbits by mass spectrum GLC, but studies have not yet been extended into patients. Clearance of metabolites, however, is dependent on renal excretion and changes in renal function, and the value of this approach remains to be established.

Session VI:
Prevention and therapy of fungal infections

Chairman: H. C. Neu

15. Prophylaxis of fungal infections

F. Meunier

INTRODUCTION

Fungal infections are leading causes of morbidity and mortality in various categories of patients. At the bedside, physicians face frustrations owing to the difficulties in early diagnosis of these opportunistic infections, as well as due to their poor prognosis. An increasing number of patients with potentially curable underlying diseases die as a result of invasive mycoses, and optimal management of those infections remains a challenge (Meunier 1988). So preventive measures against these life-threatening infections need serious consideration.

For the last decade, numerous investigators have studied several prophylactic approaches, mainly in patients with cancer but, unfortunately, there is still a lack of consensus upon the optimal modalities as well as upon specific recommendations for each category of patient at risk. Current strategies in the prevention of fungal infections, as well as their effectiveness, are discussed from a clinical perspective.

CHALLENGING PATHOGENS

An extensive list of potential fungal pathogens should be considered when defining prevention strategies.

Candidiasis is the most common invasive fungal infection and results mainly from endogenous proliferation of yeasts leading to invasion and dissemination from haematogenous spread (Meunier 1989b). In addition to *Candida albicans*, numerous other species are responsible for similar clinical entities. In particular, *Candida tropicalis* has been recognized as highly pathogenic, mainly in neutropenic patients. Moreover, several reports have shown an increasing incidence of invasive diseases caused by *Torulopsis glabrata*, *Candida krusei* and others (Aisner et al 1976a, Merz et al 1986, Meunier et al 1991 in press, McQuillen et al 1991 in press). Rarely identified *Candida* species should not be regarded as contaminants or as non-pathogenic.

Aspergillus fumigatus, *Aspergillus flavus* and *Aspergillus niger* are also responsible for a large number of invasive fungal infections. Aspergillosis is an airborne infection and *Aspergillus* spores are ubiquitous. Susceptible patients are those with neutropenia (Gerson et al 1984) or those treated with immunosuppressive agents including corticosteroids (Gustafson et al 1983). Infection results mainly from exposure of immunocompromised patients in a highly contaminated environment. Reactivation of persistent foci of infection also occurs, mainly in patients with haematologic malignancy, requiring prolonged antineoplastic chemotherapy.

Cryptococcosis is also a common fungal infection, in patients with defects in cell-mediated-immunity, including those with the acquired immunodeficiency syndrome (AIDS) or with lymphoma as well as those undergoing organ transplantation. Infection caused by *Cryptococcus neoformans* leads mainly to meningitis but various clinical presentations such as encephalitis or disseminated infection occur, often in patients with AIDS (Gold 1986).

During the last decade, several 'newly' recognized or more unusual opportunistic fungal pathogens have been identified as responsible for life-threatening infections (Venditti et al 1988, Walsh et al 1986b, Anaissie et al 1989). Those pathogens including *Fusarium* spp., *Trichosporon* spp., *Geotrichum* spp., and *Petriellidium boydii* should be taken into account when new strategies for prevention are elaborated.

Moreover, recent developments in supportive care, as well as more aggressive therapeutic modalities for various underlying diseases, have led to severe opportunistic fungal infections in other categories of patients (Pirsch & Maki 1986, Brochstein et al 1987, Butler & Baker 1988). Infections caused by *Malassezia furfur* in neonates receiving total parenteral nutrition with Intralipid represent such a new clinical syndrome (Dankner et al 1987) as well as invasive mucormycosis in patients undergoing dialysis and receiving deferoxamine (Daly et al 1989). For these reasons there is a need to recognize all fungi, common or unusual, as challenging pathogens.

THE TARGETED PATIENTS

Until now, preventive measures against fungal infections have been evaluated mainly in neutropenic patients with haematological malignancy (Meunier 1987). The mortality rate caused by bacterial infections in immunocompromised hosts has dramatically decreased because of empiric therapy with effective antibacterial agents. This prolongs the survival of patients who are more aggressively treated and therefore are predisposed to opportunistic fungal infections (Meunier 1989c). Neutropenia is a major predisposing factor to invasive candidiasis and aspergillosis. Those opportunistic infections occur in 20–30% of patients with haematological malignancy, in 10% of patients treated for lymphoma and in 5% of patients treated for solid tumours. However, invasive and aggressive therapeutic modalities are increasingly applied to all cancer patients and a higher incidence of invasive fungal infections should be expected among patients with solid tumour. Numerous other categories of patients should also be considered as potential targets for effective prophylaxis.

Candidiasis and cryptococcosis are the most common infections in patients with AIDS, but aspergillosis, coccidioidomycosis and histoplasmosis are also encountered, depending on local epidemiological factors. The persistent defects in cell-mediated immunity of patients with AIDS, as well as their improved survival resulting from more effective antiviral chemotherapy, lead to an increasing risk of invasive fungal infections. Preventive measures as well as specific strategies for maintaining antifungal coverage, are currently being developed for these patients.

Another expanding category of patients at risk of fungal infections is those undergoing organ transplantation. Current medical technology allows organ transplantation for a greater number of patients. These procedures aim to cure various life-threatening underlying diseases, but opportunistic complications remain a challenge (Peterson & Andersen 1986, Gentry & Zeluff 1988, Kusne et al 1988).

Over the last decade, an increasing number of patients underwent organ transplantation, including bone marrow, kidney, heart, liver, lungs, pancreas and even multiple organs. In fact, indications for combined transplantations are expanding nowadays. One should stress the human catastrophe in losing a potentially curable patient to invasive fungal infections, but only limited strategies have been considered so far for preventing such complications, and practical recommendations are needed.

Nosocomial fungal infections represent a new challenge for physicians at the bedside, and also for long-term medical research. These infections often occur in patients hospitalized for prolonged periods in surgical wards or in intensive care. Recent epidemiological data show that *Candida* spp. are now more commonly encountered than Gram-negative bacilli – 10% of all nosocomial blood-stream infections being caused by *Candida* spp. Too often, physicians still underestimate these data as well as the mortality attributable to nosocomial candidiasis, which has reached 38% (Harvey & Myers 1987, Wey et al 1988). Moreover, the morbidity related to fungaemia is overlooked, and loss of vision or severe osteomyelitis should become preventable diseases by increasing the awareness of physicians facing so-called 'transient' or catheter-related fungaemia (Brooks 1989, Edwards 1982).

ROLE OF CHEMOPROPHYLAXIS

The definite benefit of chemoprophylaxis against fungal infections remains a highly controversial issue (Meunier et al 1989). Physicians are divided into 'users' and 'non-users', mainly because the specific impact of currently available chemoprophylaxis has not been clearly established among the various groups of patients at risk, and also because it is impossible to prevent all fungal infections with currently available agents.

Most studies have been performed in neutropenic cancer patients with the aim of preventing candidiasis and aspergillosis. This concept implied that optimal chemoprophylaxis should be effective against *Candida* spp. and *Aspergillus* spp. In addition, the sources and means of infection should be considered when defining effective prevention. One should not expect to prevent aspergillosis with a non-absorbable antifungal agent. These limitations explain the divergent opinions in the literature concerning the specific role of chemoprophylaxis. End points of studies should be clearly defined, and it is necessary to stress that, today, no antifungal agent should be recognized as a panacea, effective against all fungal infections in all patients. Nevertheless, the progress and achievements so far should not be underestimated.

Most 'historical' studies were performed using oral amphotericin B or nystatin (non-absorbable polyenes). Those studies have shown that high doses are necessary in order to prevent yeast colonization, but it is extremely difficult to recommend those regimens owing to the poor tolerance and compliance of patients. In addition, the impact on the incidence of disseminated candidiasis is still controversial (Meunier et al 1989). The data available on nystatin prophylaxis after liver transplantation are also limited (Kusne et al 1988, Wiesner et al 1988). Some encouraging data are available on the topical (intranasal) use of amphotericin B to prevent aspergillosis (Meunier 1989a, Conneally et al 1990, Jeffery et al 1991), but its necessity will probably decrease if an effective systemic prophylaxis is available.

Clotrimazole troches have been investigated in limited studies (Owens et al 1984, Gombert et al 1987, Colonna et al 1988). Compliance is excellent, but this topical antifungal agent only seems effective against oropharyngeal candidiasis. Chlorhexidine mouth rinses have also been advocated for prevention of oropharyngeal candidiasis in neutropenic patients (Ferretti et al 1988, Weisdorf et al 1989).

Ketoconazole was the first imidazole available for oral administration. It has been extensively investigated (Meunier et al 1983, 1989, Estey et al 1984, Jones et al 1984, Shepp et al 1985, Hansen et al 1987) and is effective in decreasing the incidence of yeast colonization, but individual variations in absorption as well as its ineffectiveness against *Aspergillus* spp. and selection of *Torulopsis glabrata* represent potential drawbacks. Antagonism between ketoconazole and amphotericin B has been observed in animal models but the clinical relevance of this observation is unclear (Schaffner & Friek 1985). Similar data have been reported with other triazoles.

The availability of ketoconazole has had a tremendous impact on further developments of new antifungal agents with improved pharmacological properties. Among them, fluconazole and itraconazole are promising agents. The use of systemic antifungal agents may be suitable in patients at high risk of invasive fungal infections but each of these agents has advantages and disadvantages.

Fluconazole is available for intravenous use, an obvious advantage for patients such as those undergoing bone marrow transplantation who are unable to swallow because of severe mucositis. Fluconazole is effective against oropharyngeal candidiasis in cancer patients (Samonis et al 1990) but its impact on the incidence of disseminated candidiasis is encouraging according to current large prospective randomized studies. In addition, being active against *Candida albicans* and *Cryptococcus neoformans*, it is currently widely administered to patients with AIDS mainly as permanent maintenance therapy. Unfortunately, it does not prevent invasive aspergillosis.

Itraconazole is not yet available for intravenous use but seems effective against aspergillosis (Hay et al 1987). No large comparative studies are yet available.

The need to evaluate chemoprophylaxis separately among all 'new' groups of patients at risk, should be stressed. Chemoprophylaxis with new promising antifungal agents should be studied for, at least, neutropenic cancer patients, organ transplantation patients, AIDS patients, and for patients at risk of nosocomial candidiasis.

A major problem faced by physicians evaluating antifungal chemoprophylaxis is the poor diagnostic means available. So far, no single agent can be recommended as a gold standard for chemoprophylaxis.

Prophylactic studies should be well designed and effective chemoprophylaxis will only result from pivotal studies performed separately in the various categories of patients at risk. These studies should include large numbers of patients, use well-defined criteria and end points such as the incidence of candidiasis, aspergillosis or other opportunistic fungal infections, and recognize the need for initiation of antifungal therapy despite the use of chemoprophylaxis. Statistical expertise is also needed. All these requirements justify the use of multi-centre studies.

Finally, new considerations such as the potential emergence of resistant fungal strains should be a matter of concern when strategies for chemoprophylaxis are discussed. Until now, this was considered rare, but recent data should alert clinicians, since species of yeasts resistant to amphotericin B have been described (Dick et al 1980, 1985, Guinet et al 1983, Powderly et al 1988, Walsh et al 1990).

OTHER PREVENTIVE MEASURES

Besides specific modalities such as antifungal agents, other potentially effective preventive measures should be considered. Education of patients and their families, and training of medical and paramedical staff seem mandatory, but are still neglected.

Each patient hospitalized for invasive procedures should be informed of the potential risk of opportunistic fungal pathogens, and their various sources should be explained, justifying the prevention measures requested by the physicians. Awareness of these risks by the patient and his/her family should considerably improve the collaboration of patients as well as their compliance with recommended prophylactic approaches. Physicians and nurses in charge of patients at risk should be updated on modern developments as well as on optimal management of invasive fungal infections in the immunocompromised host, by well-trained infectious disease specialists.

Other non-specific modalities should also be recommended, mainly for neutropenic cancer patients, such as a cooked food diet, eliminating the potential contamination of fresh fruit juice and vegetables by yeasts. Ground pepper and marijuana have also been shown to be heavily contaminated with *Aspergillus* spores.

Adequate control of the environment is also mandatory. There should be no plants in the area where there are hospitalized neutropenic patients (such as those undergoing allogeneic bone marrow transplantation). Epidemics of aspergillosis have been described in numerous centres where construction work was being done either inside or outside hospitals (Opal et al 1986, Sherertz et al 1987, Weber & Rutala 1989). High-risk patients should therefore be isolated in special units distant from excavation or construction work. In addition, an increased incidence of aspergillosis may lead to the recognition of a contaminated source such as fire proofing material (Aisner et al 1976b).

Surveillance of nasal or pulmonary colonization by *Aspergillus* species might also be useful and has even been considered as predictive for the further development of infection (Aisner et al 1979, Nalesnik et al 1980, Yu et al 1986).

Other specific preventive modalities include isolation of patients in a protected environment (laminar air flow rooms) equipped with HEPA filters filtering particles such as *Aspergillus* spores, thereby limiting the exposure of patients at risk (Sheretz et al 1987). However, these units are limited in number and are expensive to maintain. Until now, laminar air flow rooms have been used almost exclusively for neutropenic patients undergoing intensive chemotherapy for leukaemia, e.g. those undergoing bone marrow transplantation. Whether the use of these units should be recommended for other patients at risk is still a matter for discussion, considering their cost as well as the psychological impact of isolation.

Education of nurses and physicians taking care of intravenous devices and catheters is essential (Torres-Rojas et al 1982, Walsh et al 1986a). Catheter-related candidaemia is an increasing problem and should be avoidable in most situations. Severe cutaneous infections caused by *Aspergillus* species have been observed also in patients with Hickman catheters (Allo et al 1987). A well-trained IV team is needed to improve the quality of care for immunocompromised patients. The recently recognized mortality attributable to fungaemia should alert medical personnel, and result in an increased number of patients with positive blood culture(s) for yeasts receiving antifungal therapy. Treatment for fungaemia is still too often withheld because of failure to correctly interpret its clinical relevance, physicians considering a single positive blood culture for yeast to be a potential contamination, despite the fact that this situation may lead to catastrophic complications (Meunier 1991, in press). Appropriate follow up and ophthalmoscopic examination (eye grounds) should be routinely recommended. Unfortunately, guidelines for treatment of fungaemia are still lacking and clinical management remains unstandardized. The availability of new antifungal agents easier to administer than amphotericin B should overcome this problem and improve the management of catheter-related infections. In particular, the role of the new triazoles should be clearly established in these circumstances (Meunier 1990), and their limits should also be defined; for example the identification of *Candida krusei* should preclude the prescription of fluconazole.

While the predictive value of surveillance cultures is controversial (Sanford et al 1980), the identification of particular species (such as *Candida krusei*, *Candida tropicalis*, *Fusarium* or *Trichosporon*) might be helpful for the bedside management of patients (Haupt et al 1983, Merz et al 1986, Pfaller et al 1987, Anaissie et al 1989).

The history of each patient should be taken into account, especially in areas where histoplasmosis and coccidioidomycosis are endemic. These patients, when at risk, should be considered for specific prophylaxis. Patients with a history of invasive aspergillosis requiring further antineoplastic chemotherapy have been shown to be at increased risk of reactivation of aspergillosis. These patients benefit from early antifungal therapy simultaneously with administration of the antineoplastic chemotherapy (Karp et al 1988). This specific modality should now be considered as a standard prophylactic procedure to avoid recurrence of aspergillosis.

For those patients undergoing organ transplants, specific measures to prevent contamination from the donor and transmission of fungal infection to the recipient should be carefully evaluated (Migliori & Simmons 1988, Gottesdiener 1989, Soifer & Gelb 1989). Careful evaluation of the donor is mandatory. Occasionally, some organ transport medium may be the source of fungal contamination in the recipient leading to increased risks of allograft loss, anastomatic complications or fatal infections.

Among other means of preventing life-threatening fungal infections, initiation of empiric antifungal therapy should be prompt when invasive fungal infection is suspected. This concept has been evaluated in neutropenic cancer patients, with success (Pizzo et al 1982, Wingard et al 1987, EORTC 1989) but it is still controversial which agent is optimal as well as when to initiate therapy. Current studies should further evaluate the potential role of new antifungal agents taking into consideration the limitations of each as well as their spectrum. In addition, the target population should also be re-estimated, owing to the increasing number of nosocomial candidaemias as well as the high number of invasive fungal infections occurring in patients without cancer. As an example, those patients undergoing heart or liver transplantation would probably benefit from early initiation of empiric antifungal therapy, although this should be further evaluated.

PERSPECTIVES

A greater interest in invasive fungal infections will lead to their improved management. The increasing incidence of these infections has been recognized and most physicians dealing with immunocompromised hosts understand the need for optimal prophylaxis against these infections.

During the last decade, the role of 'new' opportunistic fungal pathogens has been stressed and major progress in the development of new antifungal agents has been achieved. In view of the cost of modern aggressive and highly technological medical procedures, it is essential for a team effort to improve the prognosis of patients with fungal complications. All the 'clinical' approaches and potential prophylactic strategies described above will ultimately be responsible for establishing practical modalities to prevent these complications.

Besides new antifungal drugs, other means recently developed will play a major role improving the management of patients with cancer. Growth factors (granulocyte colony stimulating factor, granulocyte-macrophage colony stimulating factor, etc.) are currently being extensively evaluated by medical oncologists to decrease the morbidity and mortality of neutropenia (Milliken & Powles 1990). Their role as a potential novel modality to prevent fungal infections during antineoplastic chemotherapy should be further investigated. So far, limited data are available on this topic and extensive studies will be performed within a few years, probably not only in neutropenic patients but also in other categories of patients at risk.

In addition, optimal control of immunosuppression in organ transplant recipients should decrease the risk of opportunistic fungal infections (Hofflin et al 1987).

Finally, the economic burden of fungal infections should lead to cost–benefit studies particularly for chemoprophylaxis. Until now, very few have been undertaken.

As the need for prolonged maintenance antifungal therapy in patients with AIDS has been clearly established, it seems urgent to implement effective prevention means against fungal infections in all categories of patients at risk. So far, uniform recommendations are not available, due to the limits of the currently available agents and also to the various challenging pathogens, particularly the new opportunistic fungi. The optimal prophylactic requirements may vary from those applied to patients with cancer, and specific modalities should be established for each category of patient at risk.

REFERENCES

Aisner J, Schimpff S, Sutherland J, Young V, Wiernick P 1976a. *Torulopsis glabrata* infections in patients with cancer: increasing incidence and relationship to colonization. The American Journal of Medicine 61: 23–28

Aisner J, Murillo J, Schimpff S C et al 1979 Invasive aspergillosis in acute leukemia: correlation with nose cultures and antibiotic use. Annals of Internal Medicine 90: 4–9

Aisner J, Schimpff S C, Bennett J E et al 1976b *Aspergillus* infection in cancer patients: association with fire proofing material in a new hospital. Journal of the American Medical Association 235: 411–412

Allo M D, Miller J, Townsend T et al 1987 Primary cutaneous aspergillosis associated with Hickman intravenous catheters. The New England Journal of Medicine 317: 1105–1108

Anaissie E, Bodey G P, Kanterjian H et al 1989 New spectrum of fungal infections in patients with cancer. Review of Infectious Diseases 2(3): 369–378

Brochstein J A, Kernan N A, Groshen S et al 1987 Allogeneic bone marrow transplantation after hyperfractionated total-body irradiation and cyclophosphamide in children with acute leukemia. The New Journal of Medicine 317: 1618–1624

Brooks R G 1989 Prospective study of *Candida* endopthalmitis in hospitalized patients with candidemia. Archives of Internal Medicine 149: 2226–2228

Butler K M, Baker C J 1988 *Candida:* an increasingly important pathogen in the nursery. Pediatric Clinics of North America 35: 543–563

Colonna J O, Winston D J, Brill J E et al 1988 Infectious complications in liver transplantation. Archives of Surgery 123: 360–364

Conneally, E, Cafferkey M T, Daly P A et al 1990 Nebulized amphotericin B as prophylaxis against invasive aspergillosis in granulocytopenic patients. Bone Marrow Transplantation 5: 403–406

Daly A L, Velazquez L A, Bradley S F, Kauffman C A 1989 Mucormycosis: association with deferoxamine therapy. The American Journal of Medicine 87: 468–471

Dankner W M, Spector S S, Fiever J et al 1987 *Malassezia* fungemia in neonates and adults: complication of hyperalimentation. Review of Infectious Diseases 9: 743–753

Dick J D, Merz W G, Saral R 1980 Incidence of polyene-resistant yeasts recovered from clinical specimens. Antimicrobial Agents and Chemotherapy 18: 158–163

Dick J D, Rosengard B R, Merz W G et al 1985 Fatal disseminated candidiasis due to amphotericin B resistant *Candida guillermondii*. Annals of Internal Medicine 102: 67–68

Edwards J E 1982 *Candida* endophthalmitis. In: Remington J S, Swartz M N (eds) Current clinical topics in infectious diseases, vol 3. McGraw Hill, New York, pp 381–397

EORTC International Antimicrobial Therapy Cooperative Group 1989 Empirical antifungal therapy in febrile granulocytopenic patients. The American Journal of Medicine 86: 668–672

Estey E, Maksymiuk A, Smith T et al 1984 Infection prophylaxis in acute leukemia. Archives of Internal Medicine 144: 1562–1568

Ferretti G A, Ash R C, Brown A T, Parr M D, Romond E H, Lillich T T 1988 Control of oral mucositis and candidiasis in marrow transplantation: a prospective double-blind trial of chlorhexidine digluconate oral rinse. Bone Marrow Transplantation 3: 483–493

Gentry L O, Zeluff B 1988 Infection in the cardiac transplant patient. In: Rubin R H, Young L S (eds) Clinical approach to infection in the compromised host. Plenum Medical, New York, pp 623–641

Gerson S L, Talbot G H, Hurwitz S et al 1984 Prolonged granulocytopenia: the major risk factor for invasive pulmonary aspergillosis in patients with acute leukemia. Annals of Internal Medicine 100: 345–351

Gold J W M 1986 Infectious complications of AIDS. In: Staquet M, Hemmer R, Baert A (eds) Clinical aspects of AIDS and AIDS-related complex. Oxford University Press, Oxford, pp 93–100

Gombert M E, duBouchet L, Aulicino T, Butt K M H 1987 A comparative trial of clotrimazole troches and oral nystatin suspension in recipients of renal transplants. Journal of the American Medical Association 258 (18): 2553–2555

Gottesdiener K M 1989 Transplanted infections: donor-to-host transmission with the allograft. Annals of Internal Medicine 110: 1001–1016

Guinet R, Chanas J, Goullier A, Bonnefoy G 1983 Fatal septicemia due to amphotericin B-resistant *Candida lusitaniae*. Journal of Clinical Microbiology 18: 433–444

Gustafson T L, Schaffner W, Lavely G B, Stratton C W, Johnson H K, Hutcheson R H 1983 Invasive aspergillosis in renal transplant recipients: correlation with corticosteroid therapy. Journal of Infectious Diseases 148: 230–238

Hansen R H, Reinerio N, Sohnle P G et al 1987 Ketoconazole in prevention of candidiasis in patients with cancer. Archives of Internal Medicine 147: 710–712

Harvey R L, Myers J P 1987 Nosocomial fungemia in a large community teaching hospital. Archives of Internal Medicine 147: 2117–2120

Haupt H M, Merz W G, Beschorner W E et al 1983 Colonization and infection with *Trichosporon* species in the immunosuppressed host. Journal of Infectious Diseases 147: 199–203

Hay R J, Dupont B, Graybill J R (eds) 1987 Proceedings of the first international symposium on itraconazole. Review of Infectious Diseases 9: S1–2152

Hofflin J M, Potasman I, Baldwin J C, Oyer P E, Stinson E B, Remington J S 1987 Infectious complications in heart transplant recipients receiving cyclosporine and corticosteroids. Annals of Internal Medicine 106: 209–216

Jeffery G M, Beard M E J, Ikram R B et al 1991 Intranasal amphotericin B reduces the frequency of invasive asperigillosis in neutropenic pateients. The American Journal of Medicine 90: 685–692

Jones P G, Kaufmann C A, McAuliffe L S, Liepman M K, Bergman A G 1984 Efficacy of ketoconazole versus nystatin in prevention of fungal infections in neutropenic patients. Archives of Internal Medicine 144: 549–551

Karp J E, Burch P, Merz M G 1988 An approach to intensive antileukemia therapy in patients with previous invasive aspergillosis. The American Journal of Medicine 85: 203–209

Kusne S, Dummer J S, Singh N et al 1988 Infections after liver transplantation. Medicine 67 (2): 132–143

McQuillen D P, Zingman B S, Meunier F, Levitz S M 1991 Report of ten cases of fungemia including three cases of endophthalmitis. Review of Infectious Diseases (in press)

Merz W G, Karp J E, Schrom D, Saral R 1986 Increase incidence of fungemia caused by *Candida krusei*. Journal of Clinical Microbiology 24: 581–584

Meunier F 1987 Prevention of opportunistic mycoses in immunocompromised patients. Review of Infectious Diseases 9: 408–416

Meunier F 1988 Fungal infections in the compromised host. In: Rubin R H, Young L S (eds) Clinical approach to infection in the compromised host. 2nd edn. Plenum Medical, New York, 193–220

Meunier F 1989a New methods for delivery of antifungal agents. Review of Infectious Disease 11: S1605–S1612

Meunier F 1989b Candidiasis. European Journal of Clinical Microbiology and Infectious Diseases 8: 438–447

Meunier F 1989c Infections in patients with acute leukemia and lymphoma. In: Mandell G L, Douglas R G, Bennett J E (eds) Principles and practice of infectious diseases, 3rd edn. Churchill Livingstone, Edinburgh, pp 2265–2275

Meunier F, Leleux A, Snoeck R, Gerain J, Lambert C, Ceuppens A M 1989 Chemoprophylaxis of fungal infections In: Holmberg K, Meyer R (eds) Diagnosis and therapy of systemic fungal infections. Raven Press, New York, pp 167–177

Meunier F 1990 Fluconazole treatment of fungal infections in the immunocompromised host. Seminars in Oncology 17 (3): 19–23

Meunier F, Aoun M, Bitar N 1991 Candidemia in immunocompromised patients. Review of Infectious Diseases (in press)

Meunier-Carpentier F, Cruciani M, Klastersky J 1983 Oral prophylaxis with miconazole or ketoconazole of invasive fungal disease in neutropenic cancer patients. European Journal of Cancer and Clinical Oncology 19: 43–48

Migliori R J, Simmons R L 1988 Infection prophylaxis after organ transplantation. Transplantation Proceedings XX (3): 395–399

Milliken S T, Powles R L 1990 Antifungal prophylaxis in bone marrow transplantation. Review of Infectious Diseases 12 (supplement 3)

Nalesnik M A, Myerowitz R L, Jenkins R et al 1980 Significance of *Aspergillus* species isolated from respiratory secretions in the diagnosis of invasive pulmonary aspergillosis. Journal of Clinical Microbiology 11: 370–376

Opal S M, Asp A A, Cannady P B et al 1986 Efficacy of infection control measures during a nosocomial outbreak of disseminated aspergillosis associated with hospital construction. Journal of Infectious Diseases 153: 634–637

Owens M, Nightingale C, Schweizer R, Schauer P, Dekker P, Quintiliani R 1984 Prophylaxis of oral candidiasis with clotrimazole troches. Archives of Internal Medicine 144: 290–293

Peterson P K, Anderson R C 1986 Infection in renal transplant recipients: current approaches to diagnosis therapy and prevention. The American Journal of Medicine 81: (suppl 1A) 2–10

Pfaller M, Cabezudo I, Koontz F, Bale M, Gingrich R 1987 Predictive value of surveillance cultures for systemic infection due to *Candida* species. European Journal of Clinical Microbiology 6 (6): 628–633

Pirsch J D, Maki D G 1986 Infectious complications in adults with bone marrow transplantation and T-cell depletion of donor marrow: increased susceptibility to fungal infections. Annals of Internal Medicine 104: 619–631

Pizzo P A, Robichaud K J, Gill F A, Witebsky F 1982 Empiric antibiotic and antifungal therapy for cancer patients with prolonged fever and granulocytopenia. American Journal of Medicine 72: 101–111

Powderly W G, Kobayashi G S, Herzig G P, Medoff G 1988 Amphotericin B-resistant yeast infection in severely immunocompromised patients. The American Journal of Medicine 84: 826–832

Samonis G, Rolston K, Karl C, Miller P, Bodey G P 1990 Prophylaxis of oropharyngeal candidiasis with fluconazole. Review of Infectious Diseases 12: (supplement 3) 369–373

Sanford G R, Merz W G, Wingard J R, Sarache P, Saral R 1980 The value of fungal surveillance cultures as predictors of systemic fungal infections. Journal of Infectious Diseases 142: 503–509

Schaffner A, Friek P G 1985 The effect of ketoconazole on amphotericin B in a model of disseminated aspergillosis. Journal of Infectious Diseases 151: 902–910

Shepp D H, Klostermann A, Siegel M S, Meyers J D 1985 Comparative trial of ketoconazole and nystatin for prevention of fungal infection in neutropenic patients treated in a protective environment. Journal of Infectious Diseases 152: 1257–1263

Sherertz R J, Belani A, Kramer B S et al 1987 Impact of air filtration of nosocomial *Aspergillus* infections: unique risk of bone marrow transplant recipients. The American Journal of Medicine 83: 709–718

Soifer B E, Gelb A W 1989 The multiple organ donor: identification and management. Annals of Internal Medicine 110: 814–823

Torres-Rojas J R, Stratton C W, Sanders C V et al 1982 Candidal suppurative peripheral thrombophlebitis. Annals of Internal Medicine 96: 431–435

Venditti M, Micozzi A, Gentile G et al 1988 Invasive *Fusarium solani* infections in patients with acute leukemia. Review of Infectious Diseases 10: 653–660

Walsh T J, Bustamente C I, Vlahov D, Standiford H C 1986a Candidal suppurative peripheral thrombophlebitis: recognition prevention and management. Infection Control 7: 16–22

Walsh T J, Newman K R, Moody M et al 1986b Trichosporonosis in patients with neoplastic disease. Medicine 65: 268–279

Walsh T J, Melcher G P, Rinaldi M G et al 1990 *Trichosporon beigelii*: an emerging pathogen resistant to amphotericin B. Journal of Clinical Microbiology 28 (7): 1616–1622

Weber D J, Rutala W A 1989 Epidemiology of hospital-acquired fungal infections. In: Holmberg K, Meyer R (eds) Diagnosis and therapy of systemic fungal infections, vol. 1. Raven Press, New York, pp 1–24

Weisdorf D J, Bostrom B, Raether D 1989 Oropharyngeal mucositis complicating bone marrow transplantation: prognostic factors and the effect of chlorhexidine mouth rinse, Bone Marrow Transplantation 4: 89–95

Wey S B, Mori M, Pfaller M A, Woolson R F, Wenzel R P 1988 Hospital-acquired candidemia, the attributable mortality and excess length of stay. Archives of Internal Medicine 148: 2642–2645

Wiesner R H, Hermans P E, Rakela J et al 1988 Selective bowel decontamination to decrease Gram-negative aerobic bacterial and *Candida* colonization and prevent infection after orthotopic liver transplantation. Transplantation 45 (3): 570–574

Wingard J R, Vaughan W P et al 1987 Prevention of fungal sepsis in patients with prolonged neutropenia: a randomized double-blind placebo-controlled trial of intravenous miconazole. The American Journal of Medicine 83: 1103–1110

Yu V L, Muder R R, Poorsattar A 1986 Significance of isolation of *Aspergillus* from the respiratory tract in diagnosis of invasive pulmonary aspergillosis. The American Journal of Medicine 81: 249–254

16. Antifungal therapy in the non-compromised host

J. R. Graybill

INTRODUCTION

Until the 1960s systemic fungal infections were quite limited in number and occurred primarily in patients who were either immunologically competent or were undergoing the immunological compromises associated with the natural course of leukaemia, lymphoma, solid tumours, autoimmune diseases, steroid treatment or malnutrition. Beginning in the 1960s there was an increased use of corticosteroid therapy and the development of cytotoxic drugs, and other agents to depress phagocyte and T-lymphocyte function. There has been increasingly aggressive use of antibacterial agents, placement of long-term intravascular catheters and other prosthetic devices. This has extended the survival of patients much longer into the course of ultimately fatal diseases. The 1980s saw the inception of the ongoing AIDS pandemic. All of these events acted together to render many patients no more resistant to fungi than culture plates. Given the large number of severely compromised patients, it is no surprise that both rare and nonpathogenic fungi exploited these large gaps in host resistance. The development of life-theatening systemic mycoses in the immune compromised patients was one of the major stimuli for development of new antifungal agents, and it drives the continuing evolution of new drugs today.

In this environment there has been relatively modest attention paid to non-compromised patients with systemic mycoses. There are two reasons for this. The first is the limited numbers of such patients, and the second is that many of them have infections caused by geographically restricted pathogens.

DEFINITIONS

Who is the non-compromised patient, and to which mycoses is he or she susceptible? For the present purpose, a non-compromised patient has no catheters or other prosthetic appliances, is not receiving immunosuppressives or broad spectrum antibacterials, is without evidence of underlying immune deficiency disease, and has no 'readily apparent' immunological abnormalities.

Definition is critical, and may be illustrated by two examples. The first is cryptococcosis. Pigeon fanciers are heavily exposed to *Cryptococcus neoformans*, and yet they do not develop cryptococcosis. Cryptococcosis is a disease associated with immune suppression: nevertheless, in the pre-AIDS era only about half of the patients who developed cryptococcosis were found to have some readily identifiable disease associated with depressed cell-mediated immunity (Lewis & Tabinovich 1972). The others had no gross evidence of immunocompromise, and were assumed to be immunologically intact. However, a study conducted in the 1970s suggested that many of these 'normal' patients may have had subtle immune defects in response to antigens of *C. neoformans* (Graybill & Alford 1974). Whether these abnormalities were antecedent to or consequences of cryptococcosis was unknown. But there was some blurring of what constituted 'normality'. Therefore, although patients without obvious immune impairment will be considered 'non-compromised', one must appreciate the limitations of this definition.

The other example is *Histoplasma capsulatum*. Histoplasmosis is the classic infection of the 'non-compromised' patient (Wheat et al 1981). Usually, disseminated histoplasmosis responds well to treatment, but occasionally even the disseminated form may relapse after treatment in normal hosts (Goodwin et al 1980, Paya et al 1987). However, a small number of patients with lymphomas, corticosteroid therapy or other underlying immune depression developed histoplasmosis; they frequently had disseminated, relapsing disease (Chua et al 1978, Dismukes et al 1978, Kauffman et al 1978, Goodwin et al 1980, Bradsher et al 1982, Paya et al 1987). These small numbers of patients were in fact the prologues of the AIDS outbreak when it reached the central United States. Nowhere is this better illustrated than in Indianapolis, which experienced in 1980 an outbreak of histoplasmosis among hundreds of mainly non-compromised residents, and less than a decade later had a large outbreak involving many patients with AIDS (Wheat et al 1990). Many patients with disseminated histoplasmosis now acquire this infection in the setting of AIDS; we shall consider herein only the smaller group without immune compromise.

Thus any definition of 'non-compromised' is flawed by our limited knowledge of the subtleties of host immune defects, and also by developments, such as AIDS, which may dramatically alter the host response to, susceptibility to, and manifestations of mycoses. Defects in granulocyte numbers and/or function, treatment with corticosteroids or broad spectrum antibacterials, and placement of catheters and other prosthetic devices all may be considered forms of compromise (Wey et al 1989).

WHERE DO WE FIND THE NON-COMPROMISED PATIENTS?

A second reason for relative inattention to mycoses in non-compromised patients is that the 'leaders' have been the so-called major endemic mycoses. The four pathogens are *Coccidioides immitis, Paracoccidioides braziliensis, H. capsulatum*, and *Blastomyces dermatitidis*. All reside in geographically defined regions of the western hemisphere, though *H. capsulatum* and *B. dermatitidis* can be found elsewhere. All four species are dimorphic, and in their mycelial form can be infectious to humans by inhalation. In areas where they are endemic many residents are infected, as measured by skin test reactivity, but relatively few develop disease and, of those, many heal spontaneously.

Amphotericin B has been generally effective against these organisms, and usual medical practice was to leave the endemic mycoses to the few mycologists with an interest in the vicissitudes of amphotericin B therapy (Philips et al 1972, Goodwin et al 1980, Wheat et al 1981, Drutz 1983, Franco et al 1989). The endemic mycoses of the 1970s were sufficiently uncommon to frustrate systematic comparative antifungal studies within single institutions. There was also at that time little interest by pharmaceutical companies in developing alternatives to amphotericin B.

The recent advances in antifungal therapy for the endemic mycoses were accomplished by the (National Institute of Allergy and Infectious Diseases) Mycoses Study Group (MSG), originally formed to evaluate treatment of a major and usually opportunistic infection, cryptococcosis. After their initial study comparing amphotericin B and amphotericin B plus flucytosine, the group elected to continue as the Mycoses Study Group (Bennett et al 1979). While one major collaboration continued with cryptococcal studies, members of the group considered that other important mycoses also warranted collaborative studies, and areas of interest were expanded to include histoplasmosis, North American blastomycosis, and coccidioidomycosis (Dismukes et al 1983, NIAID MSG 1985). Paracoccidioidomycosis was not included because its northernmost range terminates several hundred miles south of the US border. While a major thrust of the studies has remained with patients who are immunocompromised, the MSG studies have provided the first systematic evaluation of azoles for three endemic mycoses, and also have provided a system for global assessment of coccidioidomycosis (Galgiani et al 1988, Graybill et al 1990).

Investigators in South America have independently devised similar systems for assessment of paracoccidioidomycosis (Restrepo et al 1983a,b).

In addition to the major endemic mycoses, there are other mycoses usually infecting the immunologically intact host. These tend to be more scattered, though they are more commonly seen in tropical than in cold climates. Chromomycosis (chromoblastomycosis) is a chronic cutaneous and subcutaneous infection which follows the percutaneous inoculation or a variety of causative agents (in the Americas *Fonsecaea pedrosoi* and *Cladosporium carrioni* most commonly) (Londero Ramos 1976, Borelli 1987, Restrepo et al 1988). Sporotrichosis commonly occurs by the same route of percutaneous inoculation (Restrepo et al 1986), though inhalation may also be a mechanism of infection, particularly for those patients with pulmonary disease. Phaeohyphomycosis is a broad name given to infections caused by brown-pigmented (dematiaceous) fungi. Many genera are represented, though *Curvularia, Alternaria, Bipolaris, Exserohilum* and *Wangiella* are perhaps the most common (Hohl et al 1983, Adam et al 1986, Pitrak et al 1988, Washburn et al 1988, Sharkey et al 1990, Wilson et al 1991). These are commonly inoculated percutaneously, though they may be transmitted by inhalation, as suggested by sinusitis and pulmonary disease (Washburn et al 1988). Some patients can develop an allergic process somewhat like bronchopulmonary aspergillosis or allergic *Aspergillus* sinusitis (Grieble et al 1975, Halwi et al 1985, Sharkey et al 1990). Although many patients are immunocompromised, as many as half are not. Hyalohyphomycosis is the name given to infections caused by light-coloured mycelial fungi, also probably inoculated percutaneously. *Pseudallescheria boydii* and *Fusarium* are found within this group (Galgiani et al 1986, Merz et al 1988, Vendetti 1988). Unlike *Pseudallescheria, Fusarium* rarely attacks normal hosts.

In addition to these agents there is the recently appreciated entity of 'chronic invasive aspergillosis' (Gefter et al 1981, Binder et al 1982, Tack et al 1982, Pervez et al 1985, Karam & Griffin 1986, Cook et al 1990). This may follow percutaneous inoculation or inhalation of *Aspergillus* conidia, with establishment of a focal chronic progressive destructive focus in an otherwise normal host. *Aspergillus* also may be inoculated traumatically or be blood borne to a site such as an osseous focus. In addition to the classic severely immunocompromised patients, aspergillosis is a major problem in patients with cystic fibrosis, where one study has shown a 57% colonization rate, versus 6.5% in patients without cystic fibrosis. Eosinophilia accompanied colonization in 37% of patients (Nelson et al 1979). Aspergillosis is a particular problem in cystic fibrosis patients in England (Simmonds et al 1990). Perhaps this is due to the chronic damp climate which may favour growth of these fungi combined with the slow clearance from the airways. It is interesting that one United States study (Nelson et al 1979) emanated from Rochester, New York, one of the cities in the United States with the fewest days of sunshine per year.

For this discussion, therefore, we shall be restricted to a present assessment and future projections in relation to endemic fungi, sporotrichosis, phaeohyphomycosis, chromomycosis, hyalohyphomycosis, and chronic invasive aspergillosis.

A NEW GEOGRAPHICALLY RESTRICTED PATHOGEN

Penicillium marneffii has recently been appreciated to cause focal granulomatous and suppurative pulmonary and haematogenously disseminated infections in normal hosts, and may cause infection after traumatic inoculation (Deng et al 1988). The organism is restricted to Southeast Asia and China, and recently has been appearing more frequently in patients with AIDS. Amphotericin B is effective if given early.

CRYPTOCOCCOSIS

Present status
Cryptococcus neoformans infects patients by the pulmonary route; the organism may be a commensal, and its presence does not always connote disease (Warr et al 1968). Some patients develop chronic pulmonary infiltrates, empyemas and, rarely, cavities. Commonly they are not immune-compromised, and when they are, there is a higher chance of dissemination to the central nervous system (Kerkering & Duma 1981). Treatment of cryptococcal pneumonia has not been systematically studied.

Before 1980, about half of patients with cryptococcal meningitis were 'normal' hosts. The first Mycoses Study Group trial found that combination therapy with low dose amphotericin B and flucytosine was as effective as higher dose amphotericin B, and less toxic (Bennett et al 1979). The second trial found that in some patients with features predicting an uncomplicated course, 4 weeks of therapy might be as effective as 6 weeks' treatment (Dismukes et al 1987). As this study was completed the importance of cryptococcosis in HIV-infected patients became apparent, and emphasis switched to AIDS. Because these patients relapse after therapy with amphotericin B is discontinued, chronic suppressive regimens were studied, using the relatively non-toxic fluconazole versus amphotericin B (Stern et al 1988, Sugar et al 1988).

Considerations for the future

With extensive data available showing primary failure rates of more than 20%, and relapse rates of 16–25% for amphotericin B/flucytosine, it may be well worth looking for alternatives to amphotericin B in non-AIDS patients (Bennett et al 1979, Dismukes et al 1987). The presently recommended therapy is amphotericin B/flucytosine for 4–6 weeks. MSG studies in AIDS patients have identified a 'low risk' group with intact cerebration, relatively low antigen titres, and a cerebrospinal fluid leukocyte count of 20 or more cells/mm^3 (Dismukes et al 1987). The low risk group had < 10% mortality at the 10-week treatment period at the conclusion of the study, with either fluconazole or amphotericin B therapy (Dismukes et al 1989). As more experience is gained with antifungal azoles, it may be reasonable to consider a treatment with either fluconazole or perhaps a more fungicidal combination such as fluconazole and flucytosine. In such a non-nephrotoxic combination, flucytosine might be easier to administer without dose adjustment and myelotoxicity.

There is increasing evidence in mice that this combination may be useful (Allen-doerfer et al 1990, Hitchcock et al 1991), and Jones et al (1991) have suggested that fluconazole/flucytosine is a rapidly effective agent in patients with AIDS and cryptococcosis. Regimens for the first week or two of primary therapy and for rescue of patients who are failing initial therapy might also include high doses of fluconazole or other antifungal azoles. Doses of 800 mg per day have been used without major adverse sequelae, and there is a suggestion that they might benefit immune-suppressed patients in whom lower doses have failed (Berry & Graybill 1991). Likewise, combined therapy might be even more effective in patients with cryptococcosis in the absence of documented immune suppression.

There has been little attention given to those uncommon patients with fungal meningitis who undergo acute deterioration from intracranial hypertension. There is increasing evidence in children with bacterial meningitis that corticosteroids reduce cerebral hypertension in part by blocking release of TNF and possibly other mediators into the cerebrospinal fluid, with a resultant smaller inflammatory response and less obstruction to cerebrospinal fluid egress from the central nervous system (Lebel et al 1988). It may also be that mechanical decompression by ventricular drainage may be equally or more effective. There are no data directly bearing on cryptococcosis, but attention directed to this area might be worthwhile.

SYSTEMIC ENDEMIC MYCOSES

Vaccines

Of the four endemic mycoses, three are found in the United States. Hundreds of thousands of people are infected annually by these pathogens, and there has been some interest in developing vaccines against these organisms. Such research has not been generously supported, partly because many people are infected but disease occurs in relatively few. One large trial of a spherule vaccine has been conducted in coccidioidomycosis (Pappagianis 1986). This was a reasonable plan because coccidioidomycosis is the most refractory of the major endemic mycoses, and one could argue that prevention might be worthwhile in forestalling the often difficult clinical cases. Unfortunately, the vaccine was not successful. Thus I would doubt that large scale vaccine development is in the offing for blastomycosis, paracoccidioiodomycosis, histoplasmosis, or coccidioidomycosis.

Blastomycosis

Present status

Perhaps the fewest 'problems' are posed by North American blastomycosis. This is a common pathogen of the Mississippi River Valley and throughout the southeastern United States. AIDS and other immune deficiency states do not predispose to blastomycosis. Despite being in the same range as histoplasmosis, where AIDS is a major problem, only 12 patients have thus far been reported with AIDS and blastomycosis (Pappas et al 1990). Thus this is almost entirely a 'normal' host disease. The initial trials of the MSG found that ketoconazole caused more than 80% clinical responses, when given at 400 mg per day for 6 months; being about as effective as amphotericin B and much less toxic, it quickly became the drug of choice in all but the patients with acute life-threatening disease (NIAID MSG 1985). These encouraging results have been duplicated by others (Bradsher et al 1985). Subsequently, itraconazole entered clinical development, and when the NDA was filed for this drug, Janssen (1990, unpublished data) noted >90% of patients clinically responded. Itraconazole was highly effective, better tolerated than ketoconazole, and had very few adverse reactions (Saag et al 1988). Fluconazole, in unpublished anecdotes, may be less effective than itraconazole or ketoconazole (Dismukes 1990, Bradsher 1990, personal communications).

Future projection

For patients with acute life-threatening disease, amphotericin B will continue to be used for the first weeks of treatment. For chronic therapy and for initial therapy in less severely ill patients, it is hard to imagine further improvement on itraconazole, 400 mg per day for 6 months. I would not anticipate blastomycosis as being a front line for new drug development in the future.

Paracoccidioidomycosis

Present status

Paracoccidioidomycosis is somewhat similar to blastomycosis. Many people from

Mexico and throughout South America are affected, but very few patients with AIDS develop paracoccidioidomycosis. The major problem has been the chronicity of treatment and tendency to relapse. Ketoconazole, 200 mg per day for a year, has been supplanted by itraconazole 100 mg per day for 6 months, with responses in more than 90% of patients and few relapses (Negroni et al 1980, Restrepo et al 1983a, b, 1987, Negroni et al 1987, Queiroz-Telles et al 1991). Saperconazole may be even more rapid in causing responses (Franco et al 1991). Thus with both blastomycosis and paracoccidioidomycosis, response rates are high and antifungal therapy is well tolerated. The greatest problem is the length of time needed for curative treatment, but this appears to be a relatively lesser consideration.

Future projection
The therapy is sufficiently effective and non-toxic that there is unlikely to be pressure for major changes to treatment of the active disease. One of the major persisting problems of paracoccidioidomycosis is the chronic respiratory impairment which attends the pulmonary fibrosis that occurs during healing. Controlling this would be a significant advance, but only recently has there been a model for studying this process (Restrepo et al 1991).

Lessons learned for paracoccidioidomycosis might be applicable to histoplasmosis and tuberculosis as well.

Histoplasmosis

Present status
Histoplasmosis is creating increasing problems in the United States and South America. The major difficulties are with HIV-infected patients rather than non-compromised hosts (Wheat et al 1990). For the non-compromised host few data are published, but those that are available in papers and abstracts suggest that itraconazole is highly effective in histoplasmosis at 200–400 mg per day for 6 months (Negroni et al 1987, Saag et al 1988). Saperconazole was also highly effective in all five patients (all with HIV infection) reported by Franco et al (1991).

Future projection
While amphotericin B will continue to be used for the first weeks of treatment of the most critically ill patients, itraconazole at 400 mg per day for 6 months is likely to become the major treatment. Saperconazole may be a future contender, but radical changes are not likely to occur (Franco et al 1991). Chronic pulmonary fibrosis also complicates chronic pulmonary histoplasmosis, and as with paracoccidioidomycosis, there may be some advantage in looking for approaches to control it. Animal models now exist for such studies (Restrepo et al 1991).

Coccidioidomycosis

Present status
Coccidioidomycosis has long been the most problematic of the endemic mycoses. The range of the infection is broad, from the southwestern United States to Argentina. Although some patients have developed coccidioidomycosis in the

setting of immunosuppression, most recently AIDS, the majority of patients have no clear immune defect (Fish et al 1990). Coccidioidomycosis in the non-compromised patient may take the form of acute self-limited or fulminating primary disease, chronic pulmonary disease or extrapulmonary dissemination, with soft tissue disease, osteoarticular disease, and meningitis being the major manifestations. Until recent years it was difficult to assess therapeutic responses to antifungal therapy because of the varying criteria for response used by investigators, and also because of a frustrating tendency to relapse after a course of therapy. Recent developments of prospective scoring criteria have enabled collaborative dose-finding studies of a variety of antifungals. The first study, with ketoconazole, was discouraging because of fewer than 40% clinical responses, the high frequency of drug intolerance to doses above 400 mg per day, and frequent relapses (Galgiani et al 1988). For a follow-up study with itraconazole, the criteria for evaluating responses were modified somewhat. The clinical response rate was 57%, with fewer than 15% late relapses (Graybill et al 1990). A fluconazole study gave similar results for response rates, as did a SCH39304 study (Galgiani et al 1990, 1991).

Relapses were higher for fluconazole, and as yet are undetermined for SCH39304. Therefore, a 50–60% response rate in 7–12 months of therapy appears to be the best that can be expected for modern day azole therapy of non-meningeal coccidioidomycosis. It is arguable whether this is better than amphotericin B, although tolerance of the new triazoles appears much superior to amphotericin B. For the most recent drug studied, amphotericin B lipid complex (ABLC), information is not yet available for clinical responses, but it does reduce the nephro-toxicity associated with chronic amphotericin B therapy (Graybill et al, unpublished observations); but patients still have severe rigors and fever when the drug is administered, and ABLC cannot be considered non-toxic.

In contrast with this mixed picture for non-meningeal disease, the azoles appear to have made major breakthroughs in treatment of coccidioidal meningitis. Though not yet published, there is a large MSG trial of fluconazole, 400 mg per day, with fewer than 15% clinical failure in now more than 40 patients (Galgiani et al 1990, J N Galgiani, personal communication). It is of interest that 10 of these patients had co-existing immune suppression from HIV disease, and fared as well as those without AIDS. Another, smaller study (Tucker et al 1990) has also shown encouraging results.

These treatments are to be contrasted with the prior standard of intrathecally administered amphotericin B. That treatment is extremely irritating to the meninges, and is associated with transverse myelitis, vasculitis, haemorrhage, and bacterial infection when Ommaya reservoirs are used (Kelly 1980).

Future projection
C. immitis appears to be susceptible to a variety of polyenes and azoles in vitro, but in vivo there are problems on several levels of management of this vexing disease.

One level is the mechanical complication associated with osteoarticular disease, particularly in vertebral sites (Galgiani et al 1988, Graybill et al 1900). At present surgical stabilization is required for most patients, whatever their medical therapy. This may need to continue no matter what treatment is used in the future.

A second level lies in the slow speed and relatively low rate of response after treatment lasting as long as several years (Dismukes et al 1983, Galgiani et al 1988, Graybill et al 1990). Some of this may be artificial, due to the scoring systems used. Among the difficulties are the requirements to demonstrate culture conversions and to decrease the serology to zero titre for a '100%' response.

Novel medical approaches may be worth exploring for chronic coccidioidomycosis. These may include the development of even more potent azoles than those presently available. However, the similarity of responses of three different triazoles suggests that this might be fruitless. Another possibility is targeting drugs to coccidioidal lesions, perhaps using liposomes to deliver amphotericin B or combined antifungals such as polyenes and azoles. (Yates et al 1990, Graybill et al 1991).

In the past there has been strong avoidance of combined polyene/azole antifungalsc. This has been based largely on the work of Schaffner & Frick (1985) with ketoconazole and amphotericin B in a model of aspergillosis. Although amphotericin B/ketoconazole antagonism in aspergillosis has been confirmed by Polak (1978), she found that this antagonism could not be generalized to other mycoses such as cryptococcosis. Further, some of her studies actually showed a benefit. This was confirmed by Albert et al (1991) in an animal study of coccidioidomycosis in which amphotericin B was combined with the triazole SCH39304. Large initial doses of amphotericin B were found to decrease tissue counts of *C. immitis* rapidly over the course of a few days, and co-existent treatment with SCH39304 may be able to hold these counts down. The combination was superior to either drug given alone. The doses used were above what can safely be given to man, but the advent of ABLC raises the question as to whether very high amphotericin B doses, combined with an antifungal azole, might be well tolerated and rapidly effective if given early in the course of therapy.

Completely novel classes of agents might have unique value in coccidioidomycosis. *C. immitis* is a fungus containing a great deal of chitin in the spherule form. Chitin synthetase blockers such as nikkomycin, therefore, may be sufficiently potent (as already demonstrated in animals) and specific as to be fungicidal (as in mice for nikkomycin) and yet benign when given to man (Pappagianis et al 1990). Nikkomycin is late in the course of its patent, and thus might not be fully developed for marketing reasons. It might be appropriate to consider nikkomycin worthy of development for orphan drug status.

Of the four major endemic mycoses, coccidioidomycosis remains in greatest need of new therapeutic approaches.

PHAEOHYPHOMYCOSIS: PRESENT/FUTURE

Other mycoses which may invade the non-compromised host include the dematiacious fungi. There are a number of species, all of which are characterized by the production of brown pigment (Grieble et al 1975, Hohl et al 1983, Halwig et al 1985, Adam et al 1986, Pitrak et al 1988, Sharkey et al 1990, Wilson et al 1991). These are often sensitive to polyenes in vitro, but patients frequently fail to respond to therapy. Itraconazole has been used with some success, particularly in patients who have failed long courses of amphotericin B, but itraconazole treatment courses are also long, and the illness may not completely resolve (Sharkey et al 1990). Surgical resection may be necessary but is not always possible. One reason may be that some patients, particularly those with bronchitis or sinusitis, may have a major allergic component to their disease. This has been relatively recently appreciated (Grieble et al 1975, Halwig et al 1985). Such patients do not have invasion so much as mucoid masses of host inflammatory cells and fungi filling the sinuses, with plugs of peanut butter-like material expectorated from time to time. The illness is thought to be similar to allergic *Aspergillus* sinusitis (Scully et al 1991). These organisms also may be commensals or possibly cause disease in patients with cystic fibrosis (Haase et al 1990). Aspergillosis in patients with cystic fibrosis tends to be the allergic variety, and it is possible that phaeohyphomycetes may cause the same problems. The management of these patients is not completely satisfactory, and has involved largely surgical resection. When this is not successful, one might consider using chronic benign antifungals, such as itraconazole, to keep down the fungal load (as has been recently suggested for allergic bronchopulmonary aspergillosis (Du Pont 1990, Denning et al 1991) and also using antihistamines or perhaps even the judicious use of corticosteroids to reduce the host response which is at the heart of the problem.

A major problem with phaeohyphomycosis is that patients are so scattered as to limit the experience in any one institution to just a few patients. Anecdotes are likely to be the basis for any future changes in therapy.

ASPERGILLOSIS: PRESENT AND FUTURE

Allergic responses to fungi are not unique to the phaeohyphomycetes, but occur also with aspergillosis (Graybill 1988). Among the forms of this illness occurring in non-compromised patients are allergic bronchopulmonary aspergillosis and allergic sinusitis. These illnesses are much more common in England than in the USA, perhaps in part due to the more continually damp climate of the area. Aspergillosis complicating cystic fibrosis is also frequent in England, and may reflect a synergistic process in which the fungi elicit abundant secretions which cannot readily be cleared, allowing for further proliferation of fungi. In one series of 20 patients from an unselected population, 12 had bronchopulmonary allergic aspergillosis, versus fungus balls in 6 patients, and invasive disease in 2 (Edge et al 1971). There also may be specific virulence characteristics of such isolates, but this is speculative. Also, occasionally there are demonstrated inherited susceptibilities to allergic bronchopulmonary aspergillosis and sinusitis (Shah et al 1990). In both of these situations chronic treatment with amphotericin B is highly toxic and not considered likely to have much benefit.

Despite treatment with corticosteroids, allergic bronchopulmonary aspergillosis tends to progress through a stage of remissions, then corticosteroid-dependent asthma, and ultimately fibrosis (Patterson et al 1982). Treatment with cort-icosteroids given intermitently for exacerbations may prevent the progression from the asthma state to permanent fibrosis (Patterson et al). It is possible that anti-inflammatory agents combined with more benign agents, such as azoles, may be balanced to control both fungal proliferation (and antigen load) as well as host inflammatory response (Denning et al 1991). Even more speculative, antibodies to cytokines or other mediator antagonists may be used to beneficial effect in these patients. Simpler measures, such as moving out of mouldy environments, e.g. farming country, may also be helpful.

In addition to allergic aspergillosis, there are two other forms of disease which occur in non-compromised hosts. These are *Aspergillus* fungus ball (formerly aspergilloma) and chronic necrotizing (invasive, semi-invasive) aspergillosis. *Aspergillus* fungus ball is well known for its poor response to medical therapy, allegedly because the fungus ball is avascular and is not accessed readily by antifungal agents. The usual recommendation is for surgical resection (Aslam et al 1978). In one series, all of nine patients treated with resection remained free of disease. Surgical resection is readily accomplished for paranasal sinus fungus balls, but many patients have severe chronic pulmonary disease and are not surgical candidates for resection of pulmonary fungus balls (Milosev et al 1969, Smolansky 1978, Washburn et al 1988). Embolization of blood vessels supplying cavities may be done in patients with severe haemoptysis. Amphotericin B delivered intravenously has not been very efficacious. Efforts to catheterize cavities and deliver antifungal agents locally into cavities have had variable results. In one old series, of 6 patients treated with intracavitary amphotericin B, 4 responded (Hargis et al 1980). It is possible that chronic therapy with agents which are benign and effective against *Aspergillus* species might be of benefit, as might topical intracavitary delivery of new antifungals. The most hopeful studies are those of Restrepo et al (1988) in Colombia, and DuPont et al (1990) in France, using orally administered itraconazole. In the experience of both, there was a major reduction of symptoms associated with itraconazole treatment, a conversion of sputum cultures to negative, and a decrease in antibody titres. More recently, saperconazole has been studied in a few patients, with similar responses (Franco et al 1991). Symptoms resolved, *Aspergillus* antibody titres declined, and cultures converted to negative. Radiographic changes have been less impressive and difficult to interpret, as most of these patients have significant underlying disease.

The last form of the disease may respond well to medical therapy or may be almost as difficult to treat as *Aspergillus* fungus balls. This is chronic invasive or chronic necrotizing aspergillosis (Gefter et al 1981, Binder et al 1982, Tack et al 1982, Pervez et al 1985, Karam & Griffin 1986, Restrepo et al 1988, Cook et al 1990). It is increasingly frequently recognized, occurs predominantly in the lungs of non-compromised patients, and is manifested by slowly progressing infiltrates, or cavities. Chronic necrotizing aspergillosis may develop as a complication of resection of fungus balls (Rosenberg et al 1982). Traumatic percutaneous inoculation may also produce focal solid lesions in peripheral tissues (Bennett et al 1962). We have seen two such patients. Some peripheral foci may be a consequence of haematogenous dissemination from a (sometimes presumed) pulmonary focus, even in non-compromised hosts (Tack et al 1982). One series by Binder et al (1982), with a review of the literature, reported a total response rate to amphotericin B, with or without flucytosine, as 81%. Chronic treatment with antifungal azoles may help to suppress or even cure the illness. In a series reported by Denning et al (1990), of 14 patients with invasive disease (one patient with *Aspergillus* onychomycosis excluded), 5 did not have underlying immune deficiency, and all 5 responded to itraconazole. In peripheral tissues, we have seen failure with itraconazole in one patient with fungus ball and one patient with *Aspergillus* osteomyelitis (though itraconazole was given at low doses with low blood levels), and improvement in a patient with fungus ball (Phillips et al 1987). We have also seen two patients with progressive lung disease and empyemas who failed to respond to itraconazole, (Graybill, unpublished observations) though others have had a much more successful record. Both responded well to SCH39304. This year others have confirmed the value of itraconazole in treatment of invasive aspergillosis, including patients with immune compromise (LeBeau et al 1991).

Therefore, some patients with chronic necrotizing aspergillosis respond well to treatment with antifungal azoles which are active against these fungi and penetrate tissues well. Long-term treatment, perhaps for years, may be needed. Surgical resection of lesions in some patients may be feasible, but prolonged medical therapy appears to me more desirable. As this illness is quite uncommon, the direction of future antifungal therapy is at present unclear, in part because we have not had sufficient experience with presently available drugs to make a conclusive assessment of their efficacy, and thus of the necessity for further drugs.

SPOROTRICHOSIS: PRESENT AND FUTURE

Sporotrichosis is a chronic invasive mycosis that is more common than its *Aspergillus* counterpart. Chronic lymphocutaneous sporotrichosis is somewhat more common in subtropical and tropical than in temperate climates. This may relate to the intense simple agricultural basis of their economies rather than climate per se. Lymphocutaneous sporotrichosis responds to potassium iodide, which is inexpensive, effective, and sometimes poorly tolerated from gastrointestinal reactions or rash.

The less common pulmonary and osteo-articular forms do not respond well to iodides and respond variably to amphotericin B. In one series of 7 patients with articular disease, only 4 patients responded to amphotericin B and surgery (Crout et al 1977). Gladstone & Littman (1970) reported 4 of 6 responding to amphotericin B. In another series, patients with pulmonary disease appeared to respond best to surgical resection (Lynch et al 1970). However, follow-up is only given irregularly, and these diseases may relapse later.

Azole therapy of sporotrichosis had a mixed start with miconazole and ketoconazole, which appear to be mostly ineffective (Rohwedder et al 1976, Dismukes et al 1983). Fluconazole is beneficial in patients with lymphocutaneous disease treated at 400 mg per day, and less effective at 200 mg per day (Montero-Gei et al 1990). Itraconazole at 100 mg per day is effective in virtually all patients treated for 6 months for lymphocutaneous disease, with no relapses at 3 month follow-up (Restrepo et al 1986). Borelli (1987) had similar results. Baker et al (1989) have found itraconazole successful in a patient with *Sporothrix* fungaemia refractory to amphotericin B. We have found that itraconazole is also effective at 200–400 mg per day for disseminated disease as well (Sharkey et al 1991). Of 21 patients treated with 23 courses, 2 of the 4 failures were patients with chronic pulmonary disease, and one of these markedly improved, though he remains culture positive on prolonged therapy. Most recently, Franco et al (1991) have treated a series of patients with lymphocutaneous disease using saperconazole at 100 mg per day. Lesions were culture negative in most patients by the end of 2 months, and it may be possible to shorten treatment of these people to 3 months.

The major problems with all of these agents is cost, which makes them unaffordable in countries where they are most needed. Potassium iodide is likely to continue as the most commonly used drug, while azoles will likely be used in the more advanced countries, particularly for patients with extrapulmonary disease.

CHROMOMYCOSIS: PRESENT AND FUTURE

Chromomycosis is an uncommon but devastating problem seen in the tropical Americas (Londero & Ramos 1976). The most commonly encountered pathogen is pedrosi. Patients are usually inoculated cutaneously, and then very slowly develop progressively enlarging lesions. These lesions intermittently drain pus and are very destructive of tissues. The term derives from the large destructive lesions, granular masses of fungi, and characteristic spheroid bodies produced by the varied fungal pathogens when growing in tissues. Until the development of itraconazole, flucytosine and amphotericin B were only intermittently effective in prolonged courses, and they were even more intermittently available in developing nations where this disease is most common. Surgical resection provided the best chance for cure, if the lesion permitted it.

Itraconazole dramatically improved the prognosis of chromomycosis (Restrepo et al 1988). Prolonged courses of 200–600 mg per day for 1–3 years have effected marked improvements in the majority of patients treated by Restrepo et al. *C. carrioni*, the other major agent of American chromomycosis, has also responded well, if slowly, to itraconazole (Borelli 1987). Though benefits have been great, few patients have achieved true cures. A newer azole, saperconazole, may cause clinical responses in an even shorter time. Franco et al (1991) have seen culture conversions in as short as 2 months of therapy, and clearance of lesions within 6 months – truly dramatic responses.

It is my suspicion that chromomycosis will yield to medical therapy with saperconazole or a successor. Extensive scarring and disfigurement will remain as sequelae, but this disease is finally becoming amenable to antifungal therapy, and is another example where antifungal azoles are clearly more efficacious than amphotericin B.

HYALOHYPHOMYCOSIS

Finally, blending in with the above are the hyalohyphomycetes, typified by *P. boydii*. *Pseudallescheria* also tends to cause chronic destructive lesions of the extremities, including chromoblastomycosis, though they can cause pulmonary disease as well.

Pseudallescheria is characteristically resistant to amphotericin B, and may be found in both pulmonary and extrapulmonary sites. There were early responses to miconazole, but ketoconazole was much easier to take and also effective (Lutwick et al 1979, Galgiani et al 1986). My suspicion (based on speculation only) is that as we gain experience with itraconazole, saperconazole, and other broad spectrum agents, these will replace ketoconazole as treatment for *Pseudallescheria* infections. I do not envision sufficient numbers of patients to be available for more than anecdotal case collections in the foreseeable future.

OTHERS

There are at present few fungal species which could not be pathogenic to man under the 'right circumstances'. The right circumstances usually infer immune suppression, but simple inoculation may be enough to establish *Pythium*, mushroom fungi, or other agents in a niche they can exploit (Lie-Kien et al 1957, Speller & MacIver 1971). These and other such agents have appeared over a number of years, but remain uncommonly encountered. Treatment will rely on the individual application of surgical skills and the continuing reassessement of the medical therapy. Antifungal drugs may play increasing roles, though for these fungi it will be a hit or miss situation until there are enough cases reported to at least suggest a direction to follow.

SUMMARY

The above mycoses comprise a heterogeneous group which, though varied in species, are much less frequently encountered than mycoses of compromised hosts. While all can infect the non-compromised host, some, such as *C. neoformans*, *Aspergillus* species, and now *H. capsulatum* cause their greatest problems in immunodeficient patients. Others, such as *C. immitis*, and the agents of phaeo-hyphomycosis, sometimes infect immunodeficient patients, but cause most of their problems in the normal host. Others, such as *Sporothrix schenckii* and the agents causing chromomycosis attack almost always only normal subjects.

It was only 15 years ago that a group of investigators came together to search for the optimal approach to an uncommon fungal infection, *C. neoformans*. This investigation was successful and led to extensions to the endemic fungi, and now aspergillosis and candidaemia. In a sense the Mycoses Study Group has become 'too successful'. It was formed to pull together a number of investigators to study the then uncommon cryptococcosis. With distractions caused by all of the mycoses associated with AIDS and the increasing use of cytotoxic agents and broad spectrum antibacterials, cryptococcosis, histoplasmosis, candidaemia and invasive aspergillosis have become far more common recently, and are now occupying the centre stage of antifungal drug development.

It is my belief that treatment of the systemic mycoses of the non-compromised host will in general follow that developed for the compromised patient. The advances already made in development of antifungal azoles have made a great impact in therapy of the majority of these mycoses. We may extend some of our new approaches, such as fluconazole therapy of cryptococcal meningitis in AIDS patients, to those without immune compromise. Fears of late relapses, which occur in patients with AIDS, may not occur in non-compromised patients. Coccidioidomycosis, phaeohyphomycosis, allergic and saprophytic forms of aspergillosis, and chromomycosis remain problematic, but it is unlikely that major resources will be diverted to the study of these particular problems.

The government support that has sustained the Mycoses Study Group is not available to most investigators in Latin American or other countries of the Third World. Here the best option may be support from pharmaceutical companies who would be willing to see their agents tested against competitors' in well-designed studies. Competent investigators in Argentina, Brazil, Colombia, Mexico, Costa Rica, Venezuela and other countries could readily form collaborative groups to accomplish these studies.

One final suggestion is that, despite their inherent limitations, animal studies can permit us to study the effects of single agents as well as combinations of therapeutic agents before they are taken to the bedside. Specific doses and durations of therapy need to be determined clinically, but concepts can be tested in animals. Among these are whether polyenes and flucytosine can be combined usefully with azoles, and which azoles are relatively the most potent (Allendoerfer et al 1990).

REFERENCES

Adam R D, Paquin M L, Petersen E A et al 1986 Phaeohyphomycosis caused by the fungal general *Bipolaris* and *Exserohilum*. Medicine 65: 203–217
Albert M, Graybill J R et al 1991 ABLC combined with SCH39304 in treatment of murine coccidioidomycosis. Antimicrobial Agents Chemotherapy
Allendoerfer R, Marquis A J, Rinaldi M G, Graybill J R 1990 Combined therapy with fluconazole and flucytosine in murine cryptococcal meningitis. Abstract 1160. Thirtieth Interscience Conference on Antimicrobial Agents and Chemotherapy, Atlanta
Aslam P A, Eastridge C E, Hughes F A 1972 Aspergillosis of the lung – an eighteen year experience. Chest 59: 28–32
Baker J H, Godpasture H C, Kuhns H R, Rinaldi M G 1989 Fungemia caused by amphotericin B-resistant isolate of *Sporothrix schenkii*. Archives of Pathology and Laboratory Medicine 113: 1279–1281
Bennett J E, Kirby E J, Blocker T G 1962 Unusual inflammatory lesions of the face. Plastic and Reconstructive Surgery 29: 684–691
Bennett J E, Dismukes W E, Duma R J et al 1979 A comparison of amphotericin B alone and combined with 5-flucytosine in the treatment of cryptococal meningitis. New England Journal of Medicine 301: 126–131
Berry A, Graybill J R 1991 The use of high dose fluconazole in cryptocococcal meningitis in AIDS. Abstract WB2287, Seventh International Conference on AIDS, Florence, Italy
Binder R E, Falling L J, Pugatch R D, Mahasaen C, Snider G L 1982 Chronic necrotizing pulmonary aspergillosis. Medicine: 109–124
Borelli D 1987 A clinical trial of itraconazole in the treatment of deep mycoses and leishmaniasis. Reviews of Infectious Diseases 9: S57–S63
Bradsher R W 1990 Personal communication
Bradsher R W, Alford R H, Kawkins S S, Spickard W A 1982 Conditions associated with relapse of amphotericin B-treated disseminated histoplasmosis. Johns Hopkins Medical Journal 150: 127–131
Bradsher R W, Rice D C, Abernathy R S 1985 Ketoconazole therapy for endemic blastomycosis. Annals of Internal Medicine 103: 872–879
Chua W A, Krauss S, Aggio M C 1978 Disseminated histoplasmosis in advanced Hodgkin's disease. Journal of the Tennessee Medical Association 71: 748–750
Cook D J, Achong M R, King D E L 1990 Disseminated aspergillosis in an apparently healthy patient. American Journal of Medicine 88: 74–76

Crout J E, Brewer N S, Tompkins R B 1977 Sporotrichous arthritis. Annals of Internal Medicine 86: 294–297

Deng Z, Ribas J L, Gibson D W, Connor D H 1988 Infections caused by *Penicillium marneffii* in China and Southeast Asia: Review of eighteen published cases and report of four more cases. Reviews of Infectious Diseases 10: 640–652

Denning D W, Tucker R M, Hanson L H 1990 Treatment of invasive aspergillosis with itraconazole. American Journal of Medicine 86: 791–800

Denning D W, Van Wye J E, Leewiston N J, Stevens D A 1991 Adjunctive therapy of allergic bronchopulmonary aspergillosis (ABPA) with itraconazole. PS2.93. XI Congress of the International Society of Human and Animal Mycology Montreal

Dismukes W E 1990 Personal communication

Dismukes W E, Royal S A, Tynes B S 1978 Disseminated histoplasmosis in corticosteroid-treated patients. Journal of the American Medical Association 240: 1495–1498

Dismukes W E, Stamm A M, Graybill J R et al 1983 Treatment of systemic mycoses with ketoconazole; emphasis on toxicity and clinical response in 52 patients. Annals of Internal Medicine 98: 13–20

Dismukes W E, Cloud G, Gallis H A et al of the NIAID Mycoses Study Group 1987 Treatment of cryptococcal meningitis with combination amphotericin B and flucytosine for four as compared with six weeks. New England Journal of Medicine 317:334–341

Dismukes W E, Cloud G, Thompson S et al 1989 Fluconazole (FLU) versus amphotericin B (AMB) therapy (Rx) of acute cryptococcal meningitis (CM). Abstract 282. Twenty Ninth Interscience Conference on Antimicrobial Agents and Chemotherapy, Washington, DC: American Society for Microbiology

Drutz D J 1983 Amphotericin B in the treatment of coccidioidomycosis. Drugs 26: 337–346

DuPont B 1990 Itraconazole therapy in aspergillosis: study of 49 patients. Journal of American Academy of Dermatology 23: 607–614

Edge J R, Stansfield D, Fletcher D E 1971 Pulmonary aspergillosis in an unselected hospital population. Chest 59: 407–413

Fish D G, Ampel N M, Galgiani J N et al 1990 Coccidioidomycosis during human immunodeficiency virus infection. Medicine 69: 394–398

Franco L, Gomez I, Restrepo A 1991 Treatment of subcutaneous and disseminated mycoses with saperconazole. Abstract PS3.99, XI Congress of the International Society of Human and Animal Mycology, Montreal

Franco M, Mendes R, Moscardi-Bacchi M, Rezkallah-Iwasso M, Montenegro M R 1989 Para-coccidioidomycosis. Balliere's Clinical Tropical Medicine and Communicable Diseases 4: 185–220

Galgiani J N, Stevens D A, Graybill J R, Stevens D L, Tillinghast A J, Levine H B 1986 *Pseudallescheria boydii* infections treated with ketoconazole. Chest 86: 219–224

Galgiani J N, Stevens D A, Graybill J R et al 1988 Ketoconazole therapy of progressive coccidioidomycosis. Comparison of 400 and 800 mg doses and observations at higher doses. American Journal of Medicine 84: 603–610

Galgiani J N, Catanzaro A, Graybill J R, Levine B, Larsen R A, Dismukes W E, Cloud G A, and others of the NIAID Mycoses Study Group 1990 Fluconazole therapy for coccidioidomycosis. Abstract 574. Thirtieth Interscience Conference on Antimicrobial Agents and Chemotherapy, Atlanta

Galgiani J N et al 1991 Personal communication

Galgiani J N, Hostetler J, Catanzaro A et al of the NIAID Mycoses Study Group 1991 Coccidioidal infections treated with SCH39304. Abstract PS3.107. XI Congress of the International Society for Human and Animal Mycology, Montreal

Gefter W B, Weingrad T R, Epstein D M, Ochs R H, Miller W T 1981 'Semi-invasive' pulmonary aspergillosis. *Radiology* 140: 313–321

Gladstone J L, Littman M L 1970 Osseous sporotrichosis. American Journal of Medicine 51: 121–133

Goodwin R A, Shapiro J L, Thurman G H, Thurman S S, DesPrez R M 1980 Disseminated histoplasmosis: clinical and pathologic correlations. Medicine 59: 1–33

Graybill J R, Alford R H 1974 Cell-mediated immunity in cryptococcosis. Cellular Immunology 14: 12–21

Graybill J R 1988 A history of the treatment of aspergillosis. In: van den Bossche H, MacKenzie D R, Cauwenburgh G (eds) *Aspergillus* and aspergillosis. Plenum Press, New York, 229–242

Graybill J R et al 1991 Unpublished observations

Graybill J R, Stevens D A, Galgiani J N et al of the NIAID Mycoses Study Group 1990 Itraconazole treatment of coccidioidomycosis. American Journal of Medicine 89: 292–290

Graybill J R, Vincent D, Johnson E et al 1991 Amphotericin B lipid complex (ABLC) in treatment (Rx) of cryptococcal meningitis (CM) in patients with AIDS. Thirty First Interscience Conference on Antimicrobial Agents and Chemotherapy, Chicago.

Grieble H G, Rippon J W, Maliwan N, Daun V 1975 Scopulariopsis and hypersensitivity pneumonitis in an adult. Annals of Internal Medicine 83: 326–329

Haase G, Skopnik H, Kusenbach G 1990 Exophiala dermatitidis infection in cystic fibrosis (letter). Lancet 336: 188

Halwig J M, Brueske D A, Greenberger P A, Dreisen R B, Sommers H M 1985 Allergic bronchopulmonary curvulariosis. American Review of Respiratory Disease 132: 186–188

Hargis J L, Bone R C, Stewart J, Rector N, Hiller F C 1980 Intracavitary amphotericin B in the treatment of symptomatic pulmonary aspergillomas. American Journal of Medicine 68: 389–394

Hitchcock C A, Andrews R J, Pye G W, Troke P F 1991 Combination therapy of intracranial cryptococcosis in mice with fluconazole (FLU) and 5-fluorocytosine (5-FC) or amphotericin-B (Ampho B). Abstract PS3.58, XI Congress of the International Society of Human and Animal Mycology, Montreal

Hohl P E, Holley P Jr, Prevost E, Ajello L, Padhye A A 1983 Infections due to *Wangiella dermatitidis* in humans: report of the first documented case from the United States and a review of the literature. Reviews of Infectious Diseases 5: 854–864

Janssen Pharmaceutica 1990 Unpublished data

Jones B E, Larsen R A, Bozzetrte S, Haghighat D, Leedom J M, McCutchan J A 1991 A phase II trial of fluconazole plus flucytosine for cryptococcal meningitis. Abstract WB2337. Seventh International Conference on AIDS, Florence

Karam G H, Griffin F M Jr 1986 Invasive pulmonary aspergillosis in non-immunocompromised, non-neutropenic hosts. Reviews of Infectious Diseases 8: 357–362

Kauffman C A, Israel K A, Smith J W, White A C, Schwarz J, Brooks G F 1978 Histoplasmosis in immunosuppressed patients. American Journal of Medicine 64: 923–932

Kelly P C 1980 Coccidioidal meningitis. In: Stevens D A (ed) Coccidioidomycosis; a text. Plenum, New York, pp 163–194

Kerkering T M, Duma R J 1981 The evolution of pulmonary cryptoccosis. Annals of Internal Medicine 94: 611–616

LeBeau B, Pelloux H, Pinel C, Ambroise-Thomas P, Grillot R 1991 Itraconazole in the treatment of aspergillosis: 18 cases. Abstract PS3.117. XI Congress of the International Society of Human and Animal Mycology, Montreal

Lebel M H, Frreij B J, Syrogiannopoulos G A et al 1988 Dexamethasone therapy for bacterial meningitis. New England Journal of Medicine 319: 964–971

Lewis J L, Rabinovich S 1972 The wide spectrum of cryptococcal infections. American Journal of Medicine 53: 315–322

Lie-Kien J, Njo-injo T et al 1957 A new verrucous mycosis caused by *Cercospora apii*. Archives of Dermatology 75: 864–870

Londero A T, Ramos C D 1976 Chromomycosis: a clinical and mycological study of thirty-five cases observed in the hinterland of Rio Grande do sul, Brazil. American Journal of Tropical Medicine and Hygiene 25:132–135

Lutwick L L, Rytel M W, Yanez J P, Galgiani J N, Stevens D A 1979 Deep infections from *Petriellidium boydii* treated with miconazole. Journal of the American Medical Association 241: 272–273

Lynch P J, Voorhees J J, Harrell R 1970 Systemic sporotrichosis. Annals of Internal Medicine 73: 23–30

Merz W G, Karp J E, Hoagland M, Jett-Goheen M, Junkins J M, Hood A F 1988 Diagnosis and successful treatment of fusariosis in the compromised host. Journal of Infectious Diseases 158: 1046

Milosev B, Mahgoub E S, Aal O A, Hussam A E 1969 Primary aspergilloma of the paranasal sinuses in the Sudan. British Journal of Surgery 56: 132–137

Montero-Gei F, Stevens D A, Siles L 1990 Fluconazole therapy in cutaneous and lymphangitic sporotrichosis. Abstract 575. Thirtieth Interscience Conference on Antimicrobial Agents and Chemotherapy, Atlanta

National Institute of Allergy and Infectious Diseases Mycoses Study Group 1985 Treatment of blastomycosis and histoplasmosis with ketoconazole. Annals of Internal Medicine 103: 861–872

Negroni R, Robles A M, Arechavala A, Tuculet M A, Galimberti R 1980 Ketoconazole in the treatment of paracoccidioidomycosis and histoplasmosis. Reviews of Infectious Diseases 2: 643–649

Negroni R, Palmieri, Koren F, Tiraboschi N, Galimberti R 1987 Oral treatment of paracoccidioidomycosis and histoplasmosis with itraconazole in humans. Reviews of Infectious Diseases 9 (Suppl 1): S47–S50

Nelson L A, Callerame M L, Schwartz R H 1979 Aspergillosis and atopy in cystic fibrosis. American Review Respiratory Diseases 120: 863–873

Pappagianis D and the Vaccine Study Group 1986 Evaluation of the protective efficacy of the killed *Coccidioides immitis* vaccine in man. Abstract 784. Twenty-sixth Interscience Conference on Antimicrobial Agents and Chemotherapy (ICAAC)

Pappagianis D, Hector R F, Zimmer D 1990 Nikkomycin-Z induced resolution of meningocerebral coccidioidomycosis in mice. Abstract 596. Thirtieth Interscience Conference on Antimicrobial Agents and Chemotherapy, Atlanta

Pappas P G, Pottage J C, Tapper M L et al 1990 Blastomycosis in AIDS patients. Abstract 1166. Thirtieth Interscience Conference on Antimicrobial Agents and Chemotherapy, Atlanta

Patterson R, Greenberger P A, Radcin R C 1982 Allergic bronchopulmonary aspergillosis: staging as an aid to management. Annals of Internal Medicine 96: 286–291

Patterson R, Greenberger P A, Lee T M et al Prolonged evaluation of patients with corticosteroid-dependent asthma stage of allergic bronchopulmonary aspergillosis. Journal of Allergy and Clinical Immunology 80: 663–866

Paya C V, Hermans P E, vanScoy R E, Ritts R E, Hombereger H A 1987 Repeatedly relapsing disseminated histoplasmosis: clinical observations during long-term followup. Journal of Infectious Diseases 156: 308–312

Pervez N K, Kleinerman J, Kattan M et al 1985 Pseudomembranous necrotizing bronchial aspergillosis. American Review of Respiratory Disease 131: 961–963

Philips J R, Jones S, Adamson J S, Abernathy R S 1972 Long-term followup of 101 patients with blastomycosis. American Review of Respiratory Diseases 105: 1006–1007

Phillips P, Fetchick R, Weisman I, Foshee S, Graybill J R 1987 Tolerance to and efficacy of itraconazole in treatment of systemic mycoses. Reviews of Infectious Diseases 9 (Suppl 1): S87–S93

Pitrak D L, Koneman E W, Estupinan R C, Jackson J 1988 *Phialophora richardsoniae* infection in humans. Reviews of Infectious Diseases 10: 1195–1203

Polak A Combination therapy of experimental candidiasis, cryptococcosis, aspergillosis and wangiellosis in mice. Chemotherapy 33: 381–395

Queiroz-Telles F, Binshack L I, Hagi N T, Purim K S 1991 Itraconazole in the treatment of paracoccidioidomycosis. PS3.109, XI Congress of the International Society of Human and Animal Mycology, Montreal

Restrepo A, Gomez I, Cano L E et al 1983a Treatment of paracoccidioidomycosis with ketoconazole: a three year experience. American Journal of Medicine 74 (1B): 48

Restrepo A, Gomez I, Cano L E et al 1983b Post-therapy status of paracoccidioidomycosis treated with ketocanazole. American Journal of Medicine 74 (Suppl 1B): 53–57

Restrepo A, Robledo J, Gomez I, Tabares A M, Gutierrez R 1986 Itraconazole therapy in lymphangitic and cutaneous sporotrichosis. Archives of Dermatology 122: 413–417

Restrepo A, Gomez I, Robledo J, Patino M M, Cano L E 1987 Itraconazole in the treatment of paracoccidioidomycosis. Reviews of Infectious Diseases 9 (Suppl1): S51–S56

Restrepo A, Gonzalez A, Gomez I, Arango M, deBedout C 1989 Treatment of chromoblastomycosis with itraconazole. Annals of the New York Academy of Sciences 544: 504–516

Restrepo A, Munera M I, Atreaga I D et al 1988 Itraconazole in the treatment of pulmonary aspergilloma and chronic pulmonary aspergillosis. In: van den Bossche H, MacKenzie D W R, Cauwenbergh G (eds) *Aspergillus* and aspergillosis. Plenum Press, New York, pp 253–265

Restrepo S, Tobon A, Trujillo J, Restrepo A 1991 Development of pulmonary fibrosis (PF) in mice during infection with *P. braziliensis* conidia (Pbc). Abstract PS4.92. XI Congress of the International Society for Human and Animal Mycology, Montreal

Rohwedder J J, Archer G 1976 Pulmonary sporotrichosis: treatment with miconazole. American Review of Respiratory Diseases 114: 403–406

Rosenberg R S, Creviston S A, Schonfeld A J 1982 Invasive aspergillosis complicating resection of a pulmonary aspergilloma in a nonimmunocompromised host. American Review of Respiratory Diseases 126: 1113–1115

Saag M, Bradsher R, Chapman S et al and the NIAID Mycoses Study Group 1988 Itraconazole (I) therapy (Rx) for blastomycosis (B) and histoplasmosis (H) and sporotrichosis (S). Abstract 574. Twenty-eight Interscience Conference on Antimicrobial Agents and Chemotherapy, Los Angeles

Schaffner A, Frick P G 1985 The effect of ketoconazole on amphotericin B in a model of disseminated aspergillosis. Journal of Infectious Diseases 151: 902–910

Scully R E, Mark E J, McNeely W F, McNeely B U 1991 Weekly Clinicopathologic Conferences: allergic fungal sinusitis. New England Journal of Medicine 324: 1423–1429

Shah S, Khan U, Chaturvedi S, Phil M, Malik G B, Randhwa S 1990 Concomitant allergic *Aspergillus* sinusitis and allergic bronchopulmonary aspergillosis associated with familial occurrence of allergic bronchopulmonary aspergillosis. Annals of Allergy 64: 507–511

Sharkey P K, Graybill J R, Rinaldi M G et al 1990 Itraconazole treatment of phaeohyphomycosis. Journal of the American Academy of Dermatology 23: 577–586

288

Sharkey P K, Kauffman C A, Graybill J R, Dismukes W E and members of the NIAID Mycoses Study Group 1991 Abstract PS3.100. Itraconazole treatment of sporotrichosis. XI Congress of the International Society for Human and Animal Mycology, Montreal

Simmonds E J, Littlewood J M, Evans E G V 1990 Cystic fibrosis and allergic bronchopulmonary aspergillosis. Archives of Disease in Childhood 65: 507–511

Smolansky S J 1978 Aspergillosis of the paranasal sinuses. Ear, Nose, and Throat Journal 57: 6–14

Speller D C E, MacIver, A C 1971 Endocarditis caused by a *Coprinus* species: a fungus of the toadstall group. Journal of Medical Microbiology 4: 370–374

Stern J J, Hartman B J, Sharkey P K et al 1988 Oral fluconazole therapy for patients with acquired immunodeficiency syndrome and cryptococcosis: experience with 22 patients. American Journal of Medicine 85: 477–480

Sugar A M, Saunders C 1988 Oral fluconazole as suppressive therapy of disseminated cryptococcosis in patients with acquired immunodeficiency syndrome. American Journal of Medicine 85: 481–489

Tack K J, Rhame F S, Brown B, Thompson R C 1982 *Aspergillus* osteomyelitis. Report of four cases and review of the literature. American Journal of Medicine 73: 295–300

Tucker R M, Galgiani J N, Denning D W, et al 1990 Treatment of coccidioidal meningitis with fluconazole. Reviews of Infectious Diseases 12 (Suppl 3): S380–S389

Vendetti M, Micozzi A, Gentile G et al 1988 Invasive *Fusarium solani* infections in patients with acute leukemia. Reviews of Infectious Diseases 10: 653–659

Warr W, Bates J H, Stone A 1968 The spectrum of pulmonary cryptococcosis. Annals of Internal Medicine 69: 1109–1126

Washburn R G, Kennedy D W, Begley M G, Henderson D K, Bennett J E 1988 Chronic fungal sinusitis in apparently normal hosts. Medicine 67: 231–247

Wey S B, Mori M, Pfaller, M A, Woolson R F, Wenzel R P 1989 Risk factors for hospital-acquired candidemia. Archives of Internal Medicine 149: 2349–2353

Wheat L J, Slama T G, Eitzen H E, Kohler R B, French M L V, Biensecker J L 1981 A large urban outbreak of histoplasmosis: clinical features. Annals of Internal Medicine 94: 331–337

Wheat L J, Connoly-Springfield P A, Backer R L et al 1990 Disseminated histoplasmosis in the acquired immunodeficiency syndrome: clinical findings, diagnosis and treatment, and review of the literature. Medicine 69: 361–374

Wilson C M, O'Rourke E J, McGinnis M R, Salkin I F 1991 *Scedosporium inflatum*: clinical spectrum of a newly recognized pathogen. Journal of Infectious Diseases 161: 102–107

Yates R R, Allendoerfer R, Sun S H, Graybill J R 1990 Comparison of amphotericin B lipid complex (ABLC) to amphotericin B (AmB) and Schering 39304 (SCH) in treatment of murine coccidioidomycosis. Abstract 285. Thirtieth Interscience Conference on Antimicrobial Agents and Chemotherapy, Atlanta

17. Antifungal therapy in AIDS patients

B. Dupont

INTRODUCTION

In the past various factors have increased the numbers of immunocompromised patients. None, however, has had the same impact as the dramatic world-wide epidemic of AIDS. The main feature of this syndrome is a progressive decrease of cell-mediated immunity due to defective functioning of T-lymphocytes or macrophages.

For this reason, certain mycoses, particularly those contained by T-cell-mediated mechanisms of host defence, have dramatically risen in frequency: namely candidiasis, cryptococcosis, histoplasmosis and coccidioidomycosis (Table 17.1).

Table 17.1 Fungal infections in HIV-positive patients

Mucocutaneous	Systemic
Candidiasis	Cryptococcosis
Onychomycosis	Histoplasmosis
Pityrosporosis	Coccidioidomycosis
	Candidiasis, aspergillosis, penicilliosis and other rare mycoses

Most systemic infections are characterized by the absence of cure with more failure at initial therapy and persistent foci of infection causing relapses. Thus maintenance therapy after clearance of signs and symptoms and a negative mycological culture are necessary to prevent relapses. Available antifungal agents are not fungicidal in vivo and the immunosuppression that permitted the mycoses to develop progresses with time. For these reasons the efficacy of antifungal therapy is limited, and we must take into account the quality of life of the patient, and his short life expectancy. Thus we must redefine the goals of treatment in AIDS patients. Should we try to cure the disease at any cost, or could we accept a non-mycological cure if the disease is quiescent, the patient is symptomless and is in some way an asymptomatic carrier of pathogenic fungi?

Besides this rather pessimistic view about fungal diseases in AIDS, the epidemic offers the opportunity of major advances in epidemiology, in basic science and in new drug development.

MYCOSES IN HIV-POSITIVE PATIENTS

Mycotic diseases in HIV-positive patients may involve the mucosal surface and if so are relatively benign although sometimes oropharyngeal and oesophagal candidiasis may play a role in the deterioration of the patient's general condition. Other mycoses are severe, disseminated and life-threatening: cryptococcosis, histoplasmosis and coccidioidomycosis. Some diseases more rarely encountered are infections due to *Penicillium marneffei*, invasive aspergillosis, and anecdotal cases of infections due to *Alternaria*, Mucorales, *Trichosporon*, etc., which may represent difficult therapeutic problems (Stevens 1990, Diamond 1991).

A few infections in which cellular immunity seems important do not appear to be more frequent in HIV-positive patients: blastomycosis and paracoccidioidomycosis. This is also true for skin dermatophytosis, but onychomycosis due to *Trichophyton rubrum* afflicts a large number of patients. Pityriasis versicolor is not a frequent disease but *Malassezia furfur* may cause folliculitis and may be involved in the pathogenesis of seborrhoeic dermatitis.

Specific therapeutic problems encountered in HIV-positive patients

Particular problems linked to HIV infection must be taken into account in the use of topical and systemic antifungal agents.

Ketoconazole needs an acid pH to be solubilized and then absorbed. Gastric pH in HIV-positive patients is often high because of achlorhydria, leading to low absorption and thus low blood levels (Blum et al 1990). This is a possible cause of failure when treating oropharyngeal or oesophageal candidiasis with ketoconazole. Also, the use of antacids or anti-H_2 substances may lower blood levels of ketoconazole; the latter are contraindicated, and the former must be prescribed some time apart from the ingestion of ketoconazole.

Rifampin is often given in the treatment of mycobacterial infections and it can interfere with the metabolism of ketoconazole, increasing the rate of its catabolism and causing low or undetectable blood levels. There is a potential toxicity of ketoconazole on adrenal glands which can worsen a latent adrenal insufficiency due to HIV-infection.

Hepatotoxicity of ketoconazole, although very rare in our own experience, should also be considered in a population where chronic hepatitis is frequent.

Other azole derivatives used as systemic antifungals are less sensitive to gastric pH although absorption of itraconazole may be slightly impaired. Rifampin seems to have a weak interaction with fluconazole. Both of these newer antifungals do not cause adrenal insufficiency. Drug interactions are possible between the anticonvulsant agents phenytoin and phenobarbital with the triazoles itraconazole and fluconazole.

When antifungal agents are taken orally the patient's ability to take the drug reliably is questionable when the patient has impaired memory and/or cognitive disturbances due to HIV encephalopathy. Gastrointestinal problems such as diarrhoea and villous atrophy are factors likely to cause a decrease of intestinal absorption of oral drugs. The large number of different drugs prescribed at the end stage of HIV disease with preventive and curative therapy may pose a problem of priority for antifungal agents given orally as prophylaxis against candidiasis.

Antifungals used intravenously, e.g. amphotericin B, fluconazole, and flucytosine (in some countries), raise the problem of obtaining easy venous access particularly in heroin addicts. The frequent use of an intravenous catheter exposes the patients to the risk of catheter-related bacterial infection.

Cutaneous reactions, which are frequent with antibacterial and antiprotozoal agents, seem unusual with antifungals, although a few rashes due to flucytosine and itraconazole and a probable Stevens–Johnsons syndrome with fluconazole have been reported.

The cost of drugs must also be considered: protracted courses of fluconazole are very expensive. This cost-benefit analysis must take into account the quality of life of the patient who often has a limited period of survival.

Candidiasis

Candidiasis is the most frequent opportunistic infection in HIV-positive patients and 90–95% will develop clinical lesions as the retroviral disease progresses. There is a large array of clinical manifestations (oropharyngeal thrush and oesophagitis being the most frequent):

Asymptomatic oral carriage
Oropharyngeal thrush
Acute atrophic erythematous candidiasis
Perlèche (angular cheilitis)
Leucoplakia
Laryngitis
Oesophagitis
Vulvovaginitis, balanitis
(Haematogenous disseminated candidiasis)

A striking point is the rarity of haematogenous disseminated candidiasis. As a rule *Candida albicans* is the species responsible for the disease.

There is in some studies an increased proportion of B serotype which is usually resistant to 5-fluorocytosine (5-FC) in non-AIDS patients. This is of little consequence as 5-FC should not be used to treat such mucosal infections. However, the possibility of resistance to 5-FC must be kept in mind in the rare instance of disseminated or deep visceral infection, proved to be due to *Candida*, against which the classical antifungal treatment is amphotericin B plus 5-FC. In oral swabs in HIV-positive patients we found 106/214 (50%) A serotype (92% sensitive to 5-FC), and 108/214 (50%) B serotype (53% resistant to 5-FC). This high rate of 5 FC resistance seems to be characteristic of HIV-positive patients, as the usual pattern of serotype B resistance to 5-FC in France is 88%, in a large series of HIV-negative patients (Drouhet et al 1975).

In oropharyngeal candidiasis, topical non-absorbable antifungals are used as first choice of therapy (Table 17.2). Clotrimazole, which is not available in every country, is largely used. The antifungal must stay in contact with infected mucosa as long as possible, justifying four to six doses per day. When such treatment fails, or when the patient gets tired of the bad taste of many of these drugs, a systemic antifungal is used: ketoconazole (200–400 mg/day) or fluconazole (50–100 mg/day), for 7–15 days as curative therapy (Dupont & Drouhet 1988). Fluconazole seems slightly more effective and is better tolerated but much more expensive than ketoconazole. These drugs can be used daily as maintenance therapy when relapses are frequent. They also represent the drug of choice for oesophagitis which often responds poorly to non-absorbable agents. Fewer data are available on the efficacy of itraconazole; but an oral solution (200 mg/day) has been shown as effective as fluconazole (50 mg/day) for the treatment of oropharyngeal and oesophageal candidiasis in one study in 20 HIV-positive African patients (Soubry et al 1991). Itraconazole capsules, 200 mg once daily, showed equivalent clinical cure rates and similar relapse rates to ketoconazole, 400 mg daily, for 4 weeks (Blatchford 1990). Owing to its toxicity, intravenous amphotericin B should be reserved for rare cases of resistance or intolerance to azoles or in unconscious or vomiting patients. A dosage of 15–30 mg daily for 15 days is generally effective in treating *Candida* oesophagitis.

Table 17.2 Treatment schedule of oropharyngeal and oesophageal candidiasis in HIV-positive patients

Compound	Dosage per day	Duration	Remarks
Non-absorbable			
Nystatin (topical)	10^6 units $\times$ 5	2–3 weeks	These drugs can be used for
Amphotericin B (topical)	200–400 mg $\times$ 5	2–3 weeks	first episode of thrush when
Clotrimazole (troches)	10 mg $\times$ 3–5	2–3 weeks	patient's compliance is good,
Miconazole (buccal gel)	2.5 ml $\times$ 3–5	2–3 weeks	and as preventive therapy
Systemic			
Ketoconazole (orally)	200–400 mg	10–15 days	Used for relapsing or chronic
Fluconazole (orally)	50–100 mg	10–15 days	thrush or oesophagitis, and
Itraconazole (orally)	200 mg	10–15 days	for preventive therapy
Amphotericin B (i.v.)	15–20 mg	10–15 days	

We have observed in France for the last 2 years an increasing number of patients with clinical resistance to fluconazole with persisting thrush or oesophagitis despite dosage with from 50–100 mg/day up to 400 mg/day. Since the drug has been used in France since 1986, the question of the mycological resistance of *C. albicans* to fluconazole has been raised, although such occurrence is known to be exceptional with azole derivatives (Ryley et al 1984).

When clinical resistance is noticed in a patient treated with fluconazole a certain number of possibilities must be ruled out: drug not taken, or poorly absorbed with low blood levels, selection of in vitro resistant *C. albicans* or particularly selection of *C. krusei* or *C. (Torulopsis) glabrata* which are known to be less sensitive to fluconazole. We observed true clinical resistance in some patients with 50 and then 200 mg/day orally and then 200–400 mg/day intravenously. The resistance of *C. albicans* was demonstrated with MICs $\geqslant 12.5\,\mu$g/ml and up to $\geqslant 50\,\mu$g/ml in a bioassay using HR medium in microplates. In each run a reference strain sensitive to fluconazole was included and displayed its usual sensitivity: 0.36–0.72 μg/ml. In a few patients we were able to show a progressive resistance of isolates. In one experiment in mice infected intravenously with a resistant or a sensitive strain, and treated with fluconazole 20 mg/kg daily, we observed a striking difference in terms of general appearance, survival and kidney burden of *Candida* in favour of those mice infected with the sensitive strain. This resistance is being studied to find out if it is a mutation or a selection of a resistant population and to discover the incidence in our AIDS population (Groupe d'Etude des Mycoses Opportunistes: GEMO, unpublished data).

Resistance occurs generally at the end stage of full-blown AIDS with the CD4 T-cell count $< 100/mm^3$ in patients taking fluconazole at a low dosage of 50 mg/day or 50 mg every other day. We did not observe any oral thrush during maintenance therapy for cryptoccocal meningitis treated with 200 mg/d after an inital curative course of 400 mg fluconazole per day.

There are some questions pending regarding the systemic preventive treatment of candidiasis in exposed HIV-positive patients in order to suppress a fungal cause of antigenic stimulation of CD4 cells – which favours replication of HIV – and to improve nutrition.

Cryptococcosis

Cryptococcosis is the primary fungal cause of death in AIDS patients, and its incidence has ranked third or fourth among major opportunistic infections (Kovacs et al 1985, Dismukes 1988, Eng et al 1986, Clark et al 1990). In some cases it appears localized to the lung but most often it is a disseminated disease in which meningitis is the most frequent and obvious site of infection. There is no consensus about the ideal treatment of the acute phase of the disease (Zuger et al 1986, Stern et al 1988, Chuck & Sande 1989, Dupont et al 1990). Only a small number

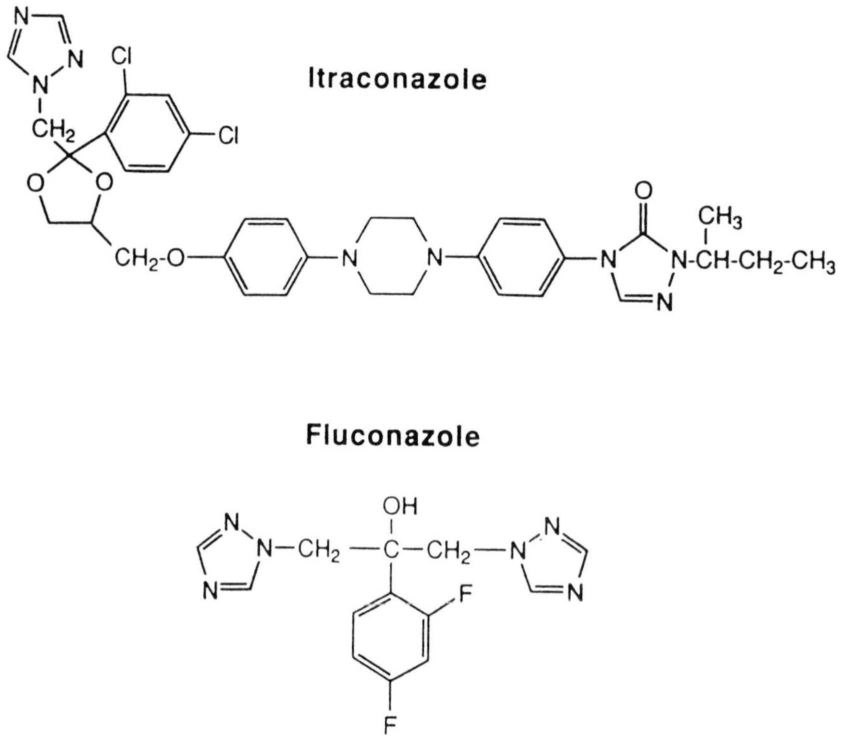

Fig. 17.1 Structural formula of two triazoles, itraconazole and fluconazole.

294

of antifungal agents are suitable to treat cryptococcal meningitis: amphotericin B, 5-FC, which must not be used as single therapy because of the risk of mutation to resistance, and in some countries the triazoles fluconazole and itraconazole (Fig. 17.1). New formulations of amphotericin B are under investigation.

The two main treatment regimens were compared in a large trial in the USA (NIAID ACTG/MSG) (Dismukes et al 1989). Patients enrolled were randomized to receive either amphotericin $B \geqslant 0.3$ mg/kg/day – with 5-FC at the discretion of the investigator – for 10 weeks, or fluconazole, 400 mg the first day and then 200 mg/day for 10 weeks. This dosage could be raised to 400 mg/day if necessary. Preliminary results did not reveal a statistically significant difference between the two regimens in success rate, with 35–40% favourable results with conversion of CSF culture to negative. There was no difference in the rate of quiescent disease (persistent positive culture of CSF in an asymptomatic patient) or of progression of the disease or death under treatment. However, there were more deaths, in the fluconazole group in patients having had less than 15 days of treatment – and therefore not being analysed – and CSF cultures converted to negative earlier in the amphotericin group. More bacteraemia and more toxicity were observed in the amphotericin-treated group. Amphotericin may have been more efficient in a subgroup of patients with pretreatment parameters of poor prognosis.

In a French multicentre study, Dupont et al (1990) have shown that fluconazole 400 mg daily was superior to 200 mg daily in terms of negative cultures of CSF. After 45–60 days treatment, 50% (7/14) of patients treated with 200 mg and 87% (27/31) of patients treated with 400 mg/day had negative CSF culture (Table 17.3).

Table 17.3 Results of microbiological study of the cerebrospinal fluid in 52 AIDS patients with cryptococcal meningitis treated with fluconazole 150–200 mg/day (17 patients) or 400 mg/day (35 patients) (after Dupont et al 1990)

	150–200 mg		400 mg	
	Day 30	Day 45–60	Day 30	Day 45–60
CSF positive				
India ink	9/16	7/14 (50%)	12/32	5/31 (16%)
Culture	8/16	7/14 (50%)	14/32	4/31 (13%)
Death	1/17	3/17	2/35	2/35
No sample	0	0	1/35	2/35

In a small number of patients, Larsen et al (1990) reported a failure in 8/14 patients with fluconazole but 100% efficacy with amphotericin B plus flucytosine in 7 patients. Staib & Seibold (1988) also published good results with this combination in a non-comparative series of patients.

Viviani et al (1990) reported clinical and mycological cures in 9/12 patients treated with itraconazole, 200–400 mg/day, and in 8/10 patients treated with itraconazole, 200–400 mg/day, plus flucytosine, 150–200 mg/kg/day (Table 17.4). Denning et al (1990) reported the efficacy of itraconazole, 200 mg/day with complete response in 16/24 patients (60%), partial response in 5/24 patients (24%) and failure in 3/24 patients (13%) (Table 17.5).

Table 17.4 Results of primary treatment of cryptococcal meningitis in AIDS patients with itraconazole (ITZ) and combined itraconazole and flucytosine (5-FC) (after Viviani et al 1990)

	No. of patients	Patients with no symptoms, negative cultures, and decrease in AG titre	Disappearance of symptoms (days)
ITZ 200–400 mg/day	12	9	7–30
ITZ 200–400 mg/day + 5-FC (1–6 weeks) 150–200 mg/kg/day	10	8	7–20

Table 17.5 Results of primary treatment with itraconazole of cryptococcal meningitis in AIDS patients (after Denning et al 1990)

24 patients treated with 200 mg/day		
16/24 (60%)	Complete response	Clinical resolution Negative cultures
5/24 (21%)	Partial response	Clinical improvement or resolution Positive culture
3/24 (13%)	Failure	

Cryptococcaemia abolished in 100%		
16/24	≥ Fourfold decline in CSF AG titre	
15/19	Clearing of initially positive CSF India ink test	
MIC Crypto	40 strains	≤ 3.13 μg/ml
	3	= 6.25 μg/ml
	1	= 12.5 μg/ml

High doses of amphotericin B, 0.8–1 mg/kg, could give better results but there are no studies to support this possibility. Because of the frequent haematological toxicity of the combination of amphotericin B plus flucytosine some authors omit flucytosine, and others prefer to use low doses of 75–100 mg/kg/day, with a measurement of blood levels.

There is a tendency to propose as the first line of treatment in cases with a poorer prognosis, primary treatment with amphotericin B (0.8–1 mg/kg) for 10–15 days, with or without flucytosine at low dose, followed by fluconazole, 400 mg/day, for up to 2 months and/or until cultures of CSF and of other positive sites of infection are negative. Fluconazole, 400 mg, could be used as single therapy

Table 17.6 Suggested treatments for cryptococcal meningitis in AIDS patients

Initial therapy
 (1) IV amphotericin B, 0.5–1 mg/kg/24 h or 48 h for ≥ 0.5 to 2 months ± flucytosine 75–100 mg/kg/day (for 10–15 days?)
 (2) IV or oral fluconazole, 400 mg/d for ≥ 2 months
 (3) Oral itraconazole 400 mg/day for ≥ 2 months
 (4) Potential treatments: itraconazole + flucytosine, fluconazole (800 mg), fluconazole + flucytosine, amphotericin B liposome, amphotericin B lipid complex, SCH 39 304
Maintenance to prevent relapse
 (1) Oral fluconazole, 200 mg/day for life
 (2) IV amphotericin B, 50 mg, twice weekly, or 50–100 mg once a week for life
 (3) Oral itraconazole, 200 mg/day for life

in less severe cases. However, no data have been published on its use as a primary treatment. Amphotericin B liposomes or amphotericin B lipid complex, which seem promising with a higher efficacy and lower toxicity than classical amphotericin, could be a very good alternative (Table 17.6).

Because of a high relapse rate after primary treatment, it is necessary to prescribe a secondary treatment called maintenance therapy to prevent relapses (Dismukes 1988, Sugar & Saunders 1988, Sugar et al 1990, Zuger et al 1988). There is a consensus on the use of 200 mg/day life-long fluconazole which was shown by Bozzette et al (1991) to be highly effective compared with placebo and more effective and less toxic than amphotericin B, 1 mg/kg weekly (Powderly et al 1990). In some studies itraconazole, 200 mg/day, seemed a good candidate for preventing relapses. Viviani et al (1990) reported 27/31 patients without relapse – most of them with declining antigen titres – with 200 mg/day itraconazole (Table 17.7). The prostate can be a residual focus of infection which may persist despite fluconazole (Bailly et al 1991) or itraconazole (Larsen et al 1989, Staib et al 1990).

Table 17.7 Maintenance therapy of cryptococcal meningitis in AIDS patients with itraconazole (ITZ) (after Viviani et al 1990)

ITZ 200 mg/d during (months)	No. of patients	No relapse	Relapse
< 6	13	3* + 6† + 1‡	3
6–12	12	7* + 3† + 1‡	1
> 12	6	3* + 3†	0
Total	31	27	4

* With negative AG titre during maintenance.
† With declining AG titre during maintenance.
‡ With persistent high AG titre during maintenance.

In patients with quiescent disease or those who have failed traditional treatment, anecdotal reports and personal cases permit us to consider as compassionate treatment a higher dose of fluconazole (800–1200 mg), the combination of fluconazole plus flucytosine, or fluconazole (400 mg) plus itraconazole (400 mg) or amphotericin B plus a triazole. The experimental compound SCH 39304, which seemed promising, was withdrawn from clinical trials because of carcinogenesis in chronically treated animals. A new vehicle for amphotericin B, liposomes and lipid complexes, gave impressive results with rapid clearing of cultures of CSF in a limited number of cases, and could also be an alternative. These compounds are under investigation (Table 17.6).

Histoplasmosis
Histoplasmosis is a major problem for HIV-positive patients living in areas where it is endemic or who have had a primary infection which can be reactivated many years after they left the endemic area (Mandell et al 1986, Johnson et al 1986, Graybill 1988, Wheat et al 1989, 1990). Wheat et al (1990) reported that 25–35%

of AIDS patients may develop disseminated histoplasmosis due to *Histoplasma capsulatum* in areas where it is endemic.

As in cryptococcosis, the treatment consists of an initial period of intensive induction therapy followed by a maintenance phase to prevent relapses from foci of residual infection. Amphotericin B gives about an 80–90% response rate with resolution of clinical manifestations of infection. McKinsey et al (1989) reported that aggressive induction treatment with a total dose of 2 g did not give better results than a total dose of 1 g, followed in both regimens by weekly or biweekly infusions of 50–80 mg continued indefinitely. Six out of seven patients in the 1 g regimen group survived without evidence of clinical or mycological relapse compared to 7/9 patients in the 2 g regimen group who survived with one histoplasmosis relapse. Thus 13 of 14 patients (93%) who did not die of other causes remained relapse free with a median follow-up period of 14 months (2–23 months). However 63% of patients developed complications related to intravascular devices. Wheat et al obtained an 80% response with initial therapy with amphotericin B in 82 episodes of histoplasmosis occurring in 69 patients; 6% of patients died of histoplasmosis despite receiving at least 500 mg of amphotericin B. Of 5 patients who did not receive maintenance treatment, 4 relapsed; of 21 patients receiving intermittent weekly or biweekly amphotericin B for maintenance therapy, 3 relapsed.

Because of the toxicity of amphotericin B and difficulties related to protracted intravenous administration it seemed worthwhile to consider azole derivatives as alternatives (Saag & Dismukes 1988, Larsen 1990). Ketoconazole was ineffective against disseminated disease in 6 cases treated by Wheat et al; of 20 patients who received ketoconazole as maintenance therapy 10 relapsed. Itraconazole seems more promising for primary treatment as well as for maintenance. Results are not yet published, but preliminary data show itraconazole to be very effective. There are fewer data with fluconazole which too is under investigation. Amphotericin B liposomes and lipid complexes are theoretically good candidates for primary treatment.

Coccidioidomycosis

Coccidioidomycosis is a frequent disease in AIDS patients living in areas where it is endemic. It seems to occur as a primary infection or reinfection rather than as a reactivation of a latent infection. Coccidioidomycosis may take the form of diffuse or localized pulmonary disease or of disseminated disease (Bronniman et al 1987, Galgiani & Ampel 1990, Fish et al 1990).

The classical treatment, as in non-AIDS patients, remains intravenous amphotericin B. However, the survival rate is low, about 42%, and has been found to be the same with the use of ketoconazole. Itraconazole was shown to be effective in coccidioidomycosis in non-AIDS patients with (Tucker et al 1990a) and without (Tucker et al 1990b) central nervous system involvement. It is currently under investigation in AIDS patients. Preliminary data are very encouraging, but data on a sufficiently large number of patients have not been published. Fluconazole is also promising and may be interesting because of its diffusion into CSF (Classen et al 1988, Tucker et al 1988, 1990c). It is also under investigation. New formulations of amphotericin B are potentially good candidates for clinical trials.

Other mycoses

Penicilliosis due to *Penicillium marneffei* is treated with intravenous amphotericin B. We had good results in three patients treated with itraconazole which could represent an alternative treatment. Aspergillosis, haematogenous candidiasis, zygomycosis and other mycoses should be treated with the same drugs as are used in non-AIDS patients.

REFERENCES

Bailly M P, Boibieux A, Biron F et al 1991 Persistence of *Cryptococcus neoformans* in the prostate: failure of fluconazole despite high doses. Journal of Infectious Diseases 164: 435–436 (letter)

Blatchford N R 1990 Treatment of oral candidosis with itraconazole: a review. Journal of the American Academy of Dermatology 23: 565–567

Blum R A, d'Andrea D T, Florentino B M et al 1991 Increased gastric pH and the bioavailability of fluconazole and ketoconazole. Annals of Internal Medicine 114: 755–757

Bozzette S A, Larsen R A, Chiu J et al 1991 A placebo-controlled trial of maintenance therapy with fluconazole after treatment of cryptococcal meningitis in the acquired immunodeficiency syndrome. New England Journal of Medicine 324: 580–584

Bronniman D A, Adam R D, Galgiani J N, Habib M P, Petersen E A, Porter B, Bloom J W 1987 Coccidioidomycosis in the acquired immunodeficiency syndrome. Annals of Internal Medicine 106: 372–379

Chuck S L, Sande M A 1989 Infections with *Cryptococcus neoformans* in the acquired immunodeficiency syndrome. New England Journal of Medicine 321: 794–799

Clark R A, Greet D, Atkinson W, Valainis G T, Hyslop N 1990 Spectrum of *Cryptococcus neoformans* infection in 68 patients infected with human immunodeficiency virus. Reviews of Infectious Diseases 12: 768–777

Classen D C, Burke J P, Smith C B 1988 Treatment of coccidioidal meningitis with fluconazole. Journal of Infectious Diseases 158: 903–904

Denning D W, Tucker R M, Hanson L H, Stevens D A 1990 Itraconazole in opportunistic mycoses: cryptococcosis and aspergillosis. Journal of the American Academy of Dermatology 23: 602–607

Diamond R D 1991 The growing problem of mycoses in patients infected with the human immunodeficiency virus. Reviews of Infectious Diseases 13: 480–488

Dismukes W E 1988 Cryptococcal meningitis in patients with AIDS. Journal of Infectious Diseases 157: 624–628

Dismukes W A, Cloud G, Thompson S et al 1989 Fluconazole versus amphotericin B therapy of acute cryptococcal meningitis. Abstract 282. Twenty Ninth Interscience Conference on Antimicrobial Agents and Chemotherapy. American Sociey for Microbiology, Washington, DC

Drouhet E, Mercier-Soucy L, Montplaisir S 1975 Sensibilité et résistance des levures pathogènes aux 5 fluoropyrimidines: relation entre les phénotypes de résistance à la 5 fluorocytosine, le sérotype de *Candida* et l'écologie de différentes espèces de *Candida* d'origine humaine. Annales de Microbiologie de l'Institut Pasteur 1263: 25–39

Dupont B, Drouhet E 1988 Fluconazole in the management of oropharyngeal candidosis in a predominantly HIV antibody-positive group of patients. Journal of Medical and Veterinary Mycology 26: 67–71

Dupont B, Hilmarsdottir I, Datry A, Gentilini M, Dellamonica P, Bernard E et al 1990 Cryptococcal meningitis in AIDS patients – a pilot study of fluconazole therapy in 52 patients. In: Vanden Bossche H, Van Cutsen J, Cauwenbergh G, Mackensie D W R, Drouhet E, Dupont B (eds) Mycoses in AIDS patients. Plenum Press, New York, pp 287–304

Eng R H K, Bisburg E, Smith S M, Kapila R 1986 Cryptococcal infections in patients with acquired immune deficiency syndrome. American Journal of Medicine 81: 19–23

Fish D G, Ampel N M, Galgiani J N et al 1990 Coccidioidomycosis during human immunodeficiency virus infection. Medicine 69: 394–398

Galgiani J N, Ampel N M 1990 Coccidioidomycosis in human immunodeficiency virus-infected patients. Journal of Infectious Diseases 162: 1165–1169

Graybill J R 1988 Histoplasmosis in AIDS. Journal of Infectious Diseases 158: 623–626

Groupe de'Etude des Mycoses Opportunistes (GEMO) 1991 Unpublished data

Johnson P C, Sarosi G A, Septimus E J, Satterwhite T K 1986 Progressive disseminated histoplasmosis in patients with the acquired immune deficiency syndrome: a report of 12 cases and a literature review. Seminars in Respiratory Infections 1: 1–8

Kovacs J A, Kovacs A A, Polis M et al 1985 Cryptococcosis in the acquired immunodeficiency syndrome. Annals of Internal Medicine 103: 533–558

Larsen R A, Bozzette S, McCutchan J A et al 1989 Persistent *Cryptococcus neoformans* infection of the prostate after successful treatment of meningitis. Annals of Internal Medicine 111: 125–128

Larsen R A 1990 Azoles and AIDS. Journal of Infectious Diseases 162: 727–730

Larsen R A, Leal M A E, Chan L S 1990 Fluconazole compared with amphotericin B plus flucytosine for cryptococcal meningitis in AIDS. A randomized trial. Annals of Internal Medicine 113: 183–187

McKinsey D S, Gupta M R, Riddler S A, Driks M R, Smith D L, Kurtin P J 1989 Long-term amphotericin B therapy for disseminated histoplasmosis in patients with the acquired immunodeficiency syndrome (AIDS). Annals of Internal Medicine 111: 655–659

Mandell W, Goldberg D M, Neu H C 1986 Histoplasmosis in patients with the acquired immune deficiency syndrome. American Journal of Medicine 81: 974–978

Powderly W, Saag M, Cloud G A, Dismukes W E, Meyer R, Robinson P 1990 NIAIDS AIDS Clinical Trials Group, NIAD Mycoses Study Group, and Pfizer Central Research. Abstract 1162. Thirtieth Interscience Conference on Antimicrobial Agents and Chemotherapy, Atlanta

Ryley J F, Wilson R G, Barett-Bee K J 1984 Azole resistance in *Candida albicans*. Sabouraudia 22: 53–63

Saag M S, Dismukes W E 1988 Azole antifungal agents: emphasis on new triazoles. Antimicrobial Agents and Chemotharapy 32: 1–8

Soubry R, Clerinx J, Banyanagiliki V et al 1991 Comparison of itraconazole oral solution and fluconazole capsules in the treatment of oral and esophageal candidiasis on HIV-infected patients. Preliminary results. Abstract M.B. 2201 VII International Conference on AIDS, p 232

Staib F, Seibold M 1988 Mycological diagnostic assessment of the efficacy of amphotericin B + flucytosine to control *Cryptococcus neoformans* in AIDS patients. Mycoses 31: 175–186

Staib F, Seibold M, L'age M 1990 Persistence of *Cryptococcus neoformans* in seminal fluid and urine under itraconazole treatment. The urogenital tract (prostate) as a niche for *Cryptococcus neoformans*. Mycoses 33: 369–373

Stern J J, Hartman B J, Sharkey P et al 1988 Oral fluconazole therapy for patients with acquired immunodeficiency syndrome and cryptococcosis: experience with 22 patients. American Journal of Medicine 85: 477–480

Stevens D A 1990 Fungal infections in AIDS patients. British Journal of Clinical Practice, Suppl. 71, 44: 11–22

Sugar A M, Saunders C 1988 Oral fluconazole as suppressive therapy of disseminated cryptococcosis in patients with acquired immunodeficiency syndrome. American Journal of Medicine 85: 481–489

Sugar A M, Stern J J, Dupont B 1990 Overview: treatment of cryptococcal meningitis. Reviews of Infectious Diseases 12: Suppl. 3 S338–S348

Tucker R M, Williams P L, Arathoon E G et al 1988 Pharmacokinetics of fluconazole in cerebrospinal fluid and serum in human coccidioidal meningitis. Antimicrobial Agents and Chemotherapy 32: 369–373

Tucker R M, Denning D W, Arathoon E G, Rinaldi M G, Stevens D A 1990a Itraconazole therapy for nonmeningeal coccidioidomycosis: clinical and laboratory observations. Journal of the American Academy of Dermatology 23: 593–601

Tucker R M, Denning D W, Dupont B, Stevens D A 1990b Itraconazole therapy for chronic coccidioidal meningitis. Annals of Internal Medcicine 112: 108–112

Tucker R M, Galgiani J N, Denning D W et al 1990c Treatment of coccidioidal meningitis with fluconazole. Reviews of Infectious Diseases 12: Suppl. 3, S380–S389

Viviani M A, Tortorano A M, Pagano A et al 1990 Euopean experience with itraconazole in systemic mycoses. Journal of the American Academy of Dermatology 23: 587–593

Wheat L J, Connolly-Stringfield P, Kohler R B, Frame P T, Gupta M R 1989 *Histoplasma capsulatum* polysaccharide antigen detection in diagnosis and management of disseminated histoplasmosis in patients with acquired immunodeficiency syndrome. American Journal of Medicine 87: 396–400

Wheat L J, Connolly-Stringfield P, Baker R L 1990 Disseminated histoplasmosis in the acquired immune deficiency syndrome: clinical findings, diagnosis and treatment. Medicine 69: 361–374

Zugar A, Louie E, Holzman R S, Simberkoff M S, Rahal J J 1986 Cryptococcal disease in patients with acquired immunodeficiency syndrome. Diagnostic features and outcome of treament. Annals of Internal Medicine 104: 234–240

Zugar A, Schuster M, Simberkoff M S, Rahal J J, Holzman R S 1988 Maintenance amphotericin B for cryptococcal meningitis in the acquired immunodeficiency syndrome (AIDS). Annals of Internal Medicine 109: 592–593

Discussion of papers presented by F. Meunier, J. R. Graybill and B. Dupont

Discussed by W. E. Dismukes
Reported by H. C. Neu

In reviewing the papers of Drs Meunier, Graybill and Dupont, Dr Dismukes selected issues relating to prophylaxis of fungal infections and antifungal therapy that are of major importance. He re-emphasized that the most important opportunistic fungal pathogens are the *Candida* species and *Aspergillus* species, and the most at-risk population of patients are the granulocytopenic cancer patients and bone marrow transplant recipients. In contrast, *Cryptococcus neoformans* and *Histoplasma* and *Coccidioides* are the reactivation fungi that present major difficulties for AIDS patients. It was noted that new pathogens such as *C. krusei, C. tropicalis, Torulopsis glabrata, Fusarium,* and *Aspergillus,* pose difficult problems regarding both prophylaxis and therapy in immunocompromised hosts.

Dr Dismukes reiterated Dr Meunier's statements that most studies of prophylaxis have been in neutropenic cancer patients, and we need similar studies in HIV-infected persons and organ transplant recipients. Only multicentre prophylactic trials which incorporate appropriate sample sizes and clearly defined criteria of disease and specific endpoints will establish what forms of prophylaxis are of value. Dr Dismukes reported that there is a trial to prevent coccidioidomycosis in HIV-infected persons living in the coccidioidal endemic area of the arid southwestern United States. It is estimated that 13% of HIV-infected individuals with a CD4 count $< 250/\text{mm}^3$ who live in areas where *Coccidioides immitis* is prevalent will develop coccidioidomycosis over a 24-month period. A double-blind placebo-controlled trial has been initiated to assess the efficacy of oral fluconazole as prophylaxis against the development of active disease in this patient population (NM Ampel, personal communication). Secondary endpoints in the trial will be the development of other systemic fungal diseases and drug toxicity.

Dr Dismukes agreed with Dr Meunier that there is a need for more focus on non-pharmacologic approaches to prevent fungal diseases. Improvement of the hospital environment, education of nurses and physicians about potential sources of fungal infection, careful screening of organ donors, and attention to prior travel or living exposures of patients will alert physicians to the potential development of fungal infection. It was agreed that it is impractical to do surveillance cultures for *Candida,* but in light of the resistance of *C. krusei* to fluconazole one should know what fungi are present. Knowledge of colonization with *C. tropicalis, C. krusei, Trichosporon* may be helpful in predicting infection in neutropenic patients.

Dr Dismukes agreed with Dr Dupont that 'cure at any cost' in the AIDS population of patients cannot be justified, and there was agreement that in this population lack of symptoms and a quiescent disease were the goals.

A number of questions were raised about resistance of certain yeasts to oral azoles, especially fluconazole. It is not established whether low-dose fluconazole, 50–100 mg/day, may predispose to emergence of resistance during therapy. It is also unclear whether the extensive use of fluconazole will cause selection of de novo resistant organisms such as *C. krusei* and *T. glabrata*. Given the widespread usage of fluconazole, these issues warrant investigation.

Dr Sobel pointed out that azoles have been used for years by the oral and vaginal route to treat vaginal candidiasis. He noted that he had not seen resistance of *C. albicans* or other *Candida* species in patients with chronic or recurrent vulvo-vaginal candidiasis even though therapy was often suboptimal. This raises the question whether the resistance of *Candida* in AIDS patients is somehow different.

The therapy of cryptococcosis in AIDS remains highly controversial. Many therapeutic options are available including single drug therapy with amphotericin B, lipid preparations of amphotericin B, fluconazole, or itraconazole, plus combination regimes such as amphotericin B and flucytosine, fluconazole and flucytosine, and amphotericin B and a triazole. There are at present limited data about combination regimens.

Dr Dismukes reported that in an effort to optimize the outcome in AIDS-associated acute cryptococcal meningitis, the NIAID AIDS Clinical Trials Group (ACTG) and Mycoses Study Group (MSG) have jointly begun a new multicentre prospective trial. Therapy for the initial 2 weeks will compare amphotericin B alone with amphotericin B plus flucytosine. After 2 weeks, patients who meet present criteria, including no neurologic deterioration, will then be re-randomized to either fluconazole or itraconazole for the next 8 weeks of therapy. The primary endpoints to be addressed at both 2 weeks and 10 weeks are culture conversion of cerebrospinal fluid (CSF) from positive to negative and death due to cryptococcosis.

Other issues which were addressed related to the use of flucytosine with fluconazole. Dr Graybill reported that such a combination in animal infection experiments showed that the number of organisms was reduced and that there was increased survival of mice. It is probable that a fluconazole–flucytosine therapy trial in man will be done sometime in the future.

Histoplasmosis has emerged as an important opportunistic mycosis in AIDS. Amphotericin B and itraconazole show good efficacy; the latter is less toxic and better tolerated. Results of three recent or ongoing trials that were not reported lend support to both amphotericin B and itraconazole as effective therapies of histoplasmosis in AIDS. McKinsey and coworkers in Kansas City (1991) evaluated 40 patients who received > 1g amphotericin B as primary therapy and received amphotericin B as maintenance therapy. In these patients, after primary therapy was completed, the central venous catheters for drug administration were removed and amphotericin B maintenance therapy was administered via peripheral venous access, resulting in a dramatic decrease in the frequency of bacterial catheter-related infections. The relapse rate was only 3% (1/36 evaluable patients).

Two ongoing studies by the NIAID MSG and/or ACTG have evaluated itraconazole therapy of histoplasmosis in AIDS patients. Among 62 patients receiving itraconazole as primary therapy, fewer than five failures have thus far been observed (L J Wheat, personal communication). In a separate trial of 42 patients receiving itraconazole as maintenance therapy, there were no relapses. Thirty of these patients were followed for > 52 weeks. These data, together with data cited by Dr Dupont, argue strongly that amphotericin B and itraconazole are highly effective therapies for AIDS-associated histoplasmosis. Accordingly, physicians and patients have a choice, and the therapy may be individualized to what is most appropriate for a satisfactory lifestyle.

Finally, most of the participants agreed that after an episode of mucosal *Candida* infection in an AIDS patient was treated, maintenance therapy was not indicated unless the patient had recurrent episodes of infection. There are no data on the maintenance therapy in AIDS patients after treatment of an initial episode.

There have been additional data on azole antifungal therapy of fungal disease in non-compromised patients. The first NIAID MSG trial evaluated itraconazole therapy of blastomycosis and histoplasmosis in a largely non-immunocompromised patient population. Only one histoplasmosis patient had AIDS. Among 48 patients with blastomycosis, itraconazole in doses of 200–400 mg/day was successful in 43, or 90%. Efficacy was even more impressive in patients treated for at least 3 months: 38 of 40, or 95%, were cured. Among 37 patients with histoplasmosis, itraconazole was successful in 30, or 82%, and in 30 of 35 (86%) treated for $\geq$ 3 months. All failures were in patients with chronic cavitary pulmonary histoplasmosis. In this trial, side-effects attributable to itraconazole were minimal. Thus itraconazole appears more efficacious and better tolerated than ketoconazole, the azole which is currently used as an alternative therapy to amphotericin B for blastomycosis and histoplasmosis.

The second MSG trial, which is ongoing, focuses on fluconazole therapy of coccidioidal meningitis. Twenty seven patients had failed previous therapy for their disease; 8 were AIDS patients. The clinical and CSF parameters indicate promising efficacy of fluconazole for this form of highly refractory chronic meningitis. If these results are sustained over time, fluconazole will become an appropriate alternative therapy to currently used intrathecal amphotericin B therapy for coccidioidal meningitis.

With regard to aspergillosis, although recent experiences with itraconazole provide encouraging results with respect to efficacy, it is clear that large, prospective, carefully designed, multicentre comparative trials are necessary to better define the role of itraconazole as therapy of aspergillosis. One such trial by the NIAID MSG will compare itraconazole with amphotericin B in patients with documented invasive aspergillosis.

It was generally agreed that azoles have become important therapeutic alternatives in blastomycosis, histoplasmosis, coccidioidomycosis, paracoccidioidomycosis, sporotrichosis, and cryptococcosis. Their role in the therapy of serious forms of candidiasis and aspergillosis remains unclear, pending the results of ongoing or planned clinical trials. The various lipid preparations of amphotericin B, which are currently being evaluated, offer potential advantages over amphotericin B, including selected tissue tropism, preferential binding to fungal cells, reduced toxicity, and increased dosage.

FURTHER READING

Galgiani J N, Catanzaro A, Graybill J R et al and the NIAID Mycoses Study Group 1990 Fluconazole therapy for coccidioidomycosis. 30th Interscience Conference of Antimicrobial Agents and Chemotherapy. Atlanta, GA. Abstract #574

Karp J E, Burch P, Merz M G 1988 An approach to intensive antileukemia therapy in patients with previous invasive aspergillosis. American Journal of Medicine 85: 203–209

McKinsey D S, Gupta M R, Smith D L, O'Connor M 1991 Histoplasmosis in acquired immunodeficiency syndrome: efficacy of maintenance amphotericin B therapy. American Journal of Medicine (in press)

Saag M, Bradshaw R, Chapman S et al and the NIAID Mycoses Study Group 1988 Itraconazole therapy for blastomycosis, histoplasmosis, and sporotrichosis. 28th Interscience Conference on Antimicrobial Agents and Chemotherapy. Los Angeles, CA. Abstract #574

Wheat L J, Hefner R E, Wulfsohn M, Johnson J, Owens S 1991 Itraconazole is effective maintenance treatment for prevention of relapse of histoplasmosis in AIDS: prospective multicenter non-comparative trial. 31st Interscience Conference on Antimicrobial Agents and Chemotherapy. Chicago, IL. Abstract #290

Index

Also published in this series

New Antiviral Strategies (Out of print)
edited by Professor S R Norrby 0 443 04166 0

New Strategies in Parasitology
edited by Professor K P W J McAdam 0 443 04257 8

New Antibacterial Strategies
edited by Professor H C Neu 0 443 04448 1

These books can be ordered through all good booksellers or, in case of difficulty, from the Sales Promotion Department, Churchill Livingstone, Robert Stevenson House, 1–3 Baxter's Place, Leith Walk, Edinburgh EH1 3AF.